# Advancing Latino, Hispanic, or of Spanish Origin+ Leadership in Academic Medicine

John Paul Sánchez • Francisco Lucio
Guadalupe Federico-Martínez • Deion Ellis
Editors

# Advancing Latino, Hispanic, or of Spanish Origin+ Leadership in Academic Medicine

Practices and Perspectives

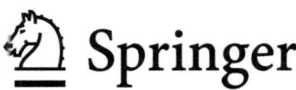

*Editors*
John Paul Sánchez
LMSA National Inc.
Chicago, IL, USA

Guadalupe Federico-Martínez
DLM Coaching, Consulting
& Wellness LLC
Paradise Valley, AZ, USA

Francisco Lucio
Health Care Advancement
University of Arizona
Phoenix, AZ, USA

Deion Ellis
Department of Physical Medicine
Anschutz Medical Campus
and Rehabilitation
University of Colorado School of Medicine
Anschutz Medical Campus
Aurora, CO, USA

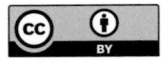

ISBN 978-3-032-07569-7          ISBN 978-3-032-07570-3   (eBook)
https://doi.org/10.1007/978-3-032-07570-3

This work was supported by Latino Medical Student Association Inc.

© The Editor(s) (if applicable) and The Author(s) 2026. This book is an open access publication.

**Open Access** This book is licensed under the terms of the Creative Commons Attribution 4.0 International License (http://creativecommons.org/licenses/by/4.0/), which permits use, sharing, adaptation, distribution and reproduction in any medium or format, as long as you give appropriate credit to the original author(s) and the source, provide a link to the Creative Commons license and indicate if changes were made.
The images or other third party material in this book are included in the book's Creative Commons license, unless indicated otherwise in a credit line to the material. If material is not included in the book's Creative Commons license and your intended use is not permitted by statutory regulation or exceeds the permitted use, you will need to obtain permission directly from the copyright holder.
The use of general descriptive names, registered names, trademarks, service marks, etc. in this publication does not imply, even in the absence of a specific statement, that such names are exempt from the relevant protective laws and regulations and therefore free for general use.
The publisher, the authors and the editors are safe to assume that the advice and information in this book are believed to be true and accurate at the date of publication. Neither the publisher nor the authors or the editors give a warranty, expressed or implied, with respect to the material contained herein or for any errors or omissions that may have been made. The publisher remains neutral with regard to jurisdictional claims in published maps and institutional affiliations.

This Springer imprint is published by the registered company Springer Nature Switzerland AG
The registered company address is: Gewerbestrasse 11, 6330 Cham, Switzerland

If disposing of this product, please recycle the paper.

# Foreword

When I reflect on my journey from a small town in Ecuador to becoming the first Latina and woman Chief Executive Officer (CEO) of NYC Health + Hospitals/Elmhurst in February 2021, I am reminded that leadership is not about titles—it is about purpose, people, and the promises we make to those who come after us.

Before becoming the CEO, I was a patient, like my father, of Elmhurst. As a patient and hospital CEO, I have seen the impact and value leadership that is inclusive, community-centered, and forward-thinking.

In academic medicine, leadership is not just a role it requires vision, courage, integrity, and a deep commitment to building a future that is equitable, innovative, and rooted in community. *Advancing Latino, Hispanic, or of Spanish Origin+ Leadership in Academic Medicine: Practices and Perspectives* arrives at a critical time. This book is more than a collection of perspectives; it is a blueprint for action. It challenges us to develop leaders who are ready for today's demands and capable of reshaping tomorrow's systems.

The future of healthcare calls for more than traditional models, it requires policies shaped by the lived experiences of the people we serve. Health equity is not solely a goal; it is a daily MUST.

I have learned that statistics do not define us—our choices and actions do.

At Elmhurst, we care for over one million people from 112 countries, speaking 138 languages, and representing 92 cultures. Of our patients, 53% report a preferred language of Spanish and 62% identify as Hispanic/Latinx [1]. We are a Level 1 Trauma Center, a Designated Stroke Center and nationally recognized in multiple specialties. We house 475 attendings and faculty. In 2024, our academic medical center trained approximately 460 medical students and 1290 residents and fellows, future doctors who carry forward our mission to care for New York City, with no exceptions. We don't just operate a hospital—we build trust, access, and opportunity in a community too often overlooked. In 2023, we became the first hospital in New York State to achieve a Health Equity Gold standard certification, based on Elmhurst's dedication to reducing disparities in healthcare access, outcomes, and experiences.

This book reflects this kind of leadership grounded in lived experience, driven by equity, and committed to transformation. It calls on us to rethink how we shape policies, grow leaders, and engage communities—not as outsiders, but as true partners.

Leadership is not about being the first. It's about ensuring you are not the last. It is about clearing the path for others, especially those told they do not belong. It is about turning pain into purpose and heart.

To every reader: lead boldly, dream big, and never forget where you came from or who you are fighting for.

Como decía mi abuela: "Ve con Dios y con fe."

Keep building, keep dreaming, and always remember that true leadership starts with the heart.

¡Adelante, siempre! (As of January 2026, Dr. Helen Arteaga stepped down as CEO Elmhurst to become the new Deputy Mayor, NYC Health and Human Services, appointed by NYC Mayor Zohran Mandani)

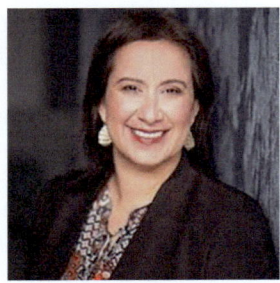

Chief Executive Officer (CEO),                                                      Helen Arteaga
NYC Health + Hospitals/Elmhurst
Queens, NY, USA

# Reference

1. Community Health Needs Assessment 2025, NYC Health + Hospitals. https://hhinternet.blob.core.windows.net/uploads/2025/06/community-health-needs-asssessment-2025.pdf, p. 90. Accessed on 3 Aug 2025.

# LIDERES: Advancing Latino, Hispanic, or of Spanish Origin+ Leadership in Academic Medicine

> **Learning Objectives**
> - Highlights Latina/o/x/e, Hispanic or of Spanish Origin+ (LHS+) individuals' representation in academic medicine leadership roles
> - Describes leadership opportunities as a faculty member, senior medical school administrator, or academic hospital leader
> - Describes the social, structural, and cultural factors that have influence LHS+ inclusion and advancement in academic medicine leadership
> - Shares engaging stories of how LHS+ identified individuals have successfully navigated and advanced within academic medicine

## Introduction

Leaders of medical schools and academic medical centers are typically charged with teaching the next generation of clinicians and researchers, developing innovations, and providing equitable health care to diverse populations. Diverse leaders can help raise awareness of specific population health issues and disparities, enhance engagement of minoritized populations, and approach problem-solving through a culturally informed lens. Since 1970, the LHS+ population has increased from 5% to nearly 20% of the US population, currently representing the largest non-white population in the United States [1]. Concomitant to the rapid LHS+ population growth are the existence of unique health-related issues of the LHS+ diaspora and the necessity for LHS+ leaders to shepherd health equity.

In discussing this population, rather than using the terms Latino or Hispanic, we use the umbrella term—Latina/o/x/e, Hispanic, or of Spanish Origin+ (LHS+) to be inclusive of communities with a common geographic (e.g., Caribbean; North, Central, and South America; and Spain) and Spanish language ancestry (Table 1); to recognize historical terms Latino, Latina, Hispanic, or of Spanish Origin (e.g., used on standardized surveys such as the AAMC Matriculating Student Questionnaire,

Table 1 Primary Spanish-speaking countries in the world

| | | | |
|---|---|---|---|
| Spain | Honduras | Puerto Rico | Ecuador, |
| Mexico | Nicaragua | Argentina | Paraguay |
| Costa Rica | Panama | Bolivia | Peru |
| El Salvador | Cuba | Chile | Uruguay |
| Guatemala | Dominican Republic | Colombia | Venezuela, and Equatorial Guinea |

AAMC Graduation Questionnaire, US Census, etc.), emerging generational/nonbinary terms (e.g., Latine, Latinx), with the plus "+" acknowledging other terms linked to national or social identity (e.g., Mexican, Afro-Latin, Nuyorican, etc.) [2]. Throughout the book a variety of terms are used to acknowledge and respect historical and current individual and communal identities. The health issues of the LHS+ population are particularly complex when one considers factors such as bilingual identity, immigration and migration patterns, level of acculturation, and generational perspectives, to name a few. For example, individuals of Mexican heritage across the United States can have lived experiences and health issues related to recent immigration or extending from 3rd+ generations in the United States.

The current proportion of LHS+ leaders at US medical schools and hospitals is significantly lower than the nearly 20% in the general US population [3]. At US LCME accredited M.D. granting medical schools, 6.3% of full-time faculty and 6.0% of departmental chairs were LHS+ in 2024 [4]. As of January 2025, there were 10 known LHS+ identified Deans of osteopathic and allopathic medical schools (Fig. 1).

The stories, lessons learned, and best practices of prior and current senior LHS+ leaders are vital to inspire, develop, empower, and inform LHS+ individuals on how to build diversity capital and achieve higher leadership positionality and promote health equity. Diversity capital is described as "wealth" owned by a minoritized person or academic organization that is contributed for the purpose of advancing a mission, strategic plan, or well-being of minoritized communities. Wealth assets can be lived experiences, competency, personal networks, money, or another form of assets.

This book highlights three important leadership tracks—faculty track, medical school senior administrator track (i.e., Dean, Chairperson), and academic hospital leadership track. Within tracks, there are even subdivisions—for example, among faculty there are clinical faculty, research faculty, or educator faculty. Readers can explore opportunities and how to thrive along one track or multiple tracks, synchronously or asynchronously.

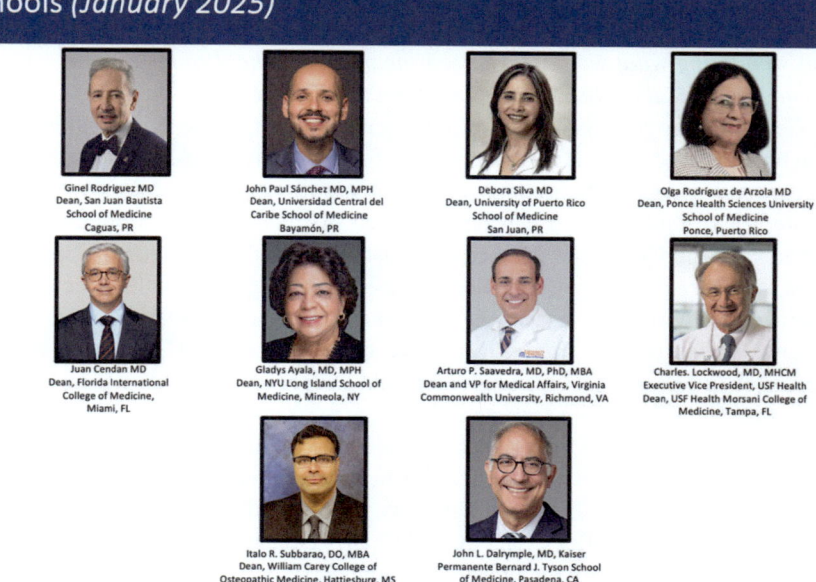

**Fig. 1** Deans of LHS+ identity at US osteopathic and allopathic medical schools (January 2025)

## Personal Reflection—John Paul Sánchez MD, MPH

My passion to serve as a healthcare leader is largely attributed to my parents, the HIV/AIDS pandemic, and experiences as a learner. My father was a Spanish teacher who excited learners through cultural mediums such as the sounds of salsa music and tastes of Puerto Rican cuisine. My mother was an English as a Second Language teacher and exhibited extraordinary empathy and skill to students learning English as a second or third language. Both were born in Puerto Rico but primarily raised and educated in New York City. They provided a learning environment that promoted curiosity, safe inquiry, and Catholic and Puerto Rican values. As an adolescent of the 1980s, the HIV/AIDS pandemic—which dominated media coverage and home discussions and precipitated my first presence at a funeral—was the most profound impact on my understanding of health inequities. Examples of inept federal efforts, the disproportionate burden of HIV among LHS+ and Black families in the Bronx, discriminatory clinical care toward LGBT community members and those infected with GRID/HIV/AIDS, and a medical emphasis on treatment over prevention, molded my future career as a clinician and public health practitioner. Being raised in the Bronx, I quickly heard, saw, and felt other health inequities—like my own emerging superpower, or today known as competency. Sitting in college, graduate school, and medical school classrooms, and infrequently experiencing a focus on the unique health issues of minoritized populations, made me reflect on the role of education in addressing health inequities. Witnessing minoritized students, with unique and powerful lived experiences, yet struggling academically rather than thriving during medical school, sharpened my journey toward academia and *wondering what would have been the medical school of my dreams and what would be an ideal medical school to address health inequities?*

Central to my professional development and growth has been my critical inquiry into how to make medical education better for future diverse generations, asking for and accepting new growth opportunities, obtaining ongoing mentorship and sponsorship, and publishing to elevate the voice of minoritized communities. At the Albert Einstein College of Medicine, Assistant Dean Soto, Senior Associate Dean Katz, Chairperson Selwyn, and Director Lee-Rey engaged me in the structure, function, and activities of the Office of Diversity Enhancement, Office of Student Affairs, Department of Family Medicine and Community Health, and Hispanic Center of Excellence … and I published. At Rutgers New Jersey Medical School, Executive Vice Dean Soto-Greene situated me to round through the roles of various SOM Associate Deans Offices and connected me to the AAMC through the Group on Diversity and Inclusion … and I published. At University of New Mexico Health Sciences Center, Vice Chancellor Diversity, Equity, and Inclusion Romero-Leggott, Associate Vice Chancellor Crandall, and Chairperson McLaughlin positioned me to align DEI efforts throughout a medical school and across health sciences centers … and I published. Leaders of the four Puerto Rico Medical Schools President Brugal, Associate Dean Perez, Dean Silva, Dean Rodriguez, and Dean Rodriguez-Arzola shared the history and challenges of bilingual medical education … and I published. The Latino Medical Student Association (LMSA) provided a safer, ongoing structure to explore LHS+ health issues and develop as a leader on a national level … and I published. Universidad Central Del Caribe President Crespo and the Board of Trustees provided me the opportunity to serve as Dean of the School Medicine (inclusive of the MD Program and Graduate Program in Biomedical Sciences) and build the next generation of practitioners to serve Puerto Rico and Hispanics on the mainland. All these experiences, focused through a DEI lens, building practical knowledge, skills, and scholarship, afforded me the opportunity to achieve Full Professor with Tenure 11 years after graduating residency and being named at age 48 (13 years after residency) as a medical school Dean. Most importantly, these experiences strengthened me to give back through my day-to-day activities and the Building the Next Generation of Academic Physicians Inc. and advance health equity for the LHS+ population and all communities.

It is the hope and purpose of the chapters' co-authors to inspire and grow the next generation of LHS+ academic leaders. We intend to introduce lessons learned so that readers can benefit early in their career journey and have success at a faster rate and higher level than our own. To quicken the momentum in addressing mounting health inequities for the LHS+ population. To inform new policies, procedures, and practices to increase LHS+ hiring, retention, and promotion rates. To maintain progress despite sociocultural influences that may stifle the voice and contributions of LHS+ identities. To remind generations to come of LHS+ current and future presence and contributions to medicine and academic medicine.

The overall learning objectives of this book are to (1) highlight Latina/o/x/e, Hispanic, or of Spanish Origin+ (LHS+) individuals' representation in academic medicine leadership roles; (2) describe leadership opportunities as a faculty member, senior medical school administrator, or academic hospital leader; (3) describe the social, structural, and cultural factors that have influenced LHS+ inclusion and advancement in academic medicine leadership; and (4) share engaging stories of how LHS+ identified individuals have successfully navigated and advanced within academic medicine.

The following is a summary of the 23 book chapters.

## Chapter 1: Why Academia Needs Faculty and Leaders with LHS+ Lived Experiences

The Latina/o/x/e, Hispanic, and/or of Spanish origin (LHS+) community represents nearly 20% of residents in the United States and a unique population to be served by academic medicine and the healthcare system. This chapter explores the critical role LHS+ faculty and leaders at medical schools play in advancing culturally informed educational, research, clinical, and service activities for LHS+ community members. They also uniquely serve as role models, mentors, and change agents, to not only support greater LHS+ representation in the medical and academic medicine workforces but also ensure LHS+ content in the curricula, foster positive learning environments for LHS+ students, and provide culturally competent, safer health care for LHS+ identified patients. To achieve health equity for LHS+ communities, it is important to understand the barriers and facilitators to LHS+ faculty and leaders' representation and advancement in academic medicine.

## Chapter 2: Hispanics and Academic Medicine: Creating an Inclusive Community, Academic Success, and Leadership Careers for Impactful Healthcare Change

Our nation is at a demographic inflection point with the Hispanic population currently being the largest minority group, and its child population set to approximate the non-Hispanic White child population within the next 30 years. To create healthy communities for our nation's Hispanic population, present and future, their health disparities will need to be addressed. Academic medicine has the responsibility to do this, but without Hispanic academic leaders involved in the process, efforts are likely to be less effective and take longer to address Hispanic health disparities. This chapter provides a roadmap for developing a greater number of Hispanic academic health leaders by drawing on the reflections of the authors, themselves senior Hispanic academic leaders, about their paths and the insights they gained about the academic environment through personal experiences. The sections cover the following: (1) Who are we and why are Hispanics important in academic medicine; (2) How do Hispanics succeed in academic medicine: the process of acculturation and inclusion; and (3) Hispanic academic leadership and creating change. The authors then provide a brief discussion of their career paths to exemplify how their academic medical leadership developed. The goal of this chapter is to help create the next generation of Hispanic academic leaders who will address the health disparities in our communities.

## Chapter 3: Making a Decision About an Academic Faculty Track

This chapter explores the integral role of personal values in selecting a professional career within academia. It begins by defining common academic tracks, including tenure-track, non-tenure track, clinical, and teaching-focused paths, highlighting their distinct expectations and opportunities. Understanding these tracks is essential for making informed decisions that align with one's career aspirations. We intend to guide you through a reflective process that helps you identify the academic track best suited to your goals and strengths. We hope that you can make choices that resonate with your LHS+ identities and professional objectives. We want to empower aspiring academicians to navigate career journeys with clarity and purpose, ensuring both fulfillment and impact.

## Chapter 4: How to Switch to an Academic Faculty Track

This chapter provides an overview of what to consider, how to begin the conversation, and what to expect when switching academic tracks. Reviewed are (a) one's professional identity alignment with faculty roles, expectations, and time allocated for the tripartite mission, (b) necessary conversations with mentors, and (c) understanding the collective needs of your department. Situating these factors into the context of considering or preparing to track switch is important. The dynamics heavily influence decision-making around the appropriateness of academic track determination with the ultimate goal of successful professorial promotion up the ranks. Reading this chapter will assist you with understanding how these core elements can assist you with individualizing your academic career path forward and weighing the pros and cons of switching tracks. A reflection segment at the end of the chapter is offered to ensure an opportunity to engage in deep introspection about your academic mindset, strengths, and alignment with interests. The goal of the chapter is to socialize you further into the academic culture of faculty affairs and improve your knowledge about not only track switching but also why getting your initial academic track in alignment with your career vision the first time around is imperative. Information in this chapter will also assuage fears that you might be "locked in" a track that is no longer a suitable fit. You will come to find that most institutions can be nimble if you know how and who can help you navigate the policies and experience. Accessing such information easily from department chairs could be particularly challenging for LHS+, experiencing poor quality attention, career development, and mentoring.

## Chapter 5: Optimizing Your Portfolio and Executive Presence in the Recruitment Process: Perspectives from the Search Firm

It is well-recognized that candidates who have been historically excluded and underrepresented in their field encounter unique experiences, perspectives, and barriers when it comes to seeking job opportunities in medicine and science. This chapter will explore how candidates—especially LHS+ faculty—can effectively work with search consultants to position themselves for their next leadership role. In addition, the chapter will outline best practices for serving on search committees where those bodies evolve their practices and processes to mitigate implicit bias and engage in respectful discourse. Search consultants can serve as thought partners in a leadership transition and serve as stewards of inclusion and equity. They simultaneously support and assist search committee members and the candidates themselves, helping both navigate the recruitment and selection process.

## Chapter 6: Optimizing CV and Portfolio for Promotion Purposes

Promotion within a medical school is dependent on the quality of your Curriculum Vitae (CV) and your Academic Portfolio. As in all of science, the organization and presentation of the key elements of your documentation matters. Early preparation and consistency, as well as timely updating of the documents, are essential. The documents must be organized according to the institution's specifications. Awareness of the criteria for promotion at your institution and familiarity with any criteria updates is the responsibility of the individual candidate. For faculty engaged in Latina/o/x/e, Hispanic, or of Spanish Origin+ (LHS+)-related activities, it is critical to learn how to build diversity capital that can support academic promotion. Formal and transparent institutional policies, processes, and practices are important to acknowledge LHS+-related activities and their promotion merit.

## Chapter 7: A National Perspective on LHS+ Leadership in US Medical Schools

This chapter will explore national perspectives on LHS+ leadership in US medical education, focusing on medical schools, colleges of osteopathic medicine, and graduate medical education programs. Leadership from these organizations will provide updates on the current landscape and highlight opportunities for advancing LHS+ faculty in leadership roles. We will first examine the rationale for enhancing LHS+ representation in leadership, the barriers hindering their progress, and the existing disparities in academic medicine.

## Chapter 8: Succeeding Along the Clinical Track from Assistant to Full Professor

Latina/o/x/e, Hispanic, or of Spanish origin (LHS+)-identified clinical faculty play a unique role in assisting academic medical centers in achieving their tripartite mission of clinical care, education, and research and should be supported in their academic promotion. Clinical faculty also serve as the primary revenue generators for the clinical enterprise and individual strategic planning for career advancement is required to prevent the demand for clinical productivity from derailing individual academic promotion. Clinical faculty are essential to the fulfillment of the patient care, education, and research commitments of the medical school's tripartite mission; however, 80% or more of clinical faculty full-time-equivalent (FTE) effort is devoted to patient care. Successful academic advancement is a key indicator of a thriving professional career. Thriving LHS+ clinical faculty are key to accelerating the improvement of healthcare access, quality, and outcomes for their respective communities. This chapter provides evidence-based and expert recommendations, with respect to faculty promotion in the clinical track, from historically marginalized leaders in academic medicine who have successfully traversed clinical pathways to promotion. By de-constructing the promotion process, and outlining the steps along the clinical promotion track, it is possible to simultaneously de-mystify and simplify this pathway for LHS+ faculty.

## Chapter 9: Succeeding Along the Educator Track from Assistant to Full Professor

An academic career is a long and rewarding journey when chosen intentionally. However, an academic career requires you to comply with specific promotion criteria to ascend from assistant professor to full professor in your department. Being cognizant of the promotion rules and regulations and understanding how to navigate your institution is vital to secure professorial progression. In this chapter, we present key elements you should consider throughout your career as an *educator*. We extend the conversation to include appropriate planning for those on educator tracks and review common pitfalls that inhibit your success toward academic advancement.

## Chapter 10: Succeeding Along the Researcher Track from Assistant to Full Professor

A career as a basic or clinical researcher is one of the most rewarding and challenging paths in academic medicine. To be successful, numerous components, including the ability to attain research grants, run a cohesive, efficient laboratory or research team, publish original, meaningful work, and reach recognition, should work efficiently and synchronously. The complexities and obstacles of this path are enhanced for underrepresented in medicine (UiM) physicians and scientists who are Latino, Hispanic, or of Spanish Origin+ (LHS+) due to specific cultural, training, and systematic barriers routinely encountered by this group. This work aims to summarize the expectations that LHS+ physicians and scientists must meet to achieve a successful career in the research track. Practical suggestions for overcoming the barriers and taking full advantage of available opportunities are discussed. There is a significant dearth of academic LHS+ physician/scientists in the United States, and supportive arguments for recruitment and retention are presented.

## Chapter 11: Striving to Become a Department Chair

As an LHS+ academic physician, even if you have never thought of becoming a department chair, perhaps you may want to reconsider your trajectory. If you think that the LHS+ physician-to-Latino patient ratio is abysmally low, the number of LHS+ identified department chairs is even lower. An LHS+ chair is likely to be quite familiar with the challenges and barriers that Latino patients encounter with the healthcare system, as the chair themselves probably originated from either that community or a similar one. The LHS+ chair may already have thought of solutions to some of these unique patient challenges and is in an ideal position to implement some of these solutions to improve the patient experience and patient care. Indeed, many highly qualified LHS+ physicians do not even consider the chair position because they are simply not aware that they are viable candidates and that it is a position with which they can have a more favorable and durable impact on their patients' health. Furthermore, they are uncertain how to proceed with the preparation and application process, in part, because there are so few LHS+ department chairs to inspire, motivate, and mentor them. This chapter outlines the roles and responsibilities of the department chair in the context of the quadripartite missions of the academic medical center and discusses personal and professional considerations that help one prepare for this important leadership position. With respect to personal qualities and motivation, LHS+ academic physicians may be further along this trajectory than one realizes and so the purpose of this chapter is to stimulate one's active consideration of the department chair position.

## Chapter 12: Being a Medical School Dean: Perspectives from Past and Current LHS+ Deans

This chapter consists of three sections on becoming a medical school dean. It is written through the lens of three Latina/o/x/e, Hispanic, or of Spanish Origin+ (LHS+) identified deans in three individuals in different stages of their careers with different experiences. Dr. Jose Manuel de la Rosa was the Founding Dean for a new medical school and served in the role of campus leadership for over 30 years. Dr. Olga Rodríguez de Arzola is a female Hispanic Dean of a medical school in Puerto Rico founded in 1977 and has been in the role for more than 13 years. Dr. Pedro José Greer Jr. is the designated Founding Dean for the new Roseman School of Medicine in Nevada. The first section describes the motivations for those who wish to be the dean, describes some traditional and nontraditional trajectories into the Dean's office, and includes the role of the dean in the school of medicine, the pathways to the dean position, and the skills required for the Dean. It delineates some formal dean training opportunities, discusses the advantages and disadvantages of each one, and finally discusses how to capitalize on informal training opportunities. Some personal reflection exercises are included to facilitate participation. The second section discusses how a Latino leadership style is different from traditional leadership and might be specifically advantageous to bring a revolution into the medical education environment. The third and final section includes three personal stories from a former Dean, a current dean and a designated dean to be. The chapter is certainly not designed to be the authoritative guide to being a medical school dean as much has been written on this topic, but in keeping with the objective of this book simply delineates some thoughts to consider on a personal level before seeking this career route.

## Chapter 13: Striving to Become a Dean of Diversity, Equity, and Inclusion

You can't achieve a dream that you've never dreamt. This chapter's goal is to broaden your trajectory and options as a leader in medicine by raising awareness and promoting introspection. Here, we share two journeys, present lessons learned via diversity, equity, and inclusion leadership, and highlight the expanse of academic medicine leadership options that exist. Our hope is that this can help you reveal options, generate new questions, and expand your possibilities. Being intentional in personal development—establishing relationships and engaging in areas of work focusing on refining your mission-based craft or niche—are all best achieved with a blueprint. This chapter shares tips and suggestions to consider along your journey. Skill building exercises will help you anchor important areas of development including strategic planning, mentorship, and relationship building. Finally, we consider the future of diversity, equity, and inclusion for those called to serve and facilitate change in academic medicine.

## Chapter 14: Striving to Become a Dean of Undergraduate Medical Education/Curriculum

Within the leadership structure of most medical schools is a role for a faculty member who oversees the medical school curriculum. This person is usually called a "curriculum dean." Depending on the size of the school and its resources, the role might include overseeing other deans or directors in charge of specific aspects of the curriculum; alternatively, it might be combined with other oversight duties under one leadership portfolio and a larger role. The variability of this role contributes to some of the mystique around it and how one becomes a curriculum dean. This chapter is intended to help demystify the curriculum dean role, starting with a brief discussion of the leadership structure in medical schools, followed by a framework in which to consider the activities of a curriculum dean, and then by an explication of typical pathways to the curriculum dean position. The chapter concludes with a discussion of how an individual (such as you!) starts preparing for a path toward becoming a curriculum dean, including incorporation of Latina/o/x/e, Hispanic, or of Spanish Origin+ (LHS+) lenses on this position and one's own LHS+ work. This chapter is offered in the hopes that it will help especially those who might have an interest but who might not have considered the role of curriculum dean to see if it might be a fit for them and lower some of the barriers to taking on this exciting role in leadership in medical education.

## Chapter 15: Striving to Become a Dean/Designated Institutional Official of Graduate Medical Education (GME)

US Medical Schools are lacking LHS+ perspectives among its leadership despite the continued growth of this population in medical school enrollees and in US residency and fellowship programs. The LHS+ population is the largest growing minority in the United States, who through their upbringing and experienced challenges to attain professional degrees are able to contribute cross-cultural wealth, bilingual skills, and social maturity. These skills, among many others, set the LHS+ identified individual in an advantageous position to lead. Graduate Medical Education (GME) comprises the training period after medical school, where physicians receive specialty and subspecialty training. GME programs undergo high accreditation standards defined by the Accreditation Council for Graduate Medical Education to assure high-quality medical training. GME programs are expected to recruit and retain a diverse workforce and foster a clinical learning environment whereby cross-cultural mentoring is provided to ensure the academic success of all. To support these efforts, LHS+ identified individuals must have a voice and a seat at the table. This chapter aims to describe the landscape of LHS+ individuals in GME leadership. It also describes opportunities to develop expertise, reputation, and leadership in GME as a means to eventually serve as a Dean of GME or DIO.

## Chapter 16: Striving to Become a Dean of Admissions

Admissions is the portal to medicine. Every practicing physician came through an admissions process where a group of stakeholders selected them for the profession. The processes have been designed, managed, and held in place by leaders in academic medicine. As leaders have endeavored to ensure a physician workforce prepared to meet the needs of a diverse nation, the need for more representation among designers, gatekeepers, and stakeholders has become critical. Academic leaders who are prepared to engage in admissions can make significant contributions to access and equity in medicine by influencing and shaping the process of selecting the next generation of physicians. This chapter will cover the fundamentals of medical school admissions and provide a foundation for engagement across various stakeholder roles: committee chair, dean, and faculty members. Each medical school has a unique and distinct admissions process, literally no two are alike. Schools have autonomy to create their guidelines, standards, processes, and committees within legal and accreditation parameters. The faculty at the medical school are tasked under the Liaison Committee on Medical Education (LCME) to establish criteria and process and select the class [1]. Faculty can influence admissions and facilitate the incorporation of more equitable, efficient, and mission-centered approaches inclusive of LHS+ individuals and communities.

## Chapter 17: Striving to Become a Dean of Faculty Affairs and Development

Academic medicine allows you to grow in your field of expertise and interest. Yet, the guidance you receive will provide you with the path toward successful professorial promotion. As a dean of faculty affairs and development, there is no greater pleasure than serving as a guide for faculty across their lifecycle from recruitment to retirement and everything in between. In this chapter, you will find information regarding the dean of faculty affairs and development role. Depending on the maturity of your institution, you will need to define who is intended for you to serve and where the greatest needs lie. As a dean of faculty affairs and development, you are the key individual that faculty turn to for their career development; do not assume that faculty are aware of institutional resources. Your role will be to develop both in-person programs and online resources that bring together topics relevant to faculty development. We also recognize that this deanship cannot be done *solo*. It is the collaboration of many other offices such as research, graduate medical education, equity, diversity, and inclusion, to name a few, to ensure successful transitions, recruitment, and retention of faculty and, more so, faculty of minoritized groups! Believe us; nobody started off thinking they would be a dean for faculty affairs and development after finishing medical school or graduate school. We hope that this chapter inspires you to consider this deanship as an opportunity to serve as an advocate for faculty and trainees as pre-faculty.

## Chapter 18: Striving to Become a Dean for Student Affairs

The Associate Dean for Students Affairs' leadership role in medical schools represents an important, critical, and extremely valuable role within the medical school leadership suite. Deans for Students Affairs work closely with the students, leaders, and faculty to ensure students' success in medical school and beyond. The Deans for Students Affairs are responsible for fostering and supporting an environment where all students thrive. The role comes with a diverse array of responsibilities that include, for the most part, career advising, academic advising, and professional and personal advising. In addition, the Dean for Student Affairs provides oversight and coordinates student events, including orientation, white coat ceremonies, match day, and graduation. The role also requires close collaboration with others within the medical school and active participation in school committees. Many rewards come with the role, including helping students achieve their goals, celebrating milestones, and helping students with personal and professional growth. For those considering this leadership role as their career path, we recommend an intentional assessment of personal values and strengths to align those with the expectations of this role. We conclude with some practical suggestions and resources.

## Chapter 19: *MedEdPORTAL*: Publishing Educational Innovations

*MedEdPORTAL* provides an important avenue for educators in the LHS+ community to actively contribute to scholarly publishing, which is crucial for advancing in academia, promoting diverse perspectives, addressing healthcare disparities, and enhancing cultural competence. Expanding teaching and learning scholarship creates more opportunities and boosts recognition for communities historically underrepresented in medicine and publishing. This chapter offers insights into educational scholarship principles and valuable tips for identifying suitable teaching activities and successful submissions. Publishing in *MedEdPORTAL* enables educators to disseminate innovative approaches, fostering excellence in medical education. For the LHS+ community in particular, publishing highlights their unique contributions, promotes inclusive teaching practices, and enhances healthcare quality for LHS+ patients.

## Chapter 20: Serving as a Reviewer, Associate Editor, or Journal Editor In Chief

Like in medicine in general, LHS+ voices are underrepresented in publishing in the medical literature. While many articles include LHS+ patients as research subjects, relatively few LHS+ physicians serve as editor-in-chief, associate editor, or reviewer roles. A recent survey of reviewers for Family Medicine reveals that less than 5% of the reviewers identify as LHS+. In this chapter, we will talk about serving in these roles, with the perspectives of three editors—Dr. Ana Nuñez, Founding Editor in Chief, *Health Equity*; Dr. José Rodríguez, Associate Editor, *Annals of Family Medicine*; and Dr. David Sklar, former Editor in Chief, *Academic Medicine*, the leading journal in medical education.

## Chapter 21: Hospital Leadership Roles and Perspectives: Promotion and Leadership Development in Academic Medicine

Diversity in leadership is essential in all sectors of healthcare delivery, especially in the context of health disparities and the national pursuit of health equity. An extensive body of research has demonstrated the impact of diversity in health care, including on the care and experience of diverse patients. As such, it is important that aspiring, diverse healthcare professionals understand the healthcare leadership landscape, including how healthcare organizations are structured and managed. Health care is provided in many different settings, but hospitals play a unique and foundational role in the United States healthcare system. This chapter will provide an overview of hospital leadership—including a description of the different types of hospitals that deliver care and key leadership positions within hospitals—as well as critical perspectives and lessons learned from the journey of experienced and successful Latino/a healthcare executives. For those considering pursuing hospital leadership opportunities or just interested in learning more about the US healthcare system, this information will provide an important orientation that can serve as the foundation for future career choices, and leadership approaches.

## Chapter 22: Considering in Switching Institutions for Career Advancement: Background of the Road Traveled

This chapter explores the complexities of switching institutions for career advancement in academic medicine, drawing on the lived experiences of a seasoned LHS+ professional who navigated multiple transitions across diverse settings. From starting in rural clinical practice to assuming leadership roles in academic medicine and diversity, equity, and inclusion (DEI) initiatives, the narrative highlights both the challenges and opportunities inherent in such career shifts. Key lessons emphasize the importance of self-awareness, adaptability, and intentionality when considering institutional changes. "Restlessness" emerges as a recurring theme—serving as both a catalyst for personal and professional growth and a motivator to seek environments that better align with evolving aspirations. The chapter details inhibitors of success, such as misaligned institutional priorities, and catalysts, including personal calls to action and the desire for meaningful impact. Ultimately, it equips readers with better practices for navigating transitions, such as contract negotiation, documenting commitments, and identifying allies early. Through reflective insights, it provides a roadmap for leveraging institutional changes to enhance career satisfaction and impact, fostering resilience and success in academic medicine.

## Chapter 23: Considerations for Lideres of Tomorrow

The future of LHS+ *lideres* is bright. The previous chapters describe the multitude of academic medicine career opportunities available for emerging *lideres*. This chapter focuses on a synthesis of some important areas and skill development for *lideres* of tomorrow. Having a clear understanding of the role of accreditation and how accreditation can impact career advancement for faculty is key. There is a special focus on hospital and clinic leadership opportunities for *lideres* to consider. A keen awareness and skill development related to law, policy, and advocacy are more and more critical for *lideres* in academic medicine to master. Community engagement is very often the best mechanism to address local issues in partnership with local communities. Developing community engagement networks helps *lideres* learn from the community and enhance the bi-directional partnership between healers and patients. All these elements are set against the horizon of technological advancements and persistent need to improve the health outcomes of the LHS+ community.

Latino Medical Student Association Inc.                                                            John Paul Sánchez
Chicago, IL, USA

Building the Next Generation of Academic
Physicians Inc.
Rye Brook, NY, USA

## References

1. U.S. Census Bureau QuickFacts. https://www.census.gov/quickfacts/. Accessed on 22 Nov 2024.
2. Sánchez JP, Poll-Hunter NI, Acosta D. Advancing the Latino physician workforce—population trends, persistent challenges, and new directions. Acad Med. 2015;90(7):849–53.
3. Brown A. The U.S. Hispanic population has increased sixfold since 1970. https://www.pewresearch.org/short-reads/2014/02/26/the-u-s-hispanic-population-has-increased-sixfold-since-1970/. Accessed on 22 Nov 2024.
4. AAMC. Faculty Roster: U.S. medical school faculty 2024. https://www.google.com/url?q=https://www.aamc.org/data-reports/faculty-institutions/report/faculty-roster-us-medical-school-faculty&sa=D&source=docs&ust=1752090602165935&usg=AOvVaw2pcVJzv1ScyCGxuJnVohOE. Accessed on 5 July 2025.

# Acknowledgments

I would like to thank the following medical students for assisting with book content and formatting: Hrishikesh Vaddineni, Medical Student, Universidad Central Del Caribe, School of Medicine; Boris Salazar Valladares, BS, MS2 Hackensack Meridian School of Medicine; and Michael Zakhary, BS, MS2 Hackensack Meridian School of Medicine.

# Contents

1 **Why Academia Needs Faculty and Leaders with LHS+ Lived Experiences** .............................. 1
Deion Ellis, Alexandra Lopez Vera, Andy Reyes Santos, and John Paul Sánchez

2 **Hispanics and Academic Medicine: Creating an Inclusive Community, Academic Success, and Leadership Careers for Impactful Healthcare Change** ................................................. 15
Fernando S. Mendoza, Eneida O. Roldan, Laura Castillo-Page, and Débora H. Silva

3 **Making a Decision About an Academic Faculty Track** ............ 29
Sylk Sotto-Santiago and Maria Milagros Garcia

4 **How to Switch an Academic Faculty Track** ..................... 45
Guadalupe Federico-Martinez

5 **Optimizing Your Portfolio and Executive Presence in the Recruitment Process: Perspectives from the Search Firm** .... 61
Julia Omotade, David Acosta, and Philip Jaeger

6 **Optimizing CV and Portfolio for Promotion Purposes** ............ 67
Lisa Moreno-Walton, Juliana Jaramillo, and Leon S. Sanders III

7 **A National Perspective on LHS+ Leadership in US Medical Schools** ... 81
David Acosta, Joel Dickerman, and David J. Skorton

8 **Succeeding Along the Clinical Track from Assistant to Full Professor** ....................................... 103
Leon McDougle, Jeannette E. South-Paul, John Paul Sánchez, and A. Orlando Ortiz

| 9 | Succeeding Along the Educator Track from Assistant to Full Professor | 131 |
|---|---|---|

Alvaro Pérez Arcila and Maria Soto-Greene

| 10 | Succeeding Along the Researcher Track from Assistant to Full Professor | 149 |
|---|---|---|

Hector Rasgado-Flores, Cristina R. Fernández, Saira A. Mehmood, John Paul Sánchez, and Ramon Gilberto Gonzalez

| 11 | Striving to Become a Department Chair | 169 |
|---|---|---|

Monica Verduzco-Gutierrez, Julie Ann Sosa, Ruben J. Azocar, Rolando De Leon, and A. Orlando Ortiz

| 12 | Being a Medical School Dean: Perspectives from Past and Current LHS+ Deans | 193 |
|---|---|---|

Jose Manuel de la Rosa, Pedro "Joe" Greer Jr., and Olga Rodríguez de Arzola

| 13 | Striving to Become a Dean of Diversity, Equity, and Inclusion | 223 |
|---|---|---|

Ana Nunez and Francisco Lucio

| 14 | Striving to Become a Dean of Undergraduate Medical Education/Curriculum | 237 |
|---|---|---|

John A. Davis Rodríguez

| 15 | Striving to Become a Dean/Designated Institutional Official of Graduate Medical Education (GME) | 249 |
|---|---|---|

Larissa Velez, John Paul Sánchez, and Maricarmen Cruz

| 16 | Striving to Become a Dean of Admissions | 269 |
|---|---|---|

Sunny Nakae

| 17 | Striving to Become a Dean of Faculty Affairs and Development | 283 |
|---|---|---|

Beatriz Tapia and Guadalupe Federico-Martinez

| 18 | Striving to Become a Dean for Student Affairs | 303 |
|---|---|---|

Leonor Corsino and Luis Alzate-Duque

| 19 | *MedEdPORTAL*: Publishing Educational Innovations | 313 |
|---|---|---|

Hannah Turner, Débora Silva, Pilar Ortega, and Sara Hunt

| 20 | Serving as a Reviewer, Associate Editor, or Journal Editor in Chief | 335 |
|---|---|---|

Ana Nuñez, David Sklar, and José Rodríguez

| 21 | Hospital Leadership Roles and Perspectives: Promotion and Leadership Development in Academic Medicine | 347 |
|---|---|---|

Joseph R. Betancourt, Denice Cora-Bramble, and J. Emilio Carrillo

| | | |
|---|---|---|
| **22** | **Considerations in Switching Institutions for Career Advancement: Background of the Road Traveled** . . . . . . . . . . . . . . . . David A. Acosta | 361 |
| **23** | **Considerations for Lideres of Tomorrow** . . . . . . . . . . . . . . . . . . . . . . Francisco Lucio, Wined Ramirez Lopez, Cristhian A. Gutierrez-Huerta, and Arturo Saavedra | 369 |

**Index**. . . . . . . . . . . . . . . . . . . . . . . . . . . . . . . . . . . . . . . . . . . . . . . . . . . . . 377

# About the Contributors

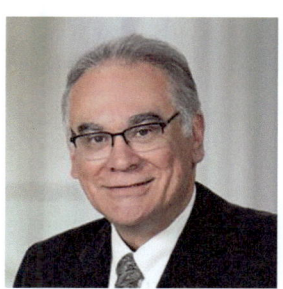

**David Acosta, MD** Former Chief Diversity and Inclusion Officer, Association of American Medical Colleges, Washington, D.C. (at the time of writing this book)

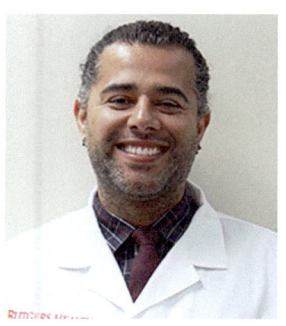

**Luis Alzate-Duque, MD, MPH** Assistant Professor, Medicine and Assistant Dean, Student Affairs
   Rutgers New Jersey Medical School, Newark, New Jersey

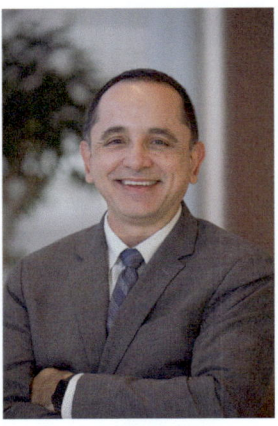

**Alvaro Pérez Arcila, MD, MS-MMEL**  Executive Dean
 Universidad Central del Caribe, Bayamon, Puerto Rico

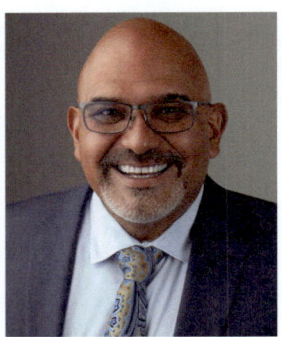

**Ruben J. Azocar, MD, MHCM, FASA, FCCM, FACHE**  Sol and Meryl Israel Chair of the Department of Anesthesiology and Perioperative Medicine
 Tulane University School of Medicine, New Orlenas, Louisiana

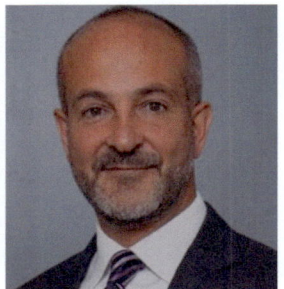

**Joseph R. Betancourt, MD, MPH**  President
 The Commonwealth Fund, New York City, New York

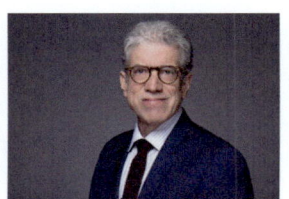

**J. Emilio Carrillo, MD, MPH**  Clinical Professor Emeritus, Epidemiology and Health Services Research
 Weill Cornell Graduate School of Medical Sciences, New York City, New York

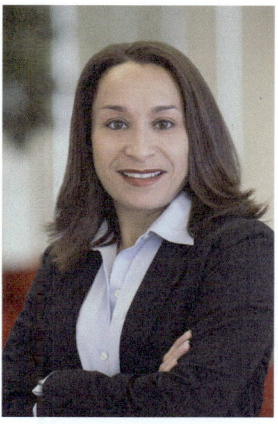

**Laura Castillo-Page, PhD**  Chief People and Culture American Board of Medical Specialties, Chicago, Illinois

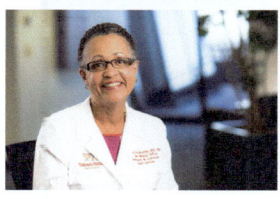

**Denice Cora-Bramble, MD, MBA**  Chief Diversity Officer, Children's National Hospital, Professor of Pediatrics George Washington University School of Medicine, Washington, D.C.

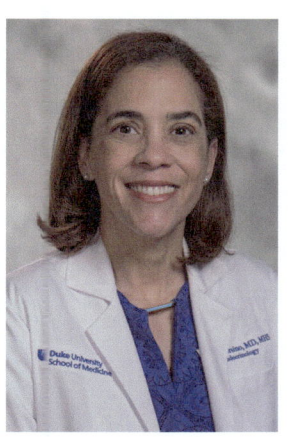

**Leonor Corsino, MD, MHS**  Associate Dean for Student Affairs, Associate Professor, Department of Medicine, Division of Endocrinology, Metabolism and Nutrition, Associate Professor, Department of Population Health Sciences, Duke School of Medicine, Durham, North Carolina

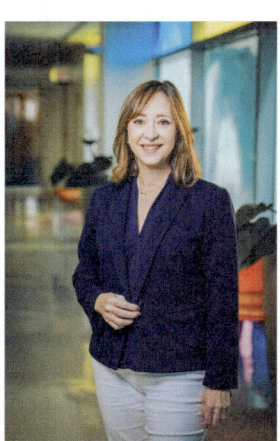

**Maricarmen Cruz, MD**  Associate Chief of Staff for Education Veteran Affairs Caribbean Healthcare System, Guaynabo, Puerto, Rico

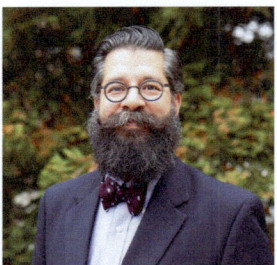

**John A. Davis Rodríguez, PhD, MD** Professor of Medicine, Vice Chancellor of Education and Student Affairs
University of California, San Francisco, San Francisco, California

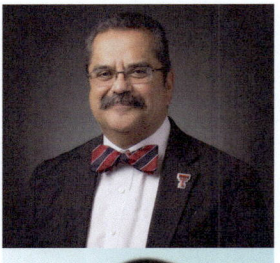

**Jose Manuel de la Rosa, MD, MSc.** Interim Chair and Tenured Professor, Department of Pediatrics, Paul L. Foster School of Medicine, Vice-President for Outreach and Community Engagement
Texas Tech University Health Sciences Center, El Paso, Texas

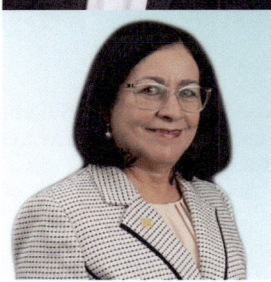

**Olga Rodríguez de Arzola, MD, FAAP** Dean
Ponce Health Sciences University School of Medicine, Ponce, Puerto Rico

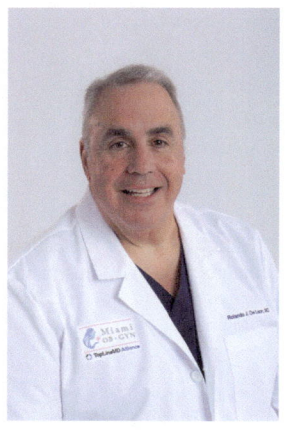

**Rolando De Leon, MD, FACOG** Founding Chair and Associate Clinical Professor, Division of Obstetrics and Gynecology,
Kiram C Patel College of Allopathic Medicine, Nova Southeastern University, Ft. Lauderdale, Florida

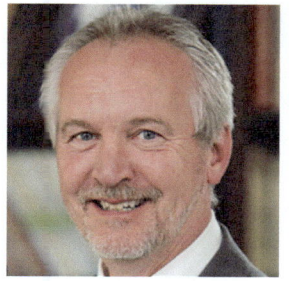

**Joel Dickerman, DO** Regional Director for Clinical Education
Rocky Vista University, Englewood, Colorado

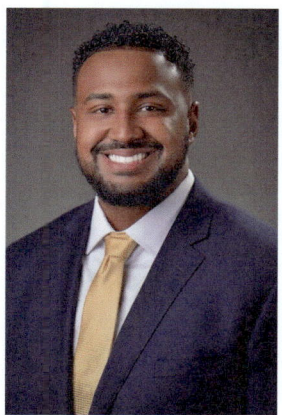

**Deion Ellis, MD, MMS** Resident, Department of Physical Medicine and Rehabilitation
University of Colorado School of Medicine, Anschutz Medical Campus

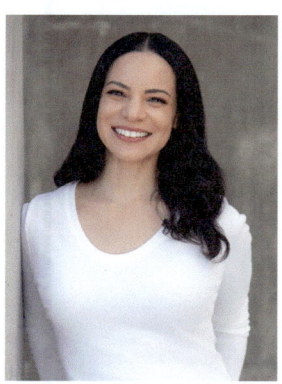

**Guadalupe Federico-Martinez, PhD** CEO, Career Coach
DLM Coaching, Consulting & Wellness LLC, Paradise Valley, Arizona

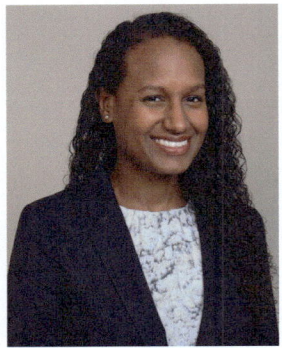

**Cristina R. Fernandez, MD, MPH, FAAP** Assistant Professor of Pediatrics, Division of Child and Adolescent Health, Department of Pediatrics
    Columbia University Vagelos College of Physicians & Surgeons, New York, New York

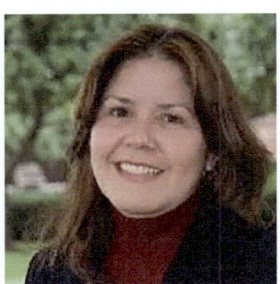

**Maria Milagros Garcia, MD** Professor of Medicine and Assistant Vice Provost for Student Success and Diversity
    University of Massachusetts Chan Medical School, Worcester, Massachusetts

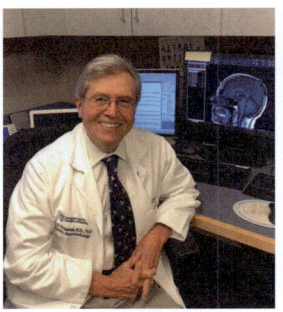

**Ramon Gilberto Gonzalez, MD, PhD** Professor and Senior Neuroradiologist, Chief of Neuroradiology, Emeritus
    Massachusetts General Hospital, Harvard Medical School, Boston, Massachusetts

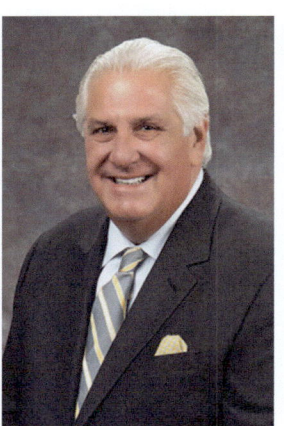

**Pedro "Joe" Greer Jr, MD** Dean and Professor
    Roseman University College of Medicine, Las Vegas, Nevada

## About the Contributors

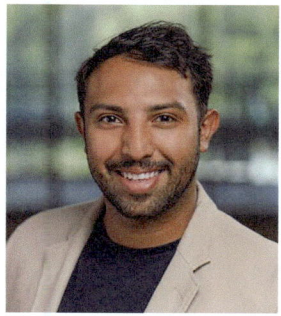

**Cristhian A. Gutierrez-Huerta** PhD, MD Candidate, Medical Scientist Training Program
  Medical College of Wisconsin, Milwaukee, Wisconsin

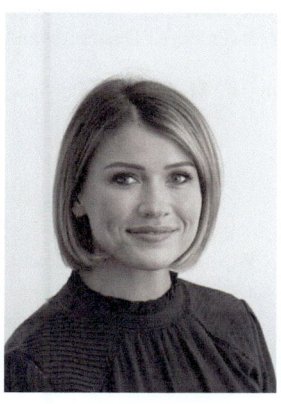

**Sara Hunt** Director, Scholarly Engagement, Association of American Medical Colleges
  Washington, D.C.

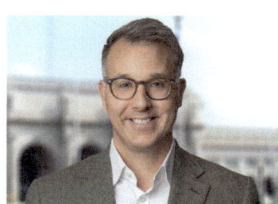

**Philip Jaeger, MBA** Consultant, Spencer Stuart
  Washington, D.C.

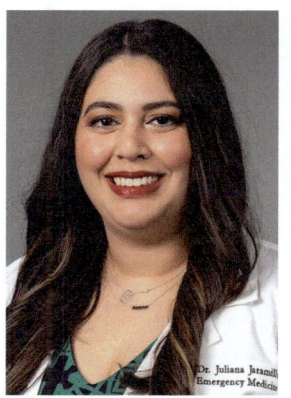

**Juliana Jaramillo, MD, FACEP** Clinical Assistant Professor, Emergency Medicine/Pediatric Emergency Medicine
  Brody School of Medicine, Greenville, North Carolina

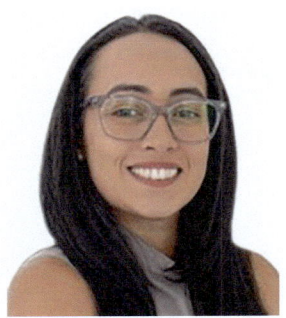

**Wined Ramirez Lopez, MPH** Director, Continuous Quality Improvement

Universidad Central Del Caribe, School of Medicine, Bayamon, Puerto Rico

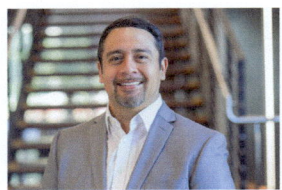

**Francisco Lucio, JD** Senior Associate Dean, Health Care Advancement, Associate Professor of Practice, Obstetrics and Gynecology

University of Arizona College of Medicine - Phoenix, Phoenix, Arizona

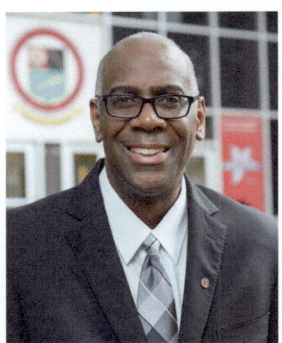

**Leon McDougle, MD, MPH, DHL** Chief Diversity Officer

The Ohio State University Wexner Medical Center. Columbus, Ohio

**Saira A. Mehmood, PhD** American Association for the Advancement of Science (AAAS), Washington, DC, USA

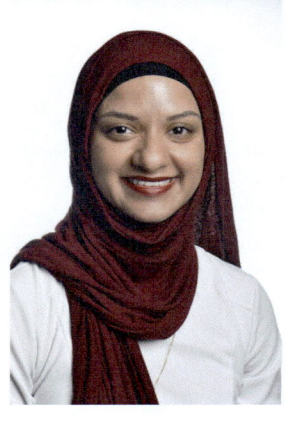

# About the Contributors

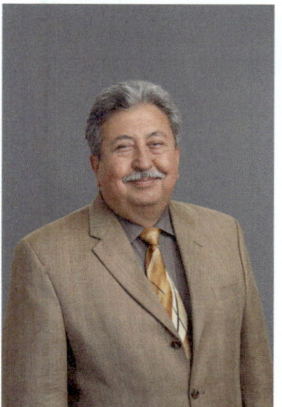

**Fernando S. Mendoza, MD, MPH** Professor of Pediatrics, Emeritus, Associate Dean of Minority Advising and Programs, Emeritus
  Stanford University School of Medicine, Stanford, California

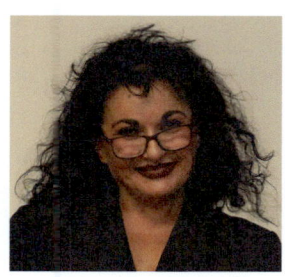

**Lisa Moreno-Walton, MD, FAAEM, FACEP, FIFEM** Professor with Tenure, Emergency Medicine
  University of South Alabama School of Medicine. Mobile Alabama

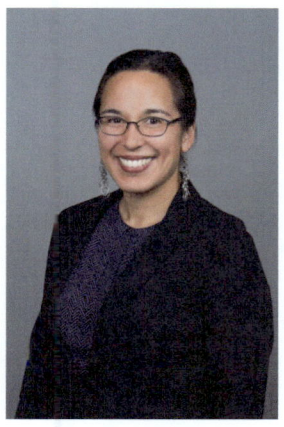

**Sunny Nakae, PhD, MSW** Senior Associate Dean for Equity, Inclusion, Diversity, and Partnership, Professor of Medical Education
  California University of Science and Medicine, Colton, CA

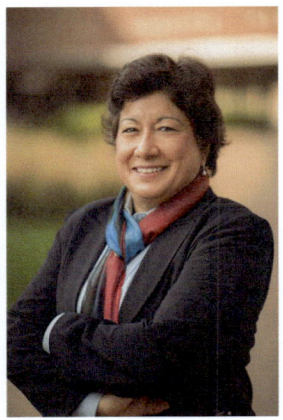

**Ana Nuñez, MD, FACP** Vice Dean, Diversity, Equity & Inclusion Professor of Medicine
University of Minnesota School of Medicine, Minneapolis, Minnesota

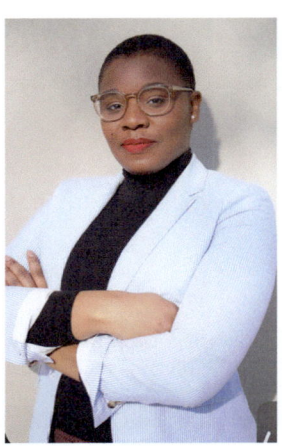

**Julia Omotade, PhD** Cellular Neuroscientist, Former Healthcare Consultant, Biomedical Science Policy Leader at Association of American Medical Colleges, Washington, D.C.

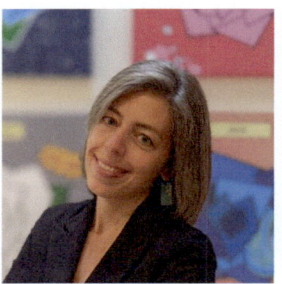

**Pilar Ortega, MD, MGM** Clinical Associate Professor, Emergency Medicine and Medical Education, University of Illinois College of Medicine, Chicago, Illinois; President/Chief Executive Officer, National Association of Medical Spanish, Chicago, Illinois

## About the Contributors

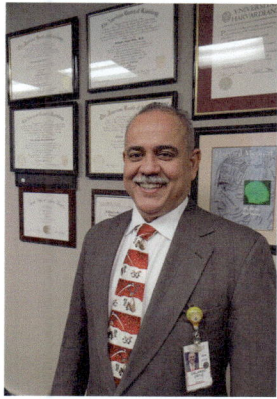

**A. Orlando Ortiz, MD, MBA, FACR, FASSR** Chairman Emeritus, Jacobi Medical Center, Professor of Radiology
Albert Einstein College of Medicine, Bronx, New York

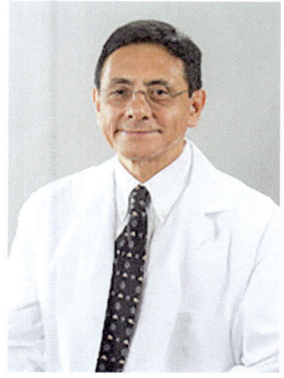

**Hector Rasgado-Flores, PhD** Professor of Physiology/Biophysics
Chicago Medical School at Rosalind Franklin University, Chicago, Illinois

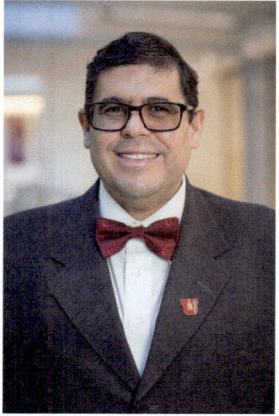

**José Rodríguez, MD** Associate Vice President, Health Equity, Diversity & Inclusion
University of Utah School of Medicine

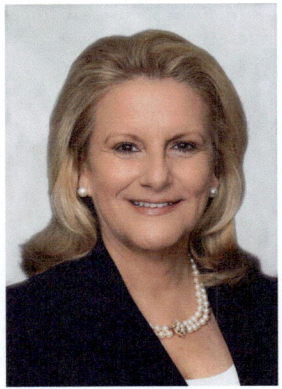

**Eneida O. Roldan, MD, MPH, MBA**  Executive Dean, College of Health and Wellness
 Barry University, Miami, Florida

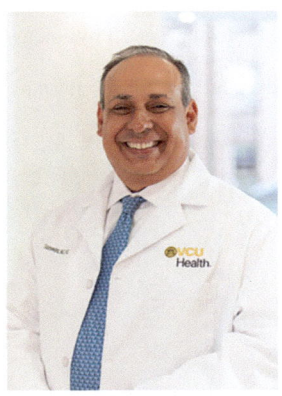

**Arturo Saavedra, MD, PhD, MBA**  Dean of the VCU School of Medicine and Executive Vice President of VCU Health System
 Richmond, Virginia

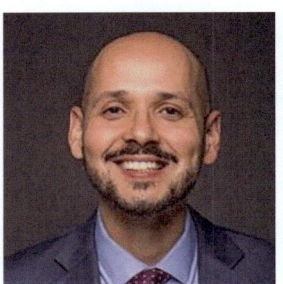

**John Paul Sánchez, MD, MPH**  Executive Director, Latino Medical Student Association Inc.
 President, Building the Next Generation of Academic Physicians Inc., Director, Elmhurst-San Juan Bautista SoM-Ponce SoM (ESP) Bilingual Med Education Program

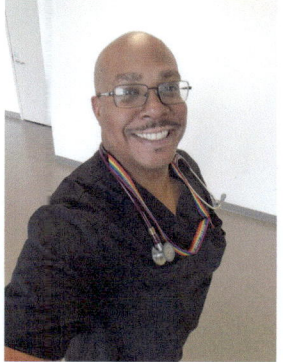

**Leon S. Sanders III, MD** Resident, Department of Internal Medicine
Tulane University School of Medicine, New Orleans, Louisiana

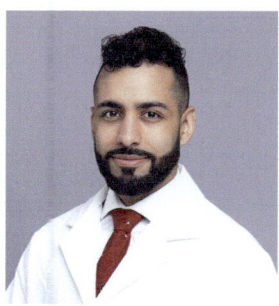

**Andy Reyes Santos, MD, FAAP** Pediatric Residency Associate Program Director, Hackensack University Medical Center Hackensack, New Jersey

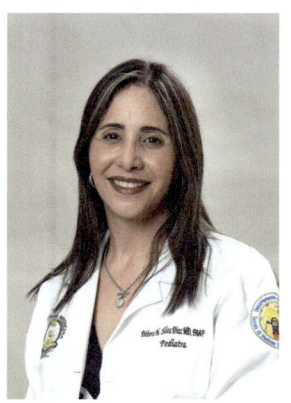

**Debora Silva, MD, MEd** Dean School of Medicine
University of Puerto Rico, San Juan, Puerto Rico

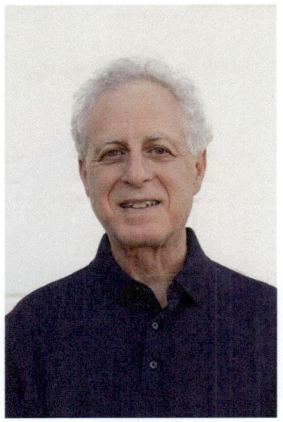

**David Sklar, MD** Senior Associate Dean Medical Education Arizona State University, Phoenix, Arizona

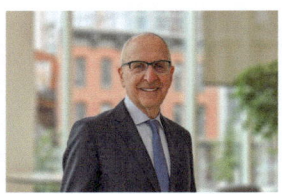

**David J. Skorton, MD** President and CEO Association of American Medical Colleges, Washington, D.C.

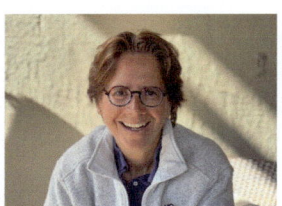

**Julie Ann Sosa, MD, MA, FACS, FSSO, MAMSE** Leon Goldman, MD Distinguished Chair and Professor of Surgery University of California San Francisco (UCSF), San Francisco, California

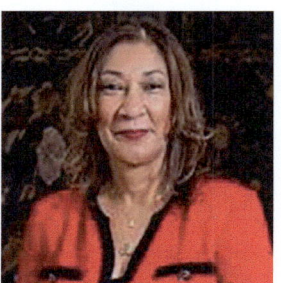

**Maria Soto-Greene, MD** Professor and Executive Vice Dean Rutgers New Jersey Medical School (NJMS), Newark, New Jersey

About the Contributors xliii

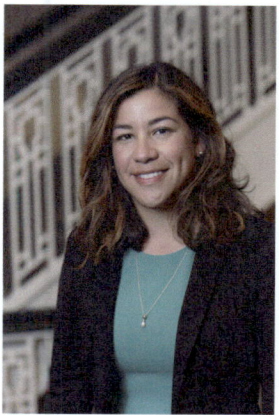

**Sylk Sotto-Santiago, EdD, MPS, MBA** Associate Vice-Chancellor for Faculty Development and Inclusive Excellence, Associate Professor of Medicine,
University of Pittsburgh School of Medicine, Health Sciences, Pittsburgh, Pennsylvania

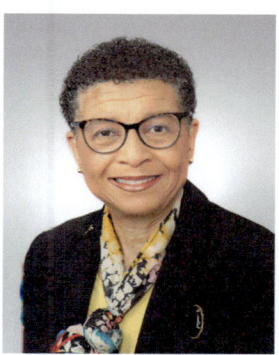

**Jeannette E. South-Paul, MD, DHL (Hon), FAAFP** EVP and Provost, Professor Emeritus Family Medicine
Meharry Medical College, Nashville, Tennessee

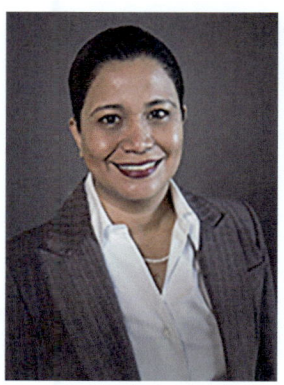

**Beatriz Tapia, MD, MPH, CPH** Associate Dean, Faculty Affairs, Associate Professor, Division of Population Health and Biostatistics
The University of Texas Rio Grande Valley School of Medicine Edinburg, Texas

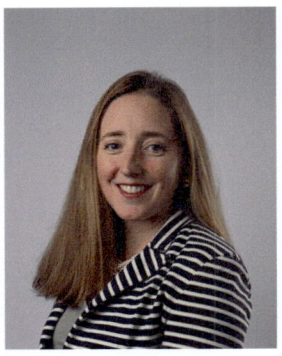

**Hannah Turner, MPH** Managing Editor, MedEdPORTAL AAMC (Association of American Medical Colleges), Washington, D.C.

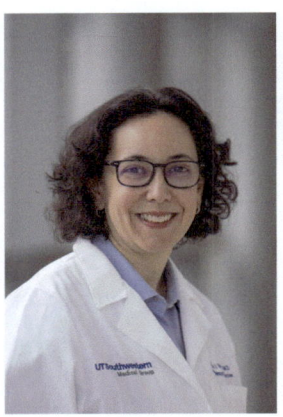

**Larissa Velez, MD** Associate Dean for Graduate Medical Education, A. Compton Broders III, MD Endowed Chair in Emergency Medicine, Professor and Vice Chair for Education, Department of Emergency Medicine, University of Texas Southwestern Medical Center, Dallas, Texas

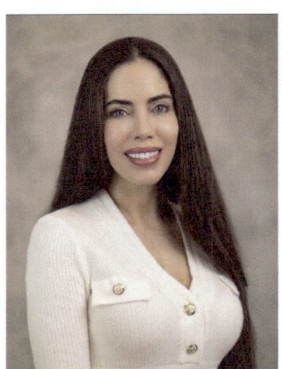

**Alexandra Lopez Vera, PhD, MPH** Assistant Professor of Medical Education, Director of Vida Medical Spanish Program, California University of Science and Medicine, Colton, California

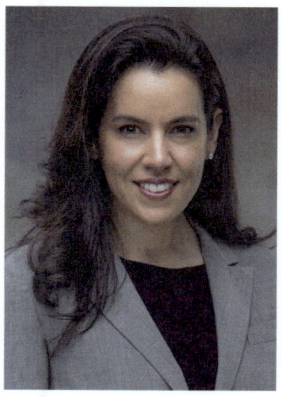

**Monica Verduzco-Gutierrez, MD** Professor and Chair, Department of Rehabilitation Medicine

Long School of Medicine at the University of Texas Health Science Center at San Antonio, San Antonio, Texas

# Chapter 1
# Why Academia Needs Faculty and Leaders with LHS+ Lived Experiences

**Deion Ellis, Alexandra Lopez Vera, Andy Reyes Santos, and John Paul Sánchez**

> **Learning Objectives**
> - Describe the LHS+ community in the USA and in the academic medicine workforce.
> - Summarize the benefits of LHS+ inclusion in medicine and academia medicine.
> - Analyze the challenges and opportunities to LHS+ advancement in academic medicine.

D. Ellis
Department of Physical Medicine and Rehabilitation, University of Colorado School of Medicine, Anschutz Medical Campus, Aurora, CO, USA

A. L. Vera
California University of Science and Medicine, Colton, CA, USA

A. R. Santos
Hackensack University Medical Center, Hackensack, NJ, USA

J. P. Sánchez (✉)
Latino Medical Student Association Inc., Chicago, IL, USA

Building the Next Generation of Academic Physicians Inc., Rye Brook, NY, USA
e-mail: exec.director@lmsa.net

© The Author(s) 2026
J. P. Sánchez et al. (eds.), *Advancing Latino, Hispanic, or of Spanish Origin+ Leadership in Academic Medicine*,
https://doi.org/10.1007/978-3-032-07570-3_1

> **Key Terms and Definitions**
> - LHS+: Latino/Latina/Latinx/Latine, Hispanic, or of Spanish origin+ (LHS+).
>   - Term to reflect the heterogeneity of terms reflective of communities with our common geographic (e.g., Caribbean; North, Central, and South America; and Spain) and Spanish language ancestry. It gives recognition to historical terms Latino, Latina, Hispanic, of Spanish origin (used on standardized surveys), emerging generational/nonbinary terms (e.g., Latinx), with the plus acknowledging other terms linked to national or sociocultural identity (e.g., Mexican, Chicano, Afro-Cuban, Honduran, Nuyorican) [1].

## The LHS+ Community in the USA

Between 1970 and 2024, the proportion of Latino/Hispanic-identified individuals in the USA increased from approximately 5 to 20% [2, 3]. Latinos/Hispanics in the USA originate from the 21 Spanish-speaking countries in the world and in 2021, 8 nationalities had greater than 1 million individuals in the US - Mexican (37.2 million), Puerto Rican (5.8), Salvadoran (2.5), Dominican (2.4), Cuban (2.4), Guatemalan (1.8), Colombian (1.4), and Hondurans (1.1) [4]. The vast majority of Latinos/Hispanics in the USA are US citizens, approximately 81% in 2021 [4]. The Latino/Hispanic population in the USA is younger than the overall US population and makes up a quarter of all children under age 18 in the USA [5]. Among the 50 states, New Mexico has the highest proportion of Latinos/Hispanics, California has the greatest number of Latinos/Hispanics, and Texas, California, and Florida have seen the greatest Latino/Hispanic population growth [6].

In terms of community, about six-in-ten Latino/Hispanic adults say what happens to other Hispanics affects what happens in their own lives [7]. In terms of language, the majority (75%) of US Latinos/Hispanics speak Spanish, and most (85%) say it is at least somewhat important for future generations of Latinos/Hispanics in the USA to speak Spanish [8]. Moreover, speaking Spanish is considered the most important part of Latino/Hispanic identity across immigrant generations, followed by having both parents of Latino/Hispanic heritage or descent, socializing with other Latinos/Hispanics, having a Spanish last name, participating or attending Latino/Hispanic cultural celebrations, and wearing attire that represents their Latino/Hispanic heritage or origin [7].

Historically, terms such as Latino, Hispanic, and of Spanish origin have been incorporated on standardized surveys, such as the Census, to determine the size of the community in the USA. For the remainder of this chapter, we will also use the term Latina/o/x/e, Hispanic, or of Spanish origin+ (LHS+) which not only reflects communities with a common geographic (e.g., Caribbean; North, Central, and

South America; and Spain) and Spanish language ancestry but also gives recognition of emerging generational/nonbinary terms (e.g., Latinx, Latine), with the plus acknowledging other terms linked to national or sociocultural identity (e.g., Mexican, Chicano, Afro-Cuban, Nuyorican) [1].

The health of the LHS+ population is well documented, and research has shown that LHS+ individuals have unique health issues and disparities. Some notable research findings include:

(a) Hispanics/Latinos are about 50% more likely to die from diabetes or liver disease than non-Hispanic whites [9].
(b) Compared to non-Hispanic whites, Hispanics/Latinos are 22% less likely to have controlled high blood pressure [9].
(c) Hispanics/Latinos have a colorectal cancer screening rate that is 28% lower than that of non-Hispanic whites [9].
(d) Hispanic/Latino children and adolescents aged 2–19 years have a higher prevalence of obesity than their non-Hispanic white and non-Hispanic Asian peers [9].
(e) The proportion of Hispanic adults with obesity is about 20% higher than non-Hispanic whites [9].
(f) Hispanics/Latinos are almost three times as likely to be uninsured as non-Hispanic whites [9].
(g) Hispanics/Latinos were more likely to die from COVID-19 than non-Hispanic whites [10].

The diversity and unique health issues and health disparities of the LHS+ population are important to consider as medical schools and academic health centers recruit, support, and promote the next generation of physicians and academic leaders to advance health equity in the USA.

## The LHS+ Community in Medicine and Academic Medicine

A brief report by the Association of American Medical Colleges in 2019 found that approximately 6% of US practicing physicians identified as LHS+, of which 43% were born in the mainland USA. Other birthplaces included South America (21%), Puerto Rico (9%), Cuba (9%), Mexico (8%), and from other parts of Central America (5%) [11].

In considering the academic medicine workforce, it primarily consists of faculty and senior administrative leaders within medical schools; however, at times medical students, residents, and fellows are also considered given their roles as pre-faculty and resident/fellow as teacher. Although in 2024 LHS+ individuals represented nearly 20% of the US population, only 11.0% of medical students who matriculated into allopathic medical schools, 6.9% of residents, and 6.3% of allopathic medical school faculty identified as LHS+ [12–14]. Among faculty who hold the rank of full professor, only 5% are LHS+ identified, and among departmental chairs, only 4.0% are LHS+ identified. It is important to note that included in these statistics are learners and faculty from the four medical schools and associated residency programs in Puerto Rico which has a population that overwhelmingly (>98%) identifies as LHS+.

Faculty with LHS+ lived experiences uniquely bring bilingualism, biculturalism, and transnational insights into their patient care, teaching, and research work. These competencies are invaluable in communities with high Spanish-speaking populations, where cultural and linguistic barriers can impede positive health outcomes [15, 16]. Yet existing academic structures—predominantly monocultural and monolingual—often do not fully recognize or reward these strengths.

## Benefits of LHS+ Inclusion in Academic Medicine

### Transforming Clinical Care Through Cultural and Linguistic Concordance

LHS+ faculty improve patient outcomes by offering culturally and linguistically congruent care, particularly for Spanish-speaking patients. Their presence fosters trust, reduces miscommunication, and enhances quality of care. Language concordance creates direct communication that deepens trust, improves compliance, and enhances the therapeutic alliance [16].

### Enriching Education and Mentorship

LHS+ faculty play a crucial role in supporting students from underrepresented backgrounds. Their mentorship can demystify academic systems, affirm cultural identity, and increase retention. Students are more likely to persist when they see faculty who reflect their identities and experiences [17]. LHS+ professionals also enrich medical education by incorporating culturally responsive curricula and community health issues that affect LHS+ populations [18].

### Advancing Diversity, Equity, and Inclusion (DEI) and Institutional Impact

Beyond patient care and education, LHS+ faculty often lead DEI efforts. They develop initiatives that address systemic racism, reimagine admissions processes, and promote social accountability. As discussed by Sánchez et al., LHS+ leaders are critical in ensuring medical institutions align with the demographic and ethical demands of contemporary medicine [19]. Their presence helps reshape how institutions define excellence, equity, and public service [20].

## Challenges and Opportunities for LHS+ Inclusion in Academic Medicine

There are numerous historical and ongoing barriers that have contributed to the current state of LHS+ representation in academic medicine. As previously noted less than half of LHS+ physicians in the USA were born in the USA. This may reflect systemic barriers for US-born LHS+-identified individuals to succeed within the educational system and gain acceptance to and graduation from US-accredited medical schools and subsequently become faculty. LHS+ applicants often have less access to financial, cultural, and social capital, which limits performance on high-stakes metrics like the MCAT [21, 22]. Disparities in test prep, advising, and exposure to healthcare roles contribute to lower matriculation rates [23]. Furthermore, institutional overreliance on test scores perpetuates inequality [24]. A lower proportion of medical school matriculants will subsequently limit the pool of candidates for faculty appointments.

URiM faculty, including those who are LHS+, produce fewer peer-reviewed publications—not due to capability but largely due to less mentorship, funding, and protected time for research [25]. Their engagement in DEI efforts, often uncompensated, takes time away from traditionally valued academic metrics [26, 27]. These disparities lead to disproportionately lower promotion rates [28].

Mentorship is crucial for navigating academia [29, 30]. Many LHS+ faculty report a lack of guidance and support, particularly in early career stages [22]. This isolation contributes to slower career advancement, decreased confidence, and burnout [23].

### *Opportunities for LHS+ Inclusion in Academic Medicine*

The previously noted challenges have been overcome by many current LHS+ faculty through various approaches. An initial step in finding opportunities for academic advancement is to understand and embrace the value LHS+-identified individuals bring to the field of medicine and academia. Research shows that nuanced cultural and linguistic differences are often better understood by those of a similar background as those served, resulting in overall improved care and patient satisfaction [15]. Cultural and linguistic assets should be framed as academic strengths, not liabilities. Bilingualism, biculturalism, and lived experience are not only examples of cultural competence but also academic capital.

Another important approach is to establish credibility in content specific to LHS+ topics. When early in a career, a LHS+ faculty member may not yet hold titles or positions that elevate their credibility. A key strategy to legitimize LHS+ lived experiences and advance in academia is by publishing in peer-reviewed journals and books. Publications are a gold standard of communication in academic medicine and serve to disseminate best or promising practices in clinical care, teaching, and research. Furthermore, most institutions require that an individual have a certain number of quality publications before being hired as a faculty member or promoted to a higher rank.

Opportunities to seek involvement in publications are abundant but may be hiding in plain sight. Individuals should not limit themselves to writing alone; it is advantageous to join writing groups or develop their own writing team of likeminded individuals. LHS+ faculty should find authors who are writing about or interested in writing about specific content that they themselves have much knowledge about given their lived experiences and discuss ways in which they could participate in the publication even if as a contributor to the publication. Although serving as first or last author is particularly valuable when seeking promotion, it is also advantageous to serve as a middle author, especially when a faculty member needs to reach a certain threshold of publications to be promoted. It is also important to consider that community-based participatory research, qualitative studies, and even perspectives or commentaries are valuable additions to the published literature and count for promotion [31, 32]. MedEdPORTAL and some other journals have provided unique spaces to publish content in Spanish, which can recognize work developed for medical Spanish electives and courses [33].

Joining and leading identity-based and/or profession-based committees, organizations, and networks can help foster identity affirmation, peer mentorship, leadership development, and sponsorship [34]. Through these entities, individuals gain access to regional and national opportunities and meet individuals who can write letters of recommendation; both are necessary for promotion.

The Faculty Physician Advisory Council (FPAC) of the Latino Medical Student Association (LMSA) is one entity which can provide opportunities to develop a sense of belonging, obtain congruent mentorship, engage in community service, and access culturally nuanced professional development [1, 34]. FPAC has two notable faculty development programs. LISTOS (LMSA Instruction, Support, Training & Orientation Session—https://fpac.lmsa.net/center/listos/) is a 1-day training to help chapter advisors and faculty mentors become updated on best and promising practices to support the academic, personal, and professional development of LHS+-identified students. LIDEReS (LHS+ Identity, Development, Empowerment, and Resources Seminar—https://fpac.lmsa.net/center/lideres/) is a multiday seminar to bring together faculty (e.g., including residents with signed contracts for faculty positions and fellows) and physician advisors from across the USA and provides participants with inspirational and practical guidance and tools for pursuing career advancement in academic medicine. The seminar helps participants develop key professional competencies that build self-efficacy, communication skills, and leadership while expanding their network.

From funding pipeline programs to rethinking promotion metrics, systemic change is necessary to address inequities. Legislative and institutional advocacy are vital for increasing LHS+ representation in medicine and academia [35].

To move from understanding to action, we invite readers to engage in the following reflection exercise designed to foster critical self-awareness and strategic thinking around LHS+ inclusion.

## Reflection Exercise

*Instructions:* Reflect on the following questions, considering your own experiences, knowledge, and biases.

1. Personal Awareness:
   - How familiar are you with the term "LHS+" and the diverse communities it represents?
   - Have you worked closely with LHS+ colleagues or mentored students from the LHS+ community? If so, reflect on that experience. If not, why might that be?
   - What cultural and language barriers have you witnessed in academic medicine or healthcare environments that impact the LHS+ community? Can you describe a specific situation where you encountered these barriers?

2. Cultural Competency:
   - Reflect on how cultural competency has played a role in your interactions with LHS+ patients, students, or colleagues. What challenges have you encountered in effectively communicating with or understanding their needs?
   - How can you actively improve your own cultural competency when working with LHS+ populations?

3. Leadership and Advocacy:
   - As you think about your future role in academic medicine, how can you use your position to advocate for greater inclusion of LHS+ individuals in both academic and clinical settings?
   - What actions can you take now to contribute to the recruitment, retention, and promotion of LHS+ individuals in your institution?

*Further instructions*: based on your reflections, create an action plan outlining steps you can take over the next 6–12 months to promote LHS+ inclusion within your professional setting. Consider the following:

1. Personal Development:
   - What cultural competency training or educational resources will you seek to better understand the LHS+ community?

- How can you mentor or sponsor LHS+ individuals in your department or institution?
2. Institutional Impact:
    - What initiatives or programs can you advocate for or develop that would promote LHS+ inclusion at your institution (e.g., mentorship programs, scholarship funds, etc.)?
    - How will you measure success in your efforts to foster inclusion and equity for the LHS+ community?

Remember that the presence of LHS+ faculty and senior administrators challenges the status quo. It disrupts the traditional, often monolithic, approaches to education and patient care by introducing diverse perspectives that reflect the reality of the world we live in. LHS+ leaders help reshape curricula to include cultural competency as a cornerstone of medical training. LHS+ faculty advocate for policies that ensure better access to care for Spanish-speaking patients [36] and mentor the next generation of healthcare providers, ensuring that our future practitioners and researchers are not only skilled but also culturally aware and empathetic. LHS+ inclusion is not a luxury but a necessity. In a world that is becoming increasingly diverse, the absence of LHS+ voices leaves a gap in both understanding and care. LHS+ leaders do not just reflect the populations they serve; they actively improve outcomes for those populations through their presence, their work, and their advocacy.

## Conclusion

LHS+ inclusion in academic medicine is essential for building systems that are representative, culturally competent, equity-driven, and impactful. Faculty and leaders from LHS+ backgrounds bring critical skills, insights, and commitments that shape more responsive medical education and healthcare systems. Institutions must move beyond performative diversity and toward structural transformation, ensuring that the lived experiences of LHS+ professionals are not only valued but integrated into daily academic activities to ensure learner success and better patient outcomes.

## Personal Narratives

### Deion Ellis, MD, MMS

As an Afro-Mexicano, with both African American and Mexican American roots, my identity has been the driving force behind my journey in medicine. Growing up in a multicultural household where two historically marginalized cultures intersect,

I witnessed firsthand the systemic barriers my immigrant grandparents faced navigating the healthcare system. These challenges became the fuel that ignited my desire to pursue medicine and address healthcare disparities in underserved communities.

From an early age, I recognized the necessity for healthcare providers who reflect the diversity of the populations they serve. My heritage instilled in me the passion and empathy to bridge cultural divides in medicine. It was clear to me that representation isn't just about filling spaces—it's about leading change, breaking down barriers, and creating systems that uplift those who've been overlooked for far too long.

Throughout my academic journey, I embraced leadership roles that allowed me to advocate for diversity and inclusion. As part of the Student National Medical Association (SNMA) and the Latino Medical Student Association (LMSA), I made it my mission to uplift individuals from underrepresented backgrounds. These roles were not just titles—they were platforms where I could push for real change. Serving as Director of the Faculty Physician Advisory Council for LMSA gave me a front-row seat to the critical need for LHS+ (Latina/o/x/e, Hispanic, and Spanish origin) representation in academic medicine.

LHS+ inclusion in academia is not just a goal—it's a necessity. Faculty and leaders from LHS+ backgrounds bring perspectives that are vital to improving patient care and fostering a medical environment where all voices are heard. The power of inclusion lies in its ability to transform systems from the inside out, creating lasting change that goes beyond diversity metrics. It's about embedding cultural competence and understanding into the core of healthcare delivery. This is how we address the disparities that disproportionately affect Black and Latino communities—by ensuring the decision-makers reflect the people they serve.

In my current residency in Physical Medicine and Rehabilitation, I am constantly reminded of the importance of these values. Every day, I strive to embody the principles of equity, inclusion, and leadership that my Afro-Mexicano heritage has taught me. I am committed to delivering culturally competent care while mentoring and inspiring the next generation of physicians to continue this work. My journey has not been without challenges, but every obstacle has strengthened my resolve to build a more inclusive medical field.

The path to LHS+ inclusion in academic medicine is filled with opportunities for those ready to lead. As LHS+ professionals, we are uniquely positioned to create systems that work for everyone. Our diverse experiences are assets that fuel innovation, empathy, and excellence in healthcare. The future of medicine depends on leaders who are willing to step up, push boundaries, and create change. Together, we will build a healthcare system that reflects the best of who we are and ensures better outcomes for the communities that need it most. The time to lead is now.

**Alexandra Lopez Vera, PhD, MPH**

My professional journey as an LHS+-identified individual has been shaped by a deep commitment to addressing healthcare disparities, particularly within Spanish-speaking communities. As an educator and researcher, I have had the privilege of working at the intersection of language, healthcare, and public health. This work has allowed me to address many of the challenges and opportunities highlighted in this chapter, including the need for increased representation and cultural competence in academic medicine. Growing up in a Spanish-speaking household, I quickly became aware of how critical language is for effective communication and understanding. This awareness would later become a driving force in my work to improve healthcare outcomes for underserved populations. I recognized early on that language barriers often prevent patients from receiving the quality care they deserve, which is why I dedicated my career to improving language concordance between healthcare providers and patients. One of the most significant aspects of my work is my role as the Director of the Medical Spanish Program at the California University of Science and Medicine (CUSM). In this role, I have developed a comprehensive curriculum designed to equip future physicians with the necessary language and cultural skills to communicate effectively with Spanish-speaking patients. This curriculum directly addresses the chapter's focus on the importance of LHS+ inclusion in the medical workforce, as it prepares students to provide more culturally competent care and reduce healthcare disparities. As this chapter emphasizes, increasing the representation of LHS+ individuals in academic medicine is essential for improving healthcare outcomes and addressing chronic health conditions within our communities. My own experiences in developing the Vida Medical Spanish Curriculum have reinforced the idea that language concordance is not only beneficial for patient care but also critical for building trust and ensuring that patients feel understood and respected. When providers can communicate with their patients in a shared language, they are better able to address sensitive topics, gather accurate information, and provide more effective care. In my research, such as "A Case Study of the Impact of Language Concordance on Patient Care" [16], I have explored the profound effects that language alignment has on patient satisfaction and healthcare outcomes. This research supports the chapter's argument that LHS+ individuals bring unique perspectives to academic medicine, which can enrich both education and patient care. By increasing LHS+ representation, we can foster a more inclusive healthcare environment that addresses the specific needs of underserved populations. Throughout my career, I have faced many of the challenges described in this chapter, including underrepresentation and the need to advocate for greater inclusion of LHS+ individuals in leadership roles. However, these challenges have also provided opportunities to create meaningful change. My work in medical education and health advocacy continues to focus on promoting equity and cultural competency, ensuring that future healthcare providers are well-equipped to serve diverse communities. What has contributed to my success as an LHS+ individual is not only my dedication to improving healthcare for Spanish-speaking patients but also the support and collaboration of colleagues and mentors who share a commitment to diversity and inclusion. As I look ahead, my goal is to continue building pathways for LHS+ individuals in academic medicine, creating opportunities for future generations to contribute to a more equitable and culturally competent healthcare system. In conclusion, my professional journey aligns closely with the chapter's focus on the importance of increasing LHS+ inclusion in academic medicine. By continuing to address the language and cultural barriers that persist in healthcare, I aim to contribute to a more inclusive and effective healthcare system that serves the needs of all patients, particularly those from underserved communities.

**Andy Reyes Santos, MD, FAAP**

I was born in the Dominican Republic and moved to the United States just before turning 4 years old. Growing up, I traveled back to the Dominican Republic frequently, which helped me stay connected to my roots as an LHS+-identified individual. Both of my parents speak little English, and I experienced the challenges that come with this, including translating for them at doctor visits when I was still very young when I myself had little understanding of medical implications. These experiences have given me a deep perspective on humanistic patient care and fueled my passion for advocating for Diversity, Equity, and Inclusion (DEI).

My connection to my history has led me to serve as a chapter advisor for the Latino Medical Student Association at Hackensack Meridian School of Medicine, where I am also an Assistant Professor of Pediatrics. Additionally, I am the Associate Program Director (APD) of the Pediatric Residency Program at Hackensack University Medical Center (HUMC), New Jersey's highest-ranked children's hospital. I earned my undergraduate degree from Rutgers University and my medical degree from Rutgers New Jersey Medical School, followed by residency and chief residency at HUMC. Being early in my career and culturally curious is something I use to my advantage. My proximity to the residents and students I mentor allows me to build trust and understand their needs, which has helped me launch key initiatives like a resident wellness program and creation of a resident survival handbook recommended to me by an LHS+ resident who felt lost in the system.

Collaboration is central to my work. I worked on designing an interdisciplinary project allowing pediatric and OB/GYN residents to collaborate on post-operative home visits, providing comprehensive care in underserved communities. I also co-lead the New Jersey Pediatric Residency Advocacy Collaborative, which unites residency programs across the state to advance advocacy efforts and share resources.

Teaching is a passion of mine, and I have remained at my training institution as a faculty member to lead small group teaching sessions for chief residents and clinical skills exams for medical students. These roles allow me to give back to the next generation of physicians and contribute to the medical education community.

My own experiences with overcoming obstacles shape my approach to mentorship. My parents were very loving but did not have the academic background to support my education. Reading was never emphasized and "bedtime stories" were only something I heard of on television. My parents did not enjoy attending parent-teacher conferences for fear of not understanding what teachers had to say. When I failed my USMLE Step 2 exam in medical school, it was a difficult setback. With the help of friends and 6 months of excellent mentorship, I was able to pass the exam and go on to succeed in later board exams. Now, residents who face similar challenges feel comfortable approaching me for advice, and I am committed to helping them succeed.

Throughout my career, I've been grateful for the opportunities others have given me and the mentorship I've received. My goal is to continue paying it forward by fostering an environment where residents and medical trainees feel supported, confident, and prepared to excel. By building a workforce that reflects the diverse populations we serve, I hope to contribute to a more inclusive and equitable healthcare system.

# References

1. Sánchez JP, Rodriguez D, editors. Latino, Hispanic, or of Spanish origin+ identified student leaders in medicine: recognizing more than 50 years of presence, activism, and leadership. Springer; 2024.
2. Funk C, Hugo Lopez M. A brief statistical portrait of U.S. Hispanics. Pew Research Center. https://www.pewresearch.org/science/2022/06/14/a-brief-statistical-portrait-of-u-s-hispanics/#:~:text=Since%201970%2C%20when%20Hispanics%20made,has%20grown%20more%20than%20sixfold. Accessed on 5 July 2025.
3. Quickfacts. U.S. census. https://www.census.gov/quickfacts/fact/table/US/RHI725223. Accessed on 5 July 2025.
4. Moslimani M, Hugo Lopez M, Noe-Bustamente O. 11 facts about Hispanic origin. Pew Research Center. https://www.pewresearch.org/short-reads/2023/08/16/11-facts-about-hispanic-origin-groups-in-the-us/#:~:text=Eight%20Hispanic%20origin%20groups%20had,Salvadorans:%20660%2C000. Accessed on 5 July 2025.
5. Pena J, Alvarez Figueroa M, Rios-Vargas M, Marks R. One in every four children in the United States were of Hispanic origin in 2020. US Census Bureau. https://www.census.gov/library/stories/2023/05/hispanic-population-younger-but-aging-faster.html. Accessed on 5 July 2025.
6. Krogstad JM, Passel J, Moslimani M, Noe-Bustamente L. Key facts about U.S. Latinos for National Hispanic Heritage Month. Pew Research Center. https://www.pewresearch.org/short-reads/2023/09/22/key-facts-about-us-latinos-for-national-hispanic-heritage-month/#:~:text=Three%20states'%20Hispanic%20populations%20increased,states%20with%20significant%20Hispanic%20populations. Accessed on 5 July 2025.
7. Gonzalez-Barrera A. The ways Hispanics describe their identity vary across immigrant generations. Pew Research Center. https://www.pewresearch.org/short-reads/2020/09/24/the-ways-hispanics-describe-their-identity-vary-across-immigrant-generations/. Accessed on 5 July 2025.
8. Mora L, Hugo Lopez M. Latinos' views of and experiences with the Spanish language. Pew Research Center. https://www.pewresearch.org/race-and-ethnicity/2023/09/20/latinos-views-of-and-experiences-with-the-spanish-language/. Accessed on 5 July 2025.
9. 2021 national healthcare quality and disparities report [Internet]. Rockville: Agency for Healthcare Research and Quality (US); 2021 Dec. Report No.: 21(22)-0054-EF. PMID: 35263063.
10. 2023 national healthcare quality and disparities report. Rockville: Agency for Healthcare Research and Quality (US); 2023 Dec. Report No.: 23(24)-0091-EF. PMID: 38377267.
11. Felida N, Zhuang J, Nouri Z, Dill M, Poll-Hunter N. Diversity among Hispanic/Latinx US physicians. Association of American Medical Colleges. 2021, September. https://www.aamc.org/media/56736/download. Accessed on 5 July 2025.
12. Matriculating Student Questionnaire (MSQ). https://www.aamc.org/data-reports/students-residents/report/matriculating-student-questionnaire-msq. Accessed on 5 July 2025.
13. 2024 Report on Residents. Table B5. Number of active MD residents, by race/ethnicity (alone or in combination) and GME specialty. 2023–24 active residents. Association of American Medical Colleges (AAMC). https://www.aamc.org/data-reports/students-residents/data/report-residents/2024/table-b5-md-residents-race-ethnicity-and-specialty. Accessed on 5 July 2025.

14. Table 8: U.S. medical school faculty by gender and race/ethnicity, 2024. AAMC Faculty Roster, December 31, 2024, snapshot, as of December 31, 2024. https://www.aamc.org/data-reports/faculty-institutions/report/faculty-roster-us-medical-school-faculty. Accessed on 5 July 2025.
15. Hsueh L, Hirsh AT, Maupomé G, Stewart JC. Patient–Provider language concordance and health outcomes: a systematic review, evidence map, and research agenda. Med Care Res Rev. 2021;78(1):3–23. https://doi.org/10.1177/1077558719860708.
16. Lopez Vera A, Thomas K, Trinh C, Nausheen F. A case study of the impact of language concordance on patient care, satisfaction, and comfort with sharing sensitive information during medical care. J Immigr Minor Health. 2023;25(6):1261–9. https://doi.org/10.1007/s10903-023-01463-8.
17. Lamb E, Burford B, Alberti H. The impact of role modeling on the future general practitioner workforce: a systematic review. Educ Prim Care. 2022;33(5):265–79. https://doi.org/10.1080/14739879.2022.2079097.
18. Ortega AN, Rodríguez HP, Vargas Bustamante A. Policy dilemmas in Latino health care and care delivery: ethical considerations. J Health Care Poor Underserved. 2015;26(4):1184–94. https://doi.org/10.1353/hpu.2015.0112.
19. Sánchez JP, Poll-Hunter NI, Acosta D. Advancing the Latino physician workforce—population trends, persistent challenges, and new directions. Acad Med. 2015;90(7):849–53. https://doi.org/10.1097/ACM.0000000000000618.
20. Yancy CW. Academic medicine and health equity: a time to be deliberate. J Am Coll Cardiol. 2020;75(7):839–41. https://doi.org/10.1016/j.jacc.2019.11.057.
21. Girotti J, Chanatry J, Clinchot D, McClure S, Swan Sein A, Walker I, Searcy C. Investigating group differences in examinees' preparation for and performance on the new MCAT exam. Acad Med. 2020;95(3):365–74. https://doi.org/10.1097/ACM.0000000000002940.
22. Tello C, Goode CA. Factors and barriers that influence the matriculation of underrepresented students in medicine. Front Psychol. 2023;14:1141045. https://doi.org/10.3389/fpsyg.2023.1141045.
23. Nguyen M, Desai MM, Fancher TL, Chaudhry SI, Mason HRC, Boatright D. Temporal trends in childhood household income among applicants and matriculants to medical school and the likelihood of acceptance by income, 2014–2019. JAMA. 2023;329(21):1882–4. https://doi.org/10.1001/jama.2023.5654.
24. Ko M, Henderson MC, Fancher TL, London MR, Simon M, Hardeman RR. US medical school admissions leaders' experiences with barriers to and advancements in diversity, equity, and inclusion. JAMA Netw Open. 2023;6(2):e2254928. https://doi.org/10.1001/jamanetworkopen.2022.54928.
25. Kaplan SE, Raj A, Carr PL, Terrin N, Breeze JL, Freund KM. Race/ethnicity and success in academic medicine: findings from a longitudinal multi-institutional study. Acad Med. 2018;93(4):616–22. https://doi.org/10.1097/ACM.0000000000001968.
26. Rodríguez JE, Campbell KM, Pololi LH. Addressing disparities in academic medicine: what of the minority tax? BMC Med Educ. 2015;15(1):6. https://doi.org/10.1186/s12909-015-0290-9.
27. Pololi L, Cooper LA, Carr P. Race, disadvantage and faculty experiences in academic medicine. J Gen Intern Med. 2010;25(12):1363–9. https://doi.org/10.1007/s11606-010-1478-7.
28. Ramirez AG, Lepe R, Cigarroa F. Uplifting the Latino population from obscurity to the forefront of health care, public health intervention, and societal presence. JAMA. 2021;326(7):597–8. https://doi.org/10.1001/jama.2021.11997.
29. Mahoney MR, Wilson E, Odom KL, Flowers L, Adler SR. Minority faculty voices on diversity in academic medicine: perspectives from one school. Acad Med. 2008;83(8):781–6. https://doi.org/10.1097/ACM.0b013e31817ec002.
30. Childs E, Yoloye K, Bhasin R, Benjamin E, Assoumou S. Retaining faculty from underrepresented groups in academic medicine: results from a needs assessment. South Med J. 2023;116(2):157–61. https://doi.org/10.14423/SMJ.0000000000001510.

31. Miles S, Renedo A, Marston C. Reimagining authorship guidelines to promote equity in co-produced academic collaborations. Glob Public Health. 2022;17(10):2547–59. https://doi.org/10.1080/17441692.2021.1971277.
32. Jameson C, Haq Z, Musse S, Kosar Z, Watson G, Wylde V. Inclusive approaches to involvement of community groups in health research: the co-produced CHICO guidance. Res Involv Engagem. 2023;9(1):76. https://doi.org/10.1186/s40900-023-00492-9.
33. MedEdPORTAL. MedEdPORTAL. n.d. Retrieved October 21, 2024, from https://www.mededportal.org/authorcenter?doi=10.15766%2Fmep&publicationCode=mep
34. Nakae S, Martinez S, Juarez JJ, Beltran Sanchez C. The impacts of engagement in the Latino Medical Student Association. Health Equity. 2023;7(1):109–15. https://doi.org/10.1089/heq.2022.0099.
35. Stanford FC. The importance of diversity and inclusion in the healthcare workforce. J Natl Med Assoc. 2020;112(3):247–9. https://doi.org/10.1016/j.jnma.2020.03.014.
36. Baker EA, Bouldin N, Durham M, Lowell ME, Gonzalez M, Jodaitis N, Cruz LN, Torres I, Torres M, Adams ST. The Latino Health Advocacy Program: a collaborative lay health advisor approach. Health Educ Behav. 1997;24(4):495–509. https://doi.org/10.1177/109019819702400408.

**Open Access** This chapter is licensed under the terms of the Creative Commons Attribution 4.0 International License (http://creativecommons.org/licenses/by/4.0/), which permits use, sharing, adaptation, distribution and reproduction in any medium or format, as long as you give appropriate credit to the original author(s) and the source, provide a link to the Creative Commons license and indicate if changes were made.

The images or other third party material in this chapter are included in the chapter's Creative Commons license, unless indicated otherwise in a credit line to the material. If material is not included in the chapter's Creative Commons license and your intended use is not permitted by statutory regulation or exceeds the permitted use, you will need to obtain permission directly from the copyright holder.

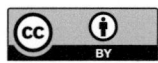

## Chapter 2
# Hispanics and Academic Medicine: Creating an Inclusive Community, Academic Success, and Leadership Careers for Impactful Healthcare Change

Fernando S. Mendoza, Eneida O. Roldan, Laura Castillo-Page, and Débora H. Silva

> **Learning Objectives**
> - Recognize the need to increase the number of Hispanics in academic medicine.
> - Advocate for mentors and sponsors to enhance successful career outcomes.
> - Understand the importance of training Hispanics in the care of this population.
> - Encourage more of the next generation of Hispanics to enter academic medicine by sharing success stories.

## Who Are We and Why Are Hispanics Important in Academic Medicine?

### The Demographic Shift in the USA

The importance of Hispanics in our country is becoming more evident as the US population demographically shifts to a larger percentage of people of color. For example, in 2020, half of all children were children of color, with the largest group

---

F. S. Mendoza (✉)
Stanford University School of Medicine, Stanford, CA, USA
e-mail: fmendoza@stanford.edu

E. O. Roldan
College of Health and Wellness, Barry University, Miami, FL, USA

L. Castillo-Page
American Board of Medical Specialties, Chicago, IL, USA

D. H. Silva
School of Medicine, University of Puerto Rico, San Juan, Puerto Rico

being Hispanic. Of all minority children (Hispanic, African American, Native American, and Asian American), 52% are Hispanic. With Hispanics having the second-highest birth rate [1], the Hispanic population group is expected to continue growing from its current 19% to 28% by 2060. Indeed, Hispanics have accounted for more than 50% of the total US population growth since 2010, with several states not typically considered to have large Hispanic populations experiencing growth of 20–40% [2]. The ten states with the highest Hispanic populations in the USA are New Mexico, Texas, California, Arizona, Nevada, Florida, Colorado, New Jersey, New York, and Illinois. Moreover, one-third of Hispanics are immigrants, with the great majority of Latino individuals being US citizens [3]. Thus, while Hispanics are and will continue to be a prominent group in the USA, lumping all Hispanics into one group obscures their distinct histories. Unique Hispanic histories stem from their countries of origin and their experiences in the USA, both shaping the various cultural nuances of the people called Hispanics. Moreover, aside from those characteristics, acculturation and political perspective also differentiate Hispanics. The literature has employed several inclusive terms to describe our community, including Hispanic, Latino/a, Latinx, and Latine. Yet, Hispanic subgroups in the US also differentiate themselves by their country of origin, such as, Mexican American (64%), Puerto Rican (10%), Central Americans (10%), South Americans (7%), Cuban Americans (4%), Dominican Americans (4%), and Spanish Americans (1%) [4].

Furthermore, the Hispanic population has the largest population of immigrants, comprising 32%, with the majority coming from Mexico, specifically 10.7 million [5]. Aside from the subgroup categories, the historical experiences and present acculturation processes, including intermarriage, make Hispanics a multiracial, multiethnic, and multidenominational group. Thus, using a single Hispanic label can cause problems when we attempt to convey our individuality. We bring this up first in our discussion because it is important to see our individuality as a strength for Hispanics, and perhaps a true model for the future of our country. Furthermore, if we can accept that we are all different yet still considered "Hispanic," then we can have a greater collective impact on our goal of improving the presence and effectiveness of Hispanic faculty, ultimately enhancing the health and well-being of our communities.

## *Equity in the Health Professions and Academic Medicine*

Given the above demographic data on the representation of Hispanics in the USA and the need to provide all people with high-quality healthcare, the presence of Hispanic physicians in healthcare is essential. This presence is particularly important in academic medicine because it is responsible for training health professionals, generating new knowledge and research to improve the health of communities, and providing leadership to ensure that effective policies are in place to meet the healthcare needs of all communities. Unfortunately, the presence of Hispanics in academic medicine has been very limited in both numbers and influence. The number of Hispanics in academic medicine has remained stagnant for the past four decades, primarily due to the limited number of Hispanic medical school graduates. Overall, the population equity (percentage of medical school matriculants to percentage of US population) for students who are underrepresented in medicine (Hispanics, African Americans, and Native Americans) increased from 1980 to 2020, from 61.1% to 71.1%, over 40 years. In 1980, 4.9% of medical school matriculants were Hispanic, and the Hispanic population was 6.4%, providing a population equity of 76.5%. In 2021, with the Hispanic population comprising 18.7% and medical school matriculants accounting for 12.0% [6], the population equity was 64.2%. Given the limited pool of Hispanic medical school matriculants, it is not surprising that the number of Hispanic faculty has been limited. In 2024, 3.6% of faculty were Hispanic. If one includes multiracial Hispanic faculty, who comprise 2.7% of all medical school faculty, then the overall percentage of Hispanic medical school faculty is 6.3%, resulting in a Hispanic population equity of 33.7% [7]. This compares with White, Asian American, and African American faculty population equities of 103%, 338%, and 30%, respectively.

## *Why Do We Need Hispanics in Academic Medicine?*

For many Hispanic medical students, the question of why they should pursue academic medicine or understand its potential to impact the health of Hispanic communities positively is often never asked or fully understood. While Hispanic communities suffer from a lack of access to and utilization of quality and equitable healthcare, their healthcare, in general, is also greatly influenced by cultural and language differences between patients and healthcare providers [8]. The premise that solely Hispanic healthcare providers can meet the health needs of the Hispanic community is unlikely to be fulfilled and is unjust. The decline in population equity for Hispanic physicians over the past four decades underscores the need for a comprehensive assessment of our healthcare system to enhance the health of Hispanic communities. A change must involve all healthcare providers, not just Hispanic providers. We believe that academic medicine can be a key component in achieving healthcare system change by influencing the training of health professionals to work with diverse populations, particularly those with different languages and cultures. Moreover, improving the health of Hispanics and other underserved populations will require influencing the training of future healthcare providers and creating new information to better serve these communities through basic, clinical, educational, and health policy research. For example, currently, 94% of genomic data is pertinent to only White European populations; however, Hispanic faculty have begun to conduct studies on the genomics of asthma among Hispanic populations, thereby creating a scientific understanding of the clear differences in asthma prevalence among Hispanics [9]. The effects of language on medical care for Hispanics have been well-documented [10]. Research on the effects of language-appropriate communication skills and language training in medical education has demonstrated improvements in clinical care [11–13]. Research has also contributed to understanding the effects of national public policy on the health of Hispanic communities, particularly those Hispanic populations that have a high prevalence (or number) of immigrant families. For example, a study on mothers who qualify for DACA demonstrated that their US-born children had 50% less adjustment and anxiety disorders than mothers who did not qualify for DACA status [14].

As noted above, research can have a significant impact on the health of the Hispanic community. Although non-Hispanic investigators research Hispanic communities, Hispanic academicians can bring cultural insights and bicultural skills to conduct nuanced, culturally specific research that advances the field of medicine to benefit Hispanic communities. Therefore, it is our purpose and goal to inspire and motivate Hispanic healthcare students and trainees to consider careers in academic medicine and encourage them to join us as LHS+ faculty.

## How Do Hispanics Succeed in Academic Medicine: The Process of Acculturation and Inclusion

### *The Acculturation Process for Academic Medicine*

The authors of this chapter have each taken a different path into academic medicine; however, in one way or another, each has had to become acculturated to the environment of academic medicine. Every culture, including the academic culture, has values, norms, and behaviors that distinguish a person's actions as positive or negative. One of the issues commonly heard among minority faculty in academic medicine is the problem of "fit," as in "we don't fit into the department or school" [15]. While mentors (those who show you the way to success) and sponsors (those who create the way to success) are important in the academic journey, it is also important to understand the process and one's role in academic acculturation.

For this discussion, we will utilize the acculturation model proposed by John Barry [16]. The main premise of this acculturation model is that two cultures interact in the acculturation process: the individual's culture and the host culture (in this case, the academic institution's culture). Each culture has its own set of values, behaviors, and rewards for specific actions. Barry's model categorizes the acculturation process into four possible outcomes, as illustrated in Fig. 2.1, depending on whether the individual retains their own cultural values and/or adopts those of the institution.

While these acculturation categories are set up as categorical outcomes, the authors of this chapter, like many other faculty, have experienced more than one of these in different areas of their careers. The understanding and support of diversity and inclusion by academic institutions enable individuals to utilize their talents to drive excellence in an academic environment while upholding their individual values. This fosters a sense of belonging to the institution's culture. Consequently, in

**Barry's Model of Acculturation**

|  |  | Individual's Culture | |
|---|---|---|---|
|  |  | Yes | No |
| Academic Culture | Yes | Integration | Assimilation |
|  | No | Separation | Marginalization |

**Fig. 2.1** Barry's modal of acculturation

the best of all worlds, a nurturing institutional environment would support individuals' values, while also conveying an understanding of what is required for success. This would be an "integrative" environment that would create the ideal environment of academic excellence for all. "Assimilation" would be an environment where all are expected to conform, but it requires someone to guide them in understanding what "falling in line" means. It doesn't necessarily require the institution to adapt to the individual's needs. Racial and ethnic minority faculty can still succeed in this type of environment, but like any assimilation process, there is a certain degree of loss of self-identity. If one fails to accept the values and "rules of the game" for the academic institution but still maintains their self-identity ("doing it my way"), then faculty will feel a sense of "separation" from the academic community, which may not lead to success. Lastly, "marginalization" occurs when, in the process of acculturation, the individual fails to adapt to the academic culture and as a result loses their professional and/or cultural self-identity. This can result in both professional and personal losses.

## *Hispanic Faculty Acculturation to the Academic Environment*

The above categories are helpful for reflection on one's career. Still, it is most likely that different components of a career (i.e., clinical care, research, teaching, and management) may each have their own acculturation categorization. As we reflect on our careers, we offer the following recommendations to support your success in the academic environment. First, try to understand the culture of the institution and promotion process by determining the category of faculty that best fits you (tenured, clinical scholar, clinician educator, etc.) and the rules for success in that faculty line (grants, publications, teaching awards, clinical time, advocacy, leadership). Culture is best understood by understanding what is valued and rewarded within it. Thus, for a faculty member, this is key if one is going to control one's fate and self-identity. A necessary aid in this process is a mentor, but the ideal aid is a sponsor, who guides you and helps open doors to achieve your goals. Hopefully, this will be another racial or ethnic minority faculty member, but since they are few and far between, it will likely be a nonminority faculty member committed to helping junior faculty. Each of the authors had individuals in their careers who served as mentors or sponsors; without them, their success would have been more challenging to achieve. So, we all encourage junior faculty to seek out these individuals.

## *Building a Hispanic Academic Community*

Beyond mentors and sponsors, it has become evident that having an academic community of "people like me" is also vital for academic success and excellence. Peer-to-peer support is essential for creating an academic space where shared cultural values and behaviors can serve as a foundation, acting as an island in the ocean of the academic institution. This makes individuals feel comfortable and nurtured as Hispanics or any group that is "minoritized." Such groups can not only support identity but also highlight members' achievements through recognitions and awards that showcase their success to both the community and outsiders. One could also label this as "team science" or "team systems" thinking, where the group can do more than one individual.

Not infrequently, successes in publications and grants have been facilitated by other members of our team, both Hispanic and non-Hispanic, who supported one's success through co-publications or by providing opportunities for being a co-PI on a grant. This is a common method of facilitating promotion for all faculty but is very influential for Hispanic and other minority faculty. Data from the NIH and grant funding indicate that the average age of a first-time NIH RO1 principal investigator is 42 years, suggesting that for junior faculty, building a portfolio with K awards and other foundation grants is crucial. While NIH institutes were trying to improve diversity in their programs and grants and are now modifying this process, the NIH is still seeking new investigators. So, as a junior faculty member, one needs to learn the "rules of the game" for the NIH institutes and centers. Junior faculty should understand the processes and opportunities of the NIH, even in the current restrictive environment. The NIH has grant officers and institute leaders who can help junior faculty become familiar with the NIH process in their area of research (List of Institutes and Centers: National Institute of Health, 2025). This is facilitated by working with mentors and sponsors who have successful NIH careers, and it will be key to advancing Hispanics in academic medicine.

## Hispanic Academic Leadership and Creating Change

As we consider how to create change in our healthcare system to improve the health of Hispanics in the USA and Puerto Rico, we have arrived at the following. The current number of Hispanic physicians in our communities and on the faculty of our medical schools is too small to significantly impact the quality of healthcare for the Hispanic population through their individual clinical, teaching, or research efforts. Consequently, we have concluded that what is necessary is to increase the number of Hispanic leaders across the spectrum of healthcare, but particularly in academic medicine. Figure 2.2 provides a schematic representation of academic leadership development. The blue boxes show the usual process or roadmap for developing academic leaders. Academically successful individuals are identified as potential leaders and then given leadership development and coaching support. This provides these selected individuals with the opportunity to become successful leaders and drive systemic change, resulting in impactful healthcare improvements in communities with health disparities. However, healthcare leaders need to understand communities' health disparities, which unfortunately is not always the case. This is why Hispanic academic leaders are key, and why academic institutions need to develop leadership development programs for Hispanic and other minority faculty.

From the authors' perspective as Hispanic academic leaders, the system changes needed to address health disparities in Hispanic populations will require modifications in the tripartite mission of academic institutions, particularly through leadership in research, medical education, and clinical delivery. This will require an increase in the number of Hispanic academic leaders. Consequently, this has led us to a "call to action" to address the need to develop Hispanic faculty leaders. Using the leadership development process in Fig. 2.2 for Hispanic faculty, there is a clear need for a shared responsibility among institutional leaders, as evidenced by the

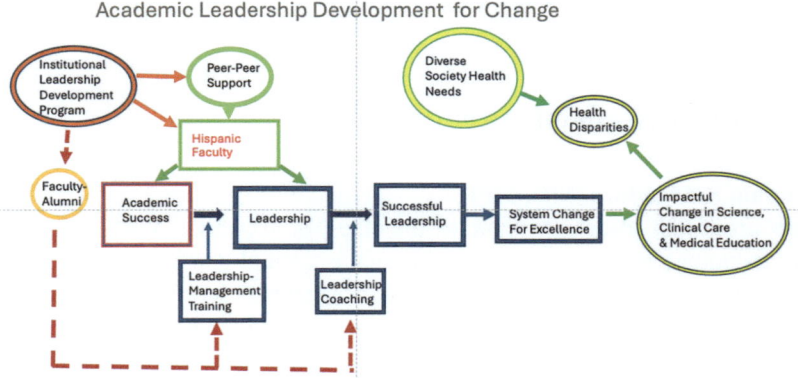

**Fig. 2.2** Academic leadership development of change

creation of leadership development programs involving senior faculty and academic center leadership. The leadership development process can be enhanced by a critical mass of academically successful Hispanic senior faculty to guide and mentor the development of junior Hispanic academic leaders. This can facilitate the sharing of paths to achievement and self-identity among Hispanic academic leaders. Leadership development and coaching should be supported by senior Hispanic and non-Hispanic faculty (with appropriate credit given) and by establishing a network of nationally recognized Hispanic academic leaders to offer a broader perspective on leadership.

The literature has documented the need to increase Hispanic leaders in academic medicine to impact the health disparities seen in our population. For all of us in senior positions, the time is now to become mentors and sponsors of the next generation of Hispanic leaders. Change will only happen if leaders dedicate their time to sharing their passion, purpose, and vision for equitable healthcare. Ultimately, senior Hispanic faculty members need to leave a legacy of understanding the importance of our Hispanic heritage in providing quality care to all. There is no better way to achieve this than by helping to create the next generation of Hispanic academic leaders.

So, while our curricula vitae tell a bit about our leadership journeys, our personal stories show different paths that led us to where we are today. Consequently, we recognize that there is more than one way to succeed in academic medicine. We hope that those of you reading this chapter will be part of the next chapter, the next generation of Hispanic healthcare leaders that will make our world a better and more equitable place. "Por La Raza":

> My leadership was best when I was helping others create their leadership futures. Fernando S. Mendoza
> 
> Leadership is best defined when there is passion and purpose. It is not a beginning or an end. It is an on-going wonderful journey. Eneida O. Roldan
> 
> Empower and support others and you will see the fruits of your labor multiply. Laura Castillo-Page
> 
> Mentors have been essential to my leadership skills development and now, I pay it forward, giving time and effort to those that are rising in academic medicine, because I know it is the only way for us to thrive. Débora H. Silva

## Our Paths to Academic Leadership

### Fernando S. Mendoza, MD, MPH

I grew up in San Jose, California, as the eldest of six children. My father was a Mexican immigrant who came to California as a child and went to a segregated school for Mexican children until sixth grade, when he left school to work with his family as a farmworker. My mother was a US citizen born in El Paso, Texas, but was deported to Mexico as a child along with her family in the 1930s. She completed high school in Juarez, Mexico, and met my father there when she was 20. After they married, they moved to San Jose, California, where their first home was a self-made room in the basement of my grandmother's house in the Gardner area of San Jose. My parents taught me to work hard, have empathy for others, and pursue my dreams. As a child, I loved science and math, and throughout my schooling, I thought I would be a chemist until one day my high school counselor changed my life. That day, she told me, "I heard you wanted to be a doctor," which was the first time I had heard I wanted to be a doctor, and I decided why not! This led me to be the first in my family to go to college, attending San Jose State University, and then to apply and enter Stanford Medical School in 1971 in the third class of affirmative action students. I subsequently completed my pediatric residency at Stanford and obtained a Master of Public Health from Harvard University. I returned to Stanford for a fellowship in academic general pediatrics. After the fellowship, I became a Stanford faculty member in the Division of General Pediatrics in 1981 and Assistant Dean of Minority Advising and Programs in 1983. I became an Associate Dean for Minority Advising and Programs (1993–2020), Division Chief of General Pediatrics at Stanford's Lucile Packard Children's Hospital, and General Pediatric Fellowship Director (1996–2014). I completed my Stanford career in 2021 as Professor Emeritus.

I always had a passion to improve the health and well-being of children, particularly those who are the most vulnerable: minority and immigrant children. Indeed, I would say it was this passion that drove my leadership. As a medical student, I helped establish the Gardner Family Health Center in San Jose, the same neighborhood of my childhood. Later, as a Division Chief of General Pediatrics, I aided in developing the Ravenswood Family Health Center in East Palo Alto. Both experiences gave me insights into the health needs of minority communities. As a faculty member, my research addressed health disparities among minority and immigrant children and diversity in the health workforce. My research on health disparities helped to identify the healthcare needs of Latino children, particularly those who were immigrants. This led to serving as an advocate on committees for the Institute of Medicine, NIH, and the American Academy of Pediatrics. In the area of diversity, I established Stanford's Center of Excellence for Diversity in Medical Education with my colleagues, Dr. Ronald Garcia and Mark Gutierrez. I was the principal investigator from 1992 to 2020 of the HRSA Center of Excellence grant that helped establish diversity efforts at Stanford Medical School. This included the establishment of the Early Matriculation/Leadership in Health Disparities program that produced minority faculty and leaders throughout the country. Nationally, I was involved with the establishment of the Hispanic Serving Health Professions Schools, was the co-chair of the Federation of Pediatric Organizations' Diversity Taskforce, and participated in diversity activities of the American Academy of Pediatrics, the American Pediatric Society, the Academic Pediatric Association, the NIH, and the Institute of Medicine. For these efforts, I was awarded the Dr. Phil De Chavez Mentor of the Year Award from the National Latino Medical Student Association, the JE Wallace Sterling "Muleshoe" Alumni Lifetime Achievement Award from Stanford Medical School Alumni Association, and the Joseph W. St. Geme Jr. Leadership Award from the Federation of Pediatric Organizations. But like all leaders, these awards do not represent my work alone, but also the work of my colleagues from over the years, and my family, who supported me throughout my career. We never do it alone!

Looking back over my 50 years of work, I reflect on how I made it. I believe it was from the core values of being Latino: hard work, empathy, respectfulness, and inclusiveness. Most of all, I had the support of *my family* and those of my extended familia, my friends, and colleagues. Yet even now, my drive for change continues to come from the children, whose faces remind me of the Latino children from my childhood. This is my passion, and this is my leadership, now even more so since I became a grandfather.

**Laura Castillo-Page, PhD**

I was born and raised in Harlem, New York. My parents came from Puerto Rico and Cuba. Growing up I saw firsthand how hard my parents worked to ensure both my brother and I would have a better life. Like many Puerto Rican women at that time, my mother worked in a factory after migrating from Puerto Rico. My father migrated from Cuba and always worked two to three jobs. Both taught me the importance of hard work, perseverance, resilience, and empathy. I grew up as a proud "New York CubaRican"! After attending Performing Arts High School, I decided that rather than pursuing the arts, I would study veterinary science. But after not receiving any mentorship or support for a successful experience in a STEMM (Science, Technology, Engineering, Mathematics, and Medicine)-related discipline, I changed paths after stumbling into a political sociology class that changed my life. This is when I fell in love with the social sciences. I felt that the social sciences allowed me to understand and explain the systemic inequities I was seeing and experiencing in my family and community. I went on to complete a doctorate and began a career as a researcher as well as a university faculty member focused on diversity, equity, and inclusion issues. I worked at the Association of American Medical Colleges as a Senior Director for Diversity, Equity, and Inclusion, where I led a portfolio of work to advance learning and workplace environments focused on achieving an inclusive culture. I currently serve as the Chief Diversity and Inclusion Officer at the National Academies of Sciences, Engineering, and Medicine.

**Débora H. Silva Díaz, MD, MEd**

I am the mother of two, a wife, a medical educator, and a pediatrician. I was born in Mexico to Puerto Rican parents who were studying medicine in Mexico City at the *Universidad Nacional Autónoma de México*. I was raised in Puerto Rico, in a family of academic physicians who instilled a sense of commitment and social responsibility to improving the health of our people. I went on to complete undergraduate studies at Tufts University, with the original plan to study Psychology but decided to become a doctor. I graduated summa cum laude and decided to go back home to study medicine at the University of Puerto Rico (UPR) School of Medicine. Once I graduated from the University of Puerto Rico School of Medicine, I completed a General Pediatrics Residency Program there and stayed as Chief Resident. During the year as Chief Resident, I had the opportunity to participate as a clinical skills preceptor for first year medical students, and this was the door to what is now my career. Since then, I have occupied multiple academic positions including Course

Director, Clinical Skills Program Director, Curriculum Office Director, Faculty Development Program Director, General Pediatrics Section Chief, Accreditation Office Director, LCME Faculty Accreditation Lead, and Associate Dean for Academic Affairs at the UPR School of Medicine, and Interim Dean of Academic Affairs (Provost) at the UPR Medical Sciences Campus. Throughout all these years and positions, I have continued to be an attending physician at the University Pediatric Hospital, which is the only pediatric tertiary care hospital of Puerto Rico and the Caribbean.

One of the most important things I have learned during these 20 plus years is that when opportunities knock on your door, you accept and proceed to make sure you are well prepared to perform to the best of your abilities. This is why I completed a Primary Care Faculty Development Fellowship, Curricular Track, at Michigan State University and a Master's in Education with emphasis on health sciences education at the University of Cincinnati. I have had the amazing opportunity to work locally, nationally, and internationally collaborating with other medical schools, including participating six times as part of an LCME survey team visiting schools during accreditation processes.

Currently, I am the Dean of the University of Puerto Rico School of Medicina and Co-editor of the *MedEdPORTAL* Language Appropriate Healthcare and Medical Language Education Collection. I have represented the Association of American Medical Colleges (AAMC) at the Pan American Federation of Associations of Medical Schools (PAFAMS) since 2016. At PAFAMS, I collaborate with numerous Latin American colleagues to enhance medical education throughout the Americas.

### Eneida O. Roldan, MD, MPH, MBA

I was born in Havana, Cuba, with Spanish from my grandparents. I was 3 years old when my family immigrated to the USA in 1960. My family frequently visited the USA for vacation. Upon my parents' marriage, they moved to New York City to start their family. However, life had a different plan. When my mother learned she was pregnant with me, the family asked for my parents to return to Cuba where they had help and family support. In 1960, months after the arrival of Fidel Castro, my family moved to Miami as residents of the USA.

I was raised in a very close family with clear values of love of family, integrity, respect, education, spirituality, hard work, and giving back. My grandmother was my first mentor. She made it her purpose to keep traditions alive and stress the family values throughout my development years. At a very young age, the curiosity of the human body incited my passion, and thus my journey as a future physician began. From a young age, the passion of lifelong learning was my foundation. As a young learner, I entered science fairs, won awards, and was fascinated by my uncles that were physicians. In high school, I volunteered at hospitals and always went well beyond my call of duty to serve.

I entered the University of Miami, and my life as a learner in the sciences began. Upon graduating from medical school, when the time arrived to choose a specialty, I searched for a specialty that integrated lifelong learning and the study of the human body. That was the specialty of pathology for me. I completed my residency in anatomic and clinical pathology and a fellowship in pediatric pathology. During this time in my professional journey, my interest in metabolic disease surfaced. I decided to focus on obesity and metabolic diseases and completed postgraduate training at Harvard, Deaconess Hospital, under Dr. George Blackburn. This was not a formal residency in obesity (bariatric medicine), but a series of postgraduate training through educational exposure for several months. Subsequently, physicians that successfully completed the work were eligible to sit for a board specialty exam and become board certified in bariatric medicine. The impact of obesity in our population's health and finances of our healthcare system drove me to attain a Master of Public Health (University of South Florida) with a focus of health policy and population health and subsequently a Master of Business Administration (Haslam School of Business, University of Tennessee Executive MBA program) with a focus on the business of healthcare. My passion for continued learning didn't stop, so in 2017, I was tapped by a specialized program at the University of Pennsylvania Wharton School of Business to be admitted in the General Management Program for Senior Executives where currently I am an alumna. I was humbled when I was appointed by Wharton's Dean and leadership to become a board member on their Advisory Board for Executive Education at Wharton.

During my long professional journey, I was blessed with the gift of mentors and sponsors that guided my personal and professional journey at opportune times. These mentors and sponsors came from all walks of life: medicine, business, and even life in general. I feel humbled and honored that I was always open for another advice, another road not only to grow personally and professionally but to share with others. I have been blessed to have attained a very senior level of leadership during my career. I am an overachiever having graduated from all my degrees with the highest honors and being honored with multiple awards in both medicine and business.

Fast forward today, what many may consider the end of a successful professional career, I still search for more. I am energized by innovation, developing new projects, and thinking outside the box. Never accepting the status quo, a lesson I learned from my first mentor, my grandmother. More importantly, I am blessed by the opportunity to give back through mentorship, sponsorship, having developed a scholarship in the medical school for Latinas that have a passion of lifelong learning, excellent academic scholarship, volunteerism, and giving back. My journey and legacy are one that began with a nurturing family that instilled values of passion for learning, giving back, never giving up, and, most importantly, gratitude. These values that I live by today and have passed on to my children and grandchildren and to those I am privileged to mentor.

*As final words of advice: seek your journey, for it is yours to enjoy: do not give up for your next move can be the most successful; find your mentors and sponsors, they are priceless; never stop learning, for life is in constant change; and finally, always start the day with gratitude, this is your best reward.*

## Questions for the Reader

1. What is your passion, and have you pursued it?
2. Do you want to make change, and do you consider yourself a leader?
3. What can you do now to help others?

## References

1. Duffin E. Total fertility rate by ethnicity U.S. 2020. Statista. 2022, September 30. Retrieved October 18, 2022, from https://www.statista.com/statistics/226292/us-fertility-rates-by-race-and-ethnicity/
2. Bureau U. S. C. Hispanic population to reach 111 million by 2060. Census.gov. 2021, October 8. Retrieved October 18, 2022, from https://www.census.gov/library/visualizations/2018/comm/hispanic-projected-pop.html
3. Krogstad JM. Hispanics have accounted for more than half of total U.S. population growth since 2010. Pew Research Center. 2020, August 14. Retrieved October 18, 2022, from https://www.pewresearch.org/fact-tank/2020/07/10/hispanics-have-accounted-for-more-than-half-of-total-u-s-population-growth-since-2010/
4. Gonzalez-Barrera A, Krogstad JM, Noe-Bustamante L. Path to legal status for the unauthorized is top immigration policy goal for Hispanics in U.S. Pew Research Center. 2020, September 22. Retrieved October 18, 2022, from https://www.pewresearch.org/fact-tank/2020/02/11/path-to-legal-status-for-the-unauthorized-is-top-immigration-policy-goal-for-hispanics-in-u-s/
5. Batalova J. Frequently requested statistics on immigrants and immigration in the United States. Migration Policy Institute. 2024, March 13. https://www.migrationpolicy.org/article/frequently-requested-statistics-immigrants-and-immigration-united-states-2024#:~:text=How%20many%20Hispanics%20in%20the,(20.4%20million)%20were%20immigrants. Accessed 20 June 25.
6. 2021 facts: applicants and matriculants data. AAMC. 2021. Retrieved October 18, 2022, from https://www.aamc.org/data-reports/students-residents/interactive-data/2021-facts-applicants-and-matriculants-data
7. Faculty Roster: U.S. medical school faculty. 2024. Retrieved June 17, 2025, from https://www.aamc.org/data-reports/faculty-institutions/report/faculty-roster-us-medical-school-faculty
8. Smedley BD, Stith AY, Nelson RA. Unequal treatment: confronting racial and ethnic disparities in health care. Recommendation 5–3. Washington, DC: National Academies Press; 2003.
9. Pino-Yanes M, Thakur N, Gignoux C, et al. Genetic ancestry influences asthma susceptibility and lung function among Latinos. J Allergy Clin Immunol. 2015;135(1):228–35.
10. Berger Z, Peled Y. Language and health (in) equity in US Latinx COMMUNITIES, AMA Journal of Ethics. 2022, April. https://journalofethics.ama-assn.org/article/language-and-health-inequity-us-latinx-communities/2022-04#:~:text=Linguistically%20discordant%20care%20often%20leads,up%2C%20and%20worse%20health%20outcomes.&text=That%20is%2C%20care%20in%20a,to%20deleterious%20or%20disparate%20outcomes. Accessed 20 June 2025.
11. Eneriz-Wiemer M, Sanders LM, Barr DA, Mendoza FS. Parental limited English proficiency and health outcomes for children with Special Health Care Needs: a systematic review. Acad Pediatr. 2014;14(2):128–36. https://doi.org/10.1016/j.acap.2013.10.003.
12. Jaramillo J, Snyder E, Dunlap JL, Wright R, Mendoza F, Bruzoni M. The Hispanic Clinic for Pediatric surgery: a model to improve parent–provider communication for Hispanic

Pediatric surgery patients. J Pediatr Surg. 2016;51(4):670–4. https://doi.org/10.1016/j.jpedsurg.2015.08.065.
13. Ortega P, Pérez N, Robles B, Turmelle Y, Acosta D. Teaching medical Spanish to improve population health: evidence for incorporating language education and assessment in U.S. medical schools. Health Equity. 2019;3(1):557–66. https://doi.org/10.1089/heq.2019.0028. PMID: 31701080; PMCID: PMC6830530.
14. Hainmueller J, Lawrence D, Martén L, Black B, Figueroa L, Hotard M, Jiménez TR, Mendoza F, Rodriguez MI, Swartz JJ, Laitin DD. Protecting unauthorized immigrant mothers improves their children's mental health. Science. 2017;357(6355):1041–4. https://doi.org/10.1126/science.aan5893.
15. Hassouneh D, Lutz KF, Beckett AK, Junkins EP, Horton LSL. The experiences of underrepresented minority faculty in schools of medicine. Med Educ Online. 2014;19(1):24768. https://doi.org/10.3402/meo.v19.24768.
16. Worthy LD, Lavigne T, Romero F. Berry's model of acculturation. Open.maricopa.edu; MMOER. 2020, July 27. https://open.maricopa.edu/culturepsychology/chapter/berrys-model-of-acculturation/

**Open Access** This chapter is licensed under the terms of the Creative Commons Attribution 4.0 International License (http://creativecommons.org/licenses/by/4.0/), which permits use, sharing, adaptation, distribution and reproduction in any medium or format, as long as you give appropriate credit to the original author(s) and the source, provide a link to the Creative Commons license and indicate if changes were made.

The images or other third party material in this chapter are included in the chapter's Creative Commons license, unless indicated otherwise in a credit line to the material. If material is not included in the chapter's Creative Commons license and your intended use is not permitted by statutory regulation or exceeds the permitted use, you will need to obtain permission directly from the copyright holder.

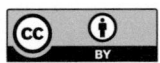

## Chapter 3
# Making a Decision About an Academic Faculty Track

**Sylk Sotto-Santiago and Maria Milagros Garcia**

**Learning Objectives**
- Consider personal values in choosing a professional career.
- Define common academic tracks.
- Decide the best academic track for you.
- Examine your place in academia.

## Introduction

LHS+ faculty represent a small percentage of the overall faculty in the United States (USA), higher education institutions, and academic medicine, making up approximately 5–6% of faculty across all ranks [1]. Although we have seen an increase in the faculty ranks over the years, the increase has remained modest. Between 1990 and 2018, the percentage of LHS+ grew from 3% to 5–6% [2]. As academic medicine works to diversify faculty, we must also note that there is an even smaller representation of LHS+ among the leadership and senior-level positions [3]. LHS+ faculty representation also varies significantly by specialty and subspecialties within the medicine realm [4].

In academic medicine, it is important to briefly communicate some of the challenges toward persistence and retention. Studies show that LHS+ faculty face

---

S. Sotto-Santiago (✉)
University of Pittsburgh School of Medicine, Health Sciences, Pittsburgh, PA, USA

M. M. Garcia
University of Massachusetts Chan Medical School, Worcester, MA, USA
e-mail: Maria.GarciaMD@umassmed.edu

barriers such as lack of mentorship, bias, fewer networking opportunities, and, for some, linguistic discrimination [5, 6]. Furthermore, disparities in funding and institutional support can impact LHS+ faculty career paths, making it difficult to secure grants or resources necessary for career advancement [7]. We state this not as discouragement, but to bring awareness of where your academic work could benefit from strategic attention.

Making the correct faculty track decision is crucial for LHS+ faculty for several reasons. LHS+ faculty bring diverse perspectives shaped by their unique cultural backgrounds, lived experiences, and the legacies of those who came before them. Their presence enriches the educational curriculum by broadening the topics discussed and ensuring more inclusive perspectives. LHS+ faculty can serve as role models and mentors not only for LHS+ students but for all historically underrepresented students. Their increased representation in academic medicine helps address systemic racism, as well as disparities in healthcare access and outcomes [8]. Their engagement and service in the community are also significant, fostering stronger connections between academic institutions and the populations they serve [5, 6].

Beyond their contributions to medicine and research, LHS+ faculty often pursue research that directly addresses issues impacting the LHS+ community [9]. This work shapes our understanding of the healthcare system and strengthens efforts to influence policies and promote equitable practices in medicine. Moreover, their contributions help pave the way for other historically underrepresented groups in medicine, fostering inclusive clinical environments and educational spaces [10].

However, the decision to join academia can be confusing, and choosing a faculty path is one of the most important decisions when considering a sustainable career. First, aligning a faculty track with personal strengths and interests significantly impacts faculty vitality, job satisfaction, and overall well-being. When faculty select a track that resonates with their skills, whether in research, teaching, service, or clinical practice, they are more likely to thrive professionally and remain in academia [11]. As LHS+ faculty, it is important to also find inclusive academic environments that reflect our common values as a community and individual interests. Our work should enhance our motivations and passions.

Throughout this chapter, we will discuss faculty tracks in general, ranks and trends, resources to support your promotion and tenure, and considerations that will help guide your decision. Let's begin.

## Guided by Your Values, Passions, and Goals

LHS+ faculty are often guided by their values, passions, and goals. We draw from our cultural heritage, background, and personal experiences to educate and care for others. This influences our teaching, service, and research interests [7]. With a strong dedication and commitment to diversity, inclusion, and health equity, we advocate for other historically underrepresented faculty and trainees, and social justice. Our enthusiasm is contagious, and we succeed by aligning our values, passions, and goals with personal aspirations. Our professional fulfillment is key to our longevity in academia. It enhances our satisfaction, increases motivation, lowers burnout rates, and helps us with work-life integration, retention, and advancement [12].

The concept of professional fulfillment seeks to draw attention to the need to go beyond simply a career. Professional fulfillment can be defined as the perception that career goals, regardless of the outcome, must be guided by the utmost importance to the individual or the positive self-evaluation of progress toward determined goals [12]. In choosing an academic path, it is important to understand these goals as part of an individual's value system [13]. Ultimately, the ability to feel professional fulfillment and satisfaction depends on the individual's ability to recognize their values, passions, and goals.

It is not often that through our educational and training paths, we pause to deliberately evaluate our priorities, much less the values that guide them. As LHS+ faculty, pausing to reflect on our career choices provides clarity of purpose, and facilitates navigating academic challenges, and our adaptation to change, again because we are particularly guided by our heritage, cultural identity, and representation.

**Exercise** What brings you *joy*? We want joy to help you guide your professional life journey. We want you to find fulfillment in your faculty role; in that way increase faculty vitality and prevent dissatisfaction.

Your career will be "a journey of growth, exploration, and transformation" [14]. Your career is one with a great impact on the healthy lives of individuals and on educating the next generation of physicians and scientists. Professional fulfillment emphasizes that healthcare professionals' ability to act in accordance with what they perceive as being core to their profession is said to be vital in attaining satisfaction and fulfillment [15]. Consider the values that guide you and what is important to you? What aspects of academia excite you most? Let that guide your career.

> **Key Terms**
> Professional fulfillment
> Professional satisfaction
> Contemplative practices
> Faculty vitality

> *Exercise: What Brings You Joy?*
> Use Table 3.1 to list the two values that are core elements in your life.
> You may consider the following values as examples: cooperation, creativity, growth, integrity, leadership, loyalty, respect, humility, etc.

(continued)

**Table 3.1** Balancing your values and passions at a professional and personal level

|  | Professional | Personal |
|---|---|---|
| Values |  |  |
| Passions |  |  |

Write a few brief sentences or phrases that articulate your professional and personal values and passions. For example, we may consider empowerment and integrity as professional values, and community engagement and mentorship as our passions. An example statement may be "Empowerment and integrity are at the core of my values, as I strive to inspire and uplift others through mentoring. Through community engagement, I aim to create meaningful connections that not only enhance individual growth but also contribute to the well-being of the communities we serve."

## Why Do You Want to Be a Faculty Member?

At the heart of a faculty member in academic medicine is the desire to prepare future generations of practitioners, to be of service to a community, and/or to be part of research innovation. The tripartite mission of academic medicine emphasizes the discovery and development of basic principles, effective policies, and best practices that advance research and education in the health sciences, ultimately improving the health and well-being of individuals and populations [16]. If this is central to your motivations, then academic medicine shall be your professional home. The social mission of academic medicine is health and health equity.

In socialization to the academic career, Austin (2002) found that faculty roles are attractive also for intrinsic reasons, such as enhancing one's knowledge in a particular discipline and finding meaning in your work [17]. Faculty roles can be attractive to LHS+ professionals because they provide the opportunity to influence future generations, especially other LHS+ students and trainees, and the opportunity to address social issues impacting underserved and under-resourced communities. Faulty roles allow us to demonstrate our resilience, that academic success is achievable, and collaboration across disciplines allows us to enhance access and equity. A faculty role may provide long-term career opportunities, such as job security, a clear path to career advancement, constant professional development, and inquiry.

The types of faculty positions are diverse. In general, faculty are expected to provide education; engage in scholarly activity through research, presentations, and publications; and serve the department and institution on committees, task forces, or workgroups. In the following section, we describe this in general.

## Faculty Appointments, Tracks, and Ranks

The changing roles of faculty members in academic medicine have been ever-evolving along with the drivers of institutional change [18]. Moreover, faculty seem to be motivated also by curiosity, creativity, and commitment and driven by the prospects of excellence [19].

In 2007, Bunton and colleagues documented tenure systems, the number and percentage of full-time faculty on tenure versus nontenure eligible tracks, and the types of financial guarantee under tenure, along with probationary periods. Results showed that although tenure systems were well established in academic medicine, the proportion of faculty on tenured or tenure-eligible tracks had continued to decline over time. Changes in the financial guarantee associated with tenure transformed the concept of tenure at many academic medical centers, and the schools that lengthened the probationary period for tenure-track faculty steadily increased during the prior 25 years. Moreover, "tenure-clock"-stopping policies exist at medical schools, though results indicate low faculty use of the policies [20]. Eleven years later, Walling and Nilsen (2018) documented that between 2006 and 2016, the number of faculty on tenure-related tracks in the clinical department declined, but nontenure appointments increased by 60.5% [21]. The number of full-time faculty in nontenure tracks can be as high as 82% [21]. According to the American Association of Medical Colleges (AAMC), the proportion of LHS+ faculty is highest among assistant professors and in nontenure tracks [22]. We discuss these trends because faculty tracks and criteria for promotion and tenure are institution specific. There are large differences, and they can relate to the uniqueness of an institution's cultures, values, and identity [21].

Although we intend to discuss these appointments, tracks, and ranks in generalities, it is important to remember to look at the criteria at each institution that you are considering. Practices and policies can have a significant impact on career progression, academic promotion, and faculty development. In addition, there is a clear trend toward nontenure track appointments, and although this chapter does not intend to argue the trend, it is important to acknowledge that career advancement is achievable within all tracks.

## Tenure-Track Faculty

Tenure generally is reserved for individuals at the Associate Professor or full Professor rank and awarded to those faculty whose contributions are considered as outstanding scholarly activity in areas of discovery, integration, application, and teaching [23, 24]. Tenure grants a secured position until resignation or retirement; however, all employment laws apply. Tenure does not guarantee a lifetime appointment. Because of the historical implications of tenure in higher education, it also may have prestige associated with tenure. Also, while tenure can be regularly under attack by both institutional practice and legislation for some public institutions, it continues to serve as the defense of academic freedom [25].

Moreover, tenure-track faculty participate in faculty governance and administration. Tenure-track faculty have responsibility for teaching, research, and service, and they are meant to make progress in these areas, annually. Not achieving the specific benchmarks for research, teaching, and service during mid-term reviews (usually third and fifth years) may indicate a difficulty in attaining tenure. These reviews are often required for tenure and promotion, and poor performance can lead to the nonrenewal of a faculty contract or a change in faculty track [26]. Titles include Professor, Associate Professor, and Assistant Professor. These titles may accompany a particular specialty, such as Professor of Medicine or Professor of Surgery. Expectations will also vary based on institutions being research-intensive or teaching-intensive.

## Clinical Faculty

The prefix "clinical" has different meanings depending on the higher education institution, but it is mostly reserved for practitioners of a particular field. In academic medicine, it is used for faculty appointments whose primary duties are teaching students and trainees and providing professional service in the clinical setting. Clinical faculty may be involved in research as well, which may derive from their specialty, clinical teaching, and professional service. Typical titles include Clinical Professor, Associate Clinical Professor, Assistant Clinical Professor, or Clinical Senior Lecturer and Clinical Lecturer.

In addition, clinical faculty may have other distinctions such as *clinician educator*—those whose roles are heavily associated with teaching—and *clinician-scholars*, those whose primary responsibilities may require scholarship production in clinical research, patient care, and medical education among others [23].

## Adjunct and Visiting Faculty

The terms "acting," "visiting," and "adjunct" may modify titles in any appointment. Generally, visiting and adjunct appointees do not have voting rights in faculty governance. Their appointment is limited and determined by a specific period.

## Lecturer/Instructors

Lecturers, instructors, and teaching professors may be assigned responsibility for teaching, and for research and service that supports teaching. The lecturer and instructor titles are also eligible for promotion such as Senior Lecturer, and Senior Instructors.

## Areas of Focus or Excellence

Individuals with the focus area of research may have additional expectations for securing funding in grants or being part of a significant research enterprise in the institution. Teaching implies the expectation of teaching, and for research and service that supports teaching. Lastly, "service," in itself, is seen as part of the faculty journey, and at some institutions, this service can be rewarded through the promotion and tenure process. Service can mean clinical service to patients. It can also refer to administrative work such as committee or workgroup activities that bolster medical education, and other activities central to the heart of the academic missions. Additionally, areas of excellence have been trending upward that emphasize contributions such as public scholarship, community engagement, and diversity, equity, and inclusion. These additional areas serve LHS+ as well, since, traditionally, LHS+ faculty have been interested in academic and health issues impacting LHS+ communities.

## Summary of Track Types

The accolades of tenure and promotion serve as mechanisms to reward faculty who perform at a high level of proficiency. However, the criteria and process for tenure and promotion are not perfect. Hence, it is increasingly important when making decisions about an academic career to have a good sense of what the requirements are for specific tracks and what the promotion and tenure process may entail for each of them. Faculty should obtain information about appointments, tracks, promotion and tenure criteria through the institution's website, faculty affairs offices, faculty handbooks, and departmental leadership. Remember that each institution and school have its own policies and processes. Table 3.2 summarizes faculty appointments per Callahan et al. [24].

**Table 3.2** Track type and definition [24]

| Track type | Definition |
|---|---|
| Traditional tenure | Faculty are expected to concentrate their efforts in the areas of teaching, research/scholarship, and patient care. Scholarship is based on original research and publication of that research in peer-reviewed medical and scientific journals |
| Clinician-educator | Faculty have primary responsibilities in teaching or in teaching and patient care. Research or scholarship may or may not be required for promotion; however, publication of original research in peer-reviewed medical and scientific journals must not be required for promotion to qualify a track for this category |
| Research | Faculty hold a primary appointment in another medical school and a secondary appointment in the reporting medical school |
| Adjunct | Faculty hold a primary appointment in another medical school and a secondary appointment in the reporting medical school |
| Emeritus | Faculty held full-time appointments at another medical school or university. At present, these faculty hold different affiliations with the medical school in an honorary or emeritus capacity |
| Visiting | Faculty hold full-time appointments at another medical school or university. Appointments in a visiting track type are of limited duration |
| Volunteer | Faculty are not paid by the medical school or associated university. These faculty engage in patient care and teaching activities in the medical school |
| Other | Faculty not fitting into any of the categories listed and defined above should be classified as other |

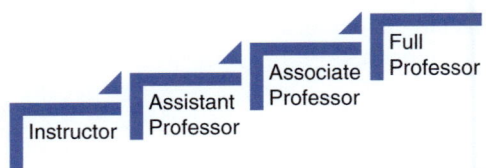

**Fig. 3.1** Faculty ranks

In general, instructor or lecturer appointments reflect a potential for academic advancement. Assistant Professors have been awarded a doctoral degree or equivalent and have exhibited a commitment to teaching, research, and scholarly productivity of high quality. Associate Professor demonstrates the same qualities but also demonstrates a national reputation as a scholar and demonstrated public, national, and emerging international reputation. Lastly, a professor includes a distinguished record of productivity and accomplishment that leads to an established national reputation or international standing (Fig. 3.1).

## Why Pay Attention to Promotion and/or Tenure Criteria?

Across institutions, the promotion and tenure guidelines include basic criteria that faculty must meet satisfactory or exceed in teaching, research, service, and scholarship and the reputation that supports it. When deciding about the appropriate faculty

**Table 3.3** Sample of accomplishment evaluations

| Evaluation of accomplishments | |
|---|---|
| Teaching | Teaching load<br>Learners' evaluation<br>Impacts on learners' successes<br>Peer review of teaching<br>Peer review of curricular materials<br>Mentoring activities |
| Clinical service | Specialty clinics developed<br>Clinical load<br>RVUs required<br>Impact of quality in patient care<br>Impact on efficiency and costs |
| Research | Assessment and significance of publications and dissemination outlets<br>Research creativity and load<br>Research funding<br>Contributions to collaborative research<br>Team science value |
| Scholarship | Publications in peer-review journals<br>Presentations at national scientific meeting |
| Service | Service to the university, professional associations, or community<br>Evaluations of speaking engagements<br>Recognition and awards |

and track appointment, it is important to understand the evaluation criteria. In Table 3.3, we provide examples to keep in mind for some key areas.

Criteria for promotion and tenure are not monolithic, but highly varied [27]. They are also highly structured and often inflexible. Therefore, deciding what faculty track to undertake requires careful career planning, continuous assessment of progress, and optimizing resources available [21]. As you begin your faculty career, remember to pay attention to the organization of your curriculum vitae and personal statement, always aim for high-quality scholarship, and be careful about a fragmented focus.

## But How Do I Choose?

We hope that the information provided here provides some clarity. The truth is that the best clarity will be provided by individuals at the institutions you are considering, or you are hired into. All institutions have offices and services devoted to faculty affairs and professional development; you may contact these offices and professionals for explicit advice. The resources at academic medicine and academic health centers can be robust but also evaluate your institution compatibility. Does it support what you value?

LHS+ individuals must recognize the importance of mentorship. Expand your definition of mentorship. There are many terms under this mentorship umbrella, reaching out to institutional agents, coaches, sponsors, allies, champions, role models, and cheerleaders. Engaging in tracks aligned with your priorities can help faculty build networks and gain visibility, which is especially important for LHS+ seeking mentorship and support. This support is critical as LHS+ may face systemic barriers in academic medicine and choosing a faculty track that speaks to your work can help counteract stereotypes, bias, and generally unpleasant interactions.

Different faculty tracks provide benefits as described above; however, keep in mind that that also means varying demands. We encourage you to also choose a track that allows for an appropriate workload, vital to your professional and personal success. LHS+ faculty may have additional personal and family commitments that impact career decisions not just about the right track or rank, but geographical location, an existing vibrant LHS+ community, and proximity to those we love and care about. It takes a community and *family* to help us navigate academia.

## Conclusion

The decision regarding faculty tracks is particularly significant for LHS+ faculty as it can influence your career trajectory, job satisfaction, and overall impact within academic medicine institutions. In summary, familiarize yourself with the differences between these tracks, and at the very least expectations for research, teaching, and service, terms of the appointment, and tenure process. In terms of clinical, research, or teaching tracks, determine which track aligns best with your skills and interests, as some institutions offer specific pathways focused on clinical practice, research, or teaching. Consider your short-term and long-term career goals. Making an informed choice can help you navigate the challenges of academia more effectively, leading to successful promotion and tenure outcomes.

## Resources (Table 3.4)

Institutional resources such as diversity, equity, and inclusion offices, community engagement, health equity, etc. These offices offer resources and advice. You may also improve your teaching effectiveness through resources in Centers for Teaching and Learning or Faculty Excellence at institutions.

Teaching resources through the National Center for Faculty Development and Diversity (NCFDD).

Professional development workshops, such as Building the Next Generation of Academic Physicians (BNGAP), National Hispanic Medical Association, and Latino Medical Student Association.

**Table 3.4** Professional goals chart, Sotto-Santiago, S. Adapted from Book: ISBN 1-58874-267-9

| Goals | Preferred | Acceptable | Deal breaker |
|---|---|---|---|
| What part of the country would you like to live in? (are there others to consider?) | | | |
| What type of institution would you like to work in? | | | |
| What academic appointment will I have? | | | |
| What type of resources will be offered to me? | | | |
| What type of supervisor will you be reporting to? | | | |
| What type of colleagues do I want? | | | |
| What faculty and professional development are available? | | | |
| Are there opportunities for administrative or leadership roles? | | | |
| What type of scholarship will I be able to focus on? | | | |
| What does the healthcare enterprise look like? Is it profitable? Does it serve the community? | | | |
| Compensation and opportunities for increases? | | | |
| What benefits are offered? Insurance? Retirement? Vacation? | | | |
| Is diversity, equity, and inclusion of importance? What is the track record of historically marginalized communities at the institution? | | | |
| Be treated with respect? | | | |

Mentoring networks available throughout the institution, but also professional societies and associations. For example, the Society for the Advancement of Chicanos/Hispanics and Native Americans in Science (SACNAS) offers mentorship programs connecting early-career faculty with experienced professionals.

Conferences with targeted professional development.

Research and funding opportunities. This comes in the form of institutional and pilot grants. NIH and NSF both offer specific funding aimed at increasing diversity in research with programs specifically designed for historically marginalized faculty in science and medicine.

Find in-person and online communities. LHS+ faculty are eager to connect either through an institutional group or through social media groups.

Book: Latino, Hispanic, or of Spanish origin identified student leaders in medicine: recognizing more than 50 years of presence, activism, and leadership.

Sánchez JP, Rodriguez D. Latino, Hispanic, or of Spanish origin+ identified student leaders in medicine: recognizing more than 50 years of presence, activism, and leadership. Cham: Springer Nature; 2024. https://doi.org/10.1007/978-3-031-35020-7.

These resources can help LHS+ faculty navigate their academic careers more effectively, find mentorship, and access professional development opportunities. Engaging with these networks and resources can contribute significantly to your success and well-being in academia.

## Personal Narratives

### Sylk Sotto Santiago, EDD, MBA, MPS
*Salud, dinero y amor.*
*(Translation: To your health, wealth, and love).*

In my Puerto Rican family, a common Spanish phrase is often used in two scenarios. First, imagine a toast—glasses raised high—where someone toasts to everyone's health, wealth, and love. [I hope this doesn't prompt you to question the order, as I do not know why it is said that way.] The second scenario occurs when someone sneezes multiple times; the witness, perhaps slightly annoyed by the repeated sneezes, wishes them *salud, dinero y amor*, one for each sneeze. [Again, what happens for those who sneeze only once or four times? You get what you get.]

This everyday act took on special meaning for me when I was about 9 years old and my mom became a single mother. I could see her sadness and worry. As a stay-at-home wife and mother without a college education and two young daughters, her concerns were palpable. I remember when someone sneezed multiple times, and she wished them "salud, dinero y amor," then looked at me, the oldest, and said, "I wish you and your sister all those things, but the truth is the only way to that money is your education. No one can take that away." Reflecting on my career path, I realize how that moment changed the meaning of that phrase for me. Now, I often think of it as *salud, educación y amor*, and it brings a smile to my face.

As a child, my motivation was to make my mom proud, which made me a stellar student. Thanks to the larger family and government support, multiple jobs, and through evictions and heartaches, my education was the one thing my mom never worried about. My curiosity and independence flourished, leading me to transfer from the University of Puerto Rico to Colorado, arriving on a January day with a Pell Grant and student loans in hand.

There were several formative moments during my college experience, too many to recount here, but one sticks with me vividly. While my professor sat in his brownish three-piece suit, I explained that I misunderstood an assignment and asked to redo it. He simply said, "No." I insisted, "It's not that I didn't do it; I just did the wrong exercises as you can see. I didn't understand." I still remember his face when he said, "If you do not understand, maybe you should go back to your country." In that moment, I felt utterly alone, but there was no way I was returning to Puerto Rico in failure. "Dame un momento pa' probar de qué estoy hecho…" I sang to myself and still do! I fought hard and graduated, making my mom proud.

I completed every graduate degree part-time because I needed full-time employment to support my family. I earned two Master's degrees and a Doctorate while raising three daughters with a fantastic partner. I delivered my hooding speech entirely in Spanish, knowing that the only person who needed to understand my words was my mom—and she was so proud. I also found my professional home easily. Remember: "Salud, educación y amor"? Salud, my professional home is in academic medicine and health sciences. I teach, conduct research, and work on health equity and access. *Educación* is obviously important to me; unfortunately, not all teaching methods and learning environments are created equally, so I strive to make them inclusive. Amor is reflected in how I treat others.

If this resonates with you, I know you are a warrior and stubborn. You are meant to prove people wrong, even when you have internalized so much doubt. Academia is the right place for you. My first academic faculty appointment was at Indiana University School of Medicine. After 1 year in the clinical track, I chose to transfer to the tenure track, focusing on service with balanced evidence in teaching and research. This chapter speaks to the decision to become a faculty member and the challenging choice of which track to pursue. Honestly, I chose the tenure track for others and because I was the only one, EdD and Latina. I was aware that only about 1% of LHS+ women hold a tenured Associate Professor appointment. I wanted to demonstrate what is possible and I achieved tenure and promotion within 5 years.

This motivation also influenced my recent appointment as Associate Vice Chancellor for Faculty Development and Inclusive Excellence at the University of Pittsburgh Health Sciences. My faculty niche and leadership roles have always aligned perfectly with my interests and scholarship. This represents the epitome of aligning values with work. I am here to support you on whatever path you choose. I will cheer you on, coach you, and celebrate you. If I can call myself a tenured, soon-to-be full professor, then so can you.

**Maria Milagros Garcia Quiñones, MD, MPH, FACP**
*No matter where I go, I know where I come from…*

I come from a strong military family. My mother was a widow when her husband was killed at the age of 19 years old in the Korean war. She had just graduated from high school. Ten years later she met my father who was also in the military and served three times during the Vietnam war. It was fun for me and my other four siblings growing up as a military family. We experienced the opportunity to travel and live abroad in countries like Germany. We also grew up being bilingual as my mother only spoke Spanish. Both of our parents only graduated from high school. My father initially started as a cook in the armed forces, but over time became a club manager. Our parents always emphasized their love for our Puerto Rico Island and keeping close connections with our Puerto Rican family. My mother was a stay-at-home mom who did not know how to drive and my father was often gone for months. However, both of my parents had seven siblings so many of our extended family were there to assist us growing up.

When I graduated from high school, I pursued a path to become a doctor. I applied to the University of Puerto Rico (UPR) and was offered a scholarship and acceptance to UPR Medical School. However, I wanted to experience living in the USA and chose to attend college at Rutgers University of New Jersey. In the beginning, it was difficult as I had no connection to the area. However, I was fortunate to have been placed in the "Casa Boricua" residence. There I met friends and "sisters" with whom I am still close today. I had no monetary support but found a job in the school library. I borrowed a suit from one of my friends and applied for a receptionist job in a dental office. The dentist who interviewed me commented smiling saying, "I am hiring you as I have never seen anyone come to a receptionist interview in a suit."

My path to medicine could have been direct, but I chose to explore my options as, coming from a military background, we were used to moving to a new location every 3 years. I was accepted to Bryn Mawr College *PostBacc Program* before attending the Medical College of Pennsylvania. This enabled me to pursue a residency in Internal Medicine at Boston Medical Center. I then worked as a Primary Care Physician at Beth Israel Deaconess Hospital. I decided to move and started as faculty at the University of Massachusetts Medical Center where I continued my Primary Care Practice. I later transitioned to working as a Hospitalist which enabled me to work and train Internal Medicine Residents. I also pursued a Master in Public Health degree.

My academic career has been guided by my passion to teach, provide the best clinical care for my patients, and make significant contributions to the area of Public Health. I have always been focused on the concepts of social justice, health equity, and opportunity for healthcare to all. Although I started as a Clinician Educator, I realized that I also wanted a health policy focus in my work. My leadership roles have enabled me to enhance institutional diversity, advance curriculum at the levels of undergraduate and graduate medical education, and develop scholarly and research interventions that guide national and state policy. The integration of all these facets of work contributes to an infrastructure at the local, state, and national level that addresses quality care, enhances medical education, impacts health policy, and fosters diversity.

# References

1. National Center for Education Statistics. Fast facts: faculty (61). U.S. Department of Education, Institute of Education Sciences. 2023. https://nces.ed.gov/fastfacts/display.asp?id=61
2. Saxena MR, Ling AY, Carrillo E, Alvarez A, Yiadom MYAB, Bennett CL, Gallegos M. Trends of academic faculty identifying as Hispanic at US medical schools, 1990-2021. J Grad Med Educ. 2023;15(2):175–9. https://doi.org/10.4300/JGME-D-22-00384.1.
3. Odei BC, Jagsi R, Diaz DA, Wilkins CH, Hinyard L. Evaluation of equitable racial and ethnic representation among departmental chairs in academic medicine, 1980–2019. JAMA Netw Open. 2021;4(5):e2110726. https://doi.org/10.1001/jamanetworkopen.2021.10726.
4. Rodríguez JE, Campbell KM, Pololi LH. Addressing disparities in academic medicine: what of the minority tax? BMC Med Educ. 2015;15:6. https://doi.org/10.1186/s12909-015-0290-9.
5. Sánchez JP, Peters L, Lee-Rey E, Garrison G, Ortega G. Racial and ethnic minority faculty perspectives on academic medicine careers: a qualitative study. J Natl Med Assoc. 2011;103(9–10):885–93. https://doi.org/10.1016/S0027-9684(15)30480-0.
6. Sotto-Santiago S, Vigil D. Racist nativism in academic medicine: an analysis of Latinx faculty experiences. Int J Qual Stud Educ. 2023;36(10):1981–95. https://doi.org/10.1080/09518398.2021.1956617.
7. Sotto-Santiago S, Moreno F. LHS+ faculty development and advancement. In: Sánchez JP, Rodriguez D, editors. Latino, Hispanic, or of Spanish Origin+ identified student leaders in medicine, Sustainable development goals series. Springer; 2024. p. 251–67. https://doi.org/10.1007/978-3-031-35020-7_13.

8. Plasencia G, Gupta R, Kaalund K, Martinez-Bianchi V, Gonzalez-Guarda R, Thoumi A. Systemic racism affecting Latinx population health during the COVID-19 pandemic and beyond: perspectives of Latinx community health workers and community-based organization leaders. Health Equity. 2023;7(1):715–21. https://doi.org/10.1089/heq.2023.0193.
9. Rodriguez JE, Campbell KM, Fogarty JP, Williams RL. Underrepresented minority faculty in academic medicine: a systematic review of URM faculty development. Fam Med. 2014;46(2):100–4.
10. Sánchez JP, Chheda SG, Negrón-Gonzales V, Torres MB, De La Cruz M, Ramos JA, Vélez J. LMSA faculty/physician advisors: a critical partner in supporting LHS+ medical students. In: Sánchez JP, Rodriguez D, editors. Latino, Hispanic, or of Spanish Origin+ identified student leaders in medicine, Sustainable development goals series. Springer; 2024. p. 165–82. https://doi.org/10.1007/978-3-031-35020-7_9.
11. Pololi L, Kern DE, Carr P, Conrad P, Knight S. The culture of academic medicine: faculty perceptions of the lack of alignment between individual and institutional values. J Gen Intern Med. 2009;24(12):1289–95. https://doi.org/10.1007/s11606-009-1131-5.
12. Oliveira-Silva LC, Porto JB, Arnold J. Professional fulfillment: concept and instrument proposition. Psico-USF. 2019;24(1):27–39. https://doi.org/10.1590/1413-82712019240103.
13. Schwartz SH, Cieciuch J, Vecchione M, Davidov E, Fischer R, Beierlein C, Ramos A, Verkasalo M, Lönnqvist JE, Demirutku K, Dirilen-Gumus O, Konty M. Refining the theory of basic individual values. J Pers Soc Psychol. 2012;103:663–88. https://doi.org/10.1037/a0029393.
14. Martin NA, Bloom JL. Career aspirations & expeditions: advancing your career in higher education administration. Stipes Publishing; 2003.
15. Gadolin C, Andersson T, Eriksson E, Hellström A. Providing healthcare through "value shops": impact on professional fulfillment for physicians and nurses. Int J Health Gov. 2020;25(2):127–36. https://doi.org/10.1108/IJHG-12-2019-0081.
16. Sotto-Santiago S, Sharp S, Mac J, Messmore N, Haywood A, Tyson M, Yi V, Lee A. Reclaiming the mission of academic medicine: an examination of institutional responses to (anti)racism. AEM Educ Train. 2021;5(Suppl 1):S33–43. https://doi.org/10.1002/aet2.10668.
17. Austin AE. Preparing the next generation of faculty: graduate school as socialization to the academic career. J High Educ. 2002;73(1):94–122.
18. Steinert Y. Faculty development in the new millennium: key challenges and future directions. Med Teach. 2000;22(1):44–50. https://doi.org/10.1080/01421590078814.
19. Steinert Y. Faculty development: core concepts and principles. In: Steinert Y, editor. Faculty development in the health professions: a focus on research and practice. Springer; 2014. p. 3–19.
20. Bunton SA, Mallon WT. The continued evolution of faculty appointment and tenure policies at U.S. medical schools. Acad Med. 2007;82(3):281–9. https://doi.org/10.1097/ACM.0b013e3180307e87.
21. Walling A, Nilsen KM. Tenure appointments for faculty of clinical departments at U.S. medical schools: does specialty designation make a difference? Acad Med. 2018;93(11):1719–26. https://doi.org/10.1097/ACM.0000000000002346.
22. Association of American Medical Colleges. Diversity in medicine: facts and figures 2023. 2023. https://www.aamc.org/data-reports/workforce/report/diversity-medicine-facts-and-figures. Accessed on 5 July 2025.
23. Buchanan GR. Academic promotion and tenure: a user's guide for junior faculty members. Hematology Am Soc Hematol Educ Program. 2009:736–41. https://doi.org/10.1182/asheducation-2009.1.736. PMID: 20008261.
24. Callahan EJ, Banks M, Medina J, Disbrow K, Soto-Greene M, Sánchez JP. Providing diverse trainees an early and transparent introduction to academic appointment and promotion processes. MedEdPORTAL. 2017;13:10661. https://doi.org/10.15766/mep_2374-8265.10661.
25. The 2022 AAUP survey of tenure practices. https://www.aaup.org/file/2022_AAUP_Survey_of_Tenure_Practices.pdf. Accessed on 5 July 2025.

26. Kniess D. Moving into a faculty role from student affairs administration. New Directions for Student Success. 2019, June 04. https://onlinelibrary.wiley.com/doi/full/10.1002/ss.20307?casa_token=M83JMpiHSeYAAAAA%3ALO9g3A7jekBtNJ0NWW1F1CufbIEM6R17ZDZVSB2Mla3sukkceQjsw1vK8rmWNBSJ6JcYcprhdVH3tg. Accessed on 5 July 2025.
27. McHale SM, Ranwala DD, DiazGranados D, Bagshaw D, Schienke E, Blank AE. Promotion and tenure policies for team science at colleges/schools of medicine. J Clin Transl Sci. 2019;3(5):245–52. https://doi.org/10.1017/cts.2019.401. PMID: 31660249; PMCID: PMC6815766.

**Open Access**  This chapter is licensed under the terms of the Creative Commons Attribution 4.0 International License (http://creativecommons.org/licenses/by/4.0/), which permits use, sharing, adaptation, distribution and reproduction in any medium or format, as long as you give appropriate credit to the original author(s) and the source, provide a link to the Creative Commons license and indicate if changes were made.

The images or other third party material in this chapter are included in the chapter's Creative Commons license, unless indicated otherwise in a credit line to the material. If material is not included in the chapter's Creative Commons license and your intended use is not permitted by statutory regulation or exceeds the permitted use, you will need to obtain permission directly from the copyright holder.

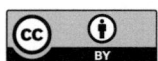

# Chapter 4
# How to Switch an Academic Faculty Track

Guadalupe Federico-Martinez

> **Learning Objectives**
> - Describe the most common contextual factors that influence a faculty member's decision to switch tracks
> - Review the risks and benefits of switching tracks
> - Outline the general administrative process of requesting and securing a track switch

**Key Terms and Definitions**
*Important Terms*

> *Professional identity*—the attitudes, values, knowledge, beliefs, and skills shared with others within a professional group, such as academic medicine. Scholars elaborate that "it is complex, personal, and shaped by contextual factors" [1]. Through the constant process of self-reflection of these attitudes and skills, in combination with institutional socialization of the faculty, individuals learn how to operate within the academic culture.
>
> *Distribution of efforts (DOE)*—a document that is illustrative of an institution's workload distribution system that informs faculty of the proportion of time dedicated to research, teaching, clinical service, and/or administrative responsibilities.
>
> *Symbolic capital*—one form of capital within the field of sociology wherein a person's resources, like a faculty member's academic title, are understood as a form that conveys prestige or recognition. Because it is laborious to accu-

---

G. Federico-Martinez (✉)
DLM Coaching, Consulting & Wellness LLC, Paradise Valley, AZ, USA

© The Author(s) 2026
J. P. Sánchez et al. (eds.), *Advancing Latino, Hispanic, or of Spanish Origin+ Leadership in Academic Medicine*,
https://doi.org/10.1007/978-3-032-07570-3_4

mulate over time, the result is demonstrative of the high value that one holds within the academic culture. Such capital (e.g., title) colors the external perception that others in your community have of you, which speaks to one's academic prowess, positionality, and credibility [2].

## Introduction

At this juncture of your career, I am sure you have noticed that the academic path is heavily saturated with complex and political-administrative processes. Further, academic medicine remains rooted in traditional hierarchies when it comes to many operations (e.g., permission, reviews, requests, and titling) that impact faculty life. It is important to have a basic understanding of these operations and organizational culture, given the competing academic cultures within your college of medicine, teaching hospital, C-suite, and broader university campus. Embedded in these operations are hidden rules and traditions that can (and will) influence your self-efficacy and decision-making processes. Ultimately, such rules have the power to define what it means to be "successful" in your field (or at least as the academic world might see it). This chapter will introduce you to these general rules and procedures when considering switching academic tracks.

## Review of the Literature

Overall, higher education data in the United States related to faculty switching tracks is scarce. Nationally, we know that tenure as an option for physicians and basic scientists plateaued before 2010 [3, 4]. Within the last decade, however, tenure opportunities have declined [5]. Interestingly, among these few studies, trends regarding track switching focus on switching off the tenure-line to any other adjunct or full-time nontenure track [6]. Additionally, studies find that minoritized faculty, across disciplines, depart tenure and/or the academic sector because of poor social integration into the academic culture during scholars' prefaculty years [7]. Research across disciplines shows that such faculty tend to have lower evaluation results and excessive teaching and service obligations, experience credibility or authority issues in boardrooms and classrooms, and often experience isolation [8]. Sensitization of such anticipated obstacles commonly experienced by such faculty with navigation skills to persist through challenges is rarely integrated into the schooling curriculum [9].

In the realm of health sciences, strides are being made in improving preparation and socialization into faculty roles [10, 11]. There is also increased federal funding to sponsor career development and skills development as part of a broader effort to enhance recruitment, cluster recruitment strategies, and retention of minoritized faculty groups over the last decade. Although critical to improving the social integration of faculty, we do not yet have robust, multiinstitutional, and longitudinal data on such programmatic efficacy as it relates to shifting within academic tracks and if and how shifts play out for minoritized groups. It takes time. Moreover, we see that over the last 30 years, academic track options have expanded, and promotion criteria have evolved [12]. Again, data around track-switching experiences for those in medicine is inadequate. Given the decline of tenure opportunities, increased competitiveness to secure funding for investigatory efforts, and ongoing self-exploration and identity formation in one's early career, there is so much at play when attempting to understand faculty decision-making and career progress trends. As such, existing medical education literature is extremely limited. There is attention to the Latina/o/x/e, Hispanic, or of Spanish Origin (LHS+) faculty composition in academic medicine when it comes to ranks. Studies show that LHS+ are less likely to be full professors (on and off tenure) and have lower rates of advancement through the ranks if LHS+ faculty do not retain (National Institute of Health) NIH funding [13]. However, data that focus on the number, frequency, and an individual's experience of switching tracks, as it relates to the LHS+ experience, are absent. Data narrowly concentrate on the shifting to clinical scholar or educator and away from clinical research pathways, life off the tenure track to keep pace with how medical education is currently delivered, and bring to the surface stigmas of titles or feelings of second-class faculty status [14]. These data are isolated to one institution, outdated, and not disaggregated by demographics or other key characteristics of broad interest.

One effective means to find general information on track switching is reviewing your department, college of medicine, or provost/chancellor's office of faculty affairs website for the promotion guidelines. You can expect these sources to be purely informational regarding the accepted procedure and basis for transfer. The experiences of faculty, particularly LHS+, with the process are unexplored. Given the ongoing evolution of the faculty role in academic medicine, studies examining a cost-benefit analysis for the member or the department are needed. Disaggregating data finely could also inform revisions to promotion and tenure policies and procedures and improve our understanding of trends across various groups. Flexibility and recalibration advising, track descriptions, and promotion criteria to assist faculty with solidifying their identity and path toward upward mobility are likely the future of retention and personalized faculty development [15, 16].

## *Contextual Factors*

Switching academic tracks is uncommon [17, 18]. However, it can be done if it is in the best interest of the faculty member's career trajectory. There are several important contextual factors, each particular to individual institutions, to understand when considering track switching. The factors we will review are (a) one's professional identity alignment with faculty roles, expectations, and time allocated for the tripartite mission, (b) critical conversations with colleagues, and (c) the collective needs of your department. These factors heavily influence decision-making around the appropriateness of academic track determination, with the ultimate goal of successful professorial promotion up the ranks [19, 20].

## Professional Identity

The alignment of your *professional identity* [21] and the strength of your skills is critical at the time of initial appointment to ensure successful integration into faculty life. Additionally, allowing your professional identity to serve as a guidepost to determine both the specific academic track you should be on (i.e., clinical educator or research scientist and where you will spend most of your time within the multiple missions. Ideally, a living and written document exists that illustrates this as a *distribution of your efforts (DOE)* in the teaching, clinical, research, and administrative realms.

## Academic Performance Reviews and Critical Conversations

Faculty performance reviews are expected in the academy. Depending on your specific institutional policies, reviews may occur midyear, annually, or midpromotion cycle. Performance reviews are often conducive to reflective dialogues between leaders and faculty [22, 23]. Such forums are most often the appropriate time and atmosphere to initiate and discuss your expectations, goals, and whether time allocations stipulated on your DOE still align with personal and departmental goals. During this time, reviewing the pros and cons of track switching is ideal and critical to your long-term success.

Performance reviews are generally conducted with the division chief or department chair. Schools of Medicine in early development phases heavily depend on the Offices of Faculty Affairs for initial guidance. While this subgroup of leaders and offices plays a central role in approving track switches, it is important to recall that, for LHS+ faculty in medicine [24], the high value of consultation through your mentors and peer professional networks when it comes to career advancement [25, 26]. Thus, consulting with additional people to inform your self-reflections is necessary. First, one may have a main mentor who serves as their "go-to" confidante. However, we now know that a panel of trusted people, inside and outside of your institution, serving in the roles of mentor, advisor, coach, role model, or sponsor, is optimal for receiving diverse guidance and feedback [15]. It is strongly recommended to establish and involve such a panel. Second, many faculty, particularly subspecialists, have administrative leadership roles. (e.g., residency association program director, clerkship director, and service line director). Given this positionality, faculty may have "dotted supervisory lines" to other leaders in addition to their immediate supervisor. These leaders and their programs may feel either the pinch or benefit from your decision to switch tracks. If this describes your current context, it is strongly recommended to include them in your internal considerations and have a prior discussion about your considerations with a dotted-line supervisor. Including the aforementioned actors has the potential to better prepare and inform your ultimate decision.

## What Is the Impetus for Switching Tracks?

Although each institution's exact titles vary, conceptually, four universal classifications track titles tend to echo within the academic medicine mission: education, research, clinical, and administrative service (See Fig. 4.1). Know your institutional promotion and tenure guidelines for knowledge of the full spectrum of available academic tracks and their descriptions. Knowing your criteria for promotion early in your career is critical.

Rarely, but at times, the following happens throughout your development as an academician: (a) individual professional identity transformations as niche interests change; (b) new educational, research, or administrative roles are added to your responsibilities; or (c) administrative, clinical, or teaching productivity needs of the division or department experience drastic change that, in the opinion of the faculty and institutional leaders, warrant switching to a track that better reflects the new landscape and workload expectations. In such cases, the faculty member's DOE may need considerable recalibration, resulting in a track switch to one that better reflects the newly anticipated needs and trajectory of the individual. Figure 4.2 illustrates how your values, passions, strengths, and preferences relate to one another. It highlights areas of overlap and distinction to help identify your "sweet spot" or ideal career track.

In sum, the impetus behind the switch is done in the spirit of improving alignment with the time allocations of your professional responsibilities.

## The Benefits and Risks of Making the Switch

When considering a track switch, it is imperative to weigh the benefits and risks of potential outcomes. The possible benefits of track switching could include the realignment of your DOE such that your roles, individual, and departmental goals more closely match collective interests and needs. In the same vein, the new track (at the same rank) will require that the faculty member be subject to a different set of performance review and promotion criteria as determined by the institution. Depending on the timing of when the switch is made and one's current body of

Institutional career tracks are universal with different labels

- Clinical Educator /Educator Scholar
- Clinical Researcher/ Research Scholar
- Primary Clinician
- Traditional Tenure Track

**Fig. 4.1** Institutional career tracks are universal, with different labels

**Fig. 4.2** Identifying the target track

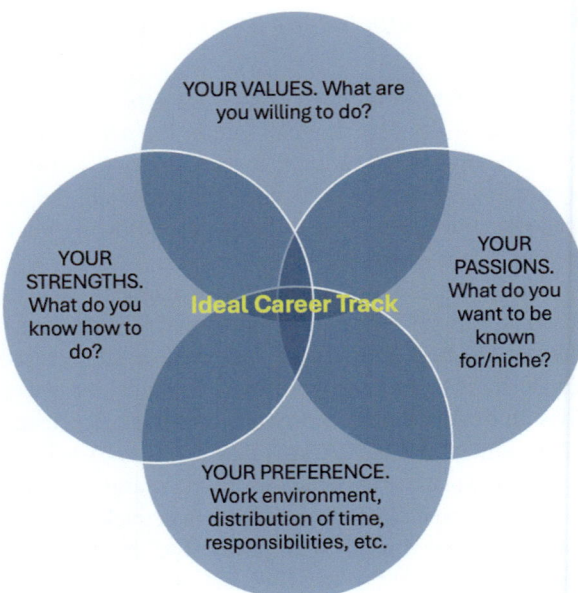

Graphic created by J.P. Sanchez MD, MPH

academic work, the result of the track change could better position one for a timely and successful promotion experience. On the other hand, as a risk, the shift to a new review or promotion criteria that results from a track switch might be a major difference that could extend the time it takes to achieve promotion to the next rank. The "time-to-promotion" will depend on the extent to which the criteria vary and the current and relevant progress the faculty member has attained. We know that LHS+ nontenure track faculty are promoted at a slower rate than their LHS+ tenure-eligible/tenured counterparts. This is mostly because tenure-eligible tracks have strictly enforced timetables to go up for midcycle reviews and promotion to the next rank as opposed to intrinsic motivation [13, 27]. However, this already delayed process can be exacerbated by switching tracks. Therefore, it is important to be highly knowledgeable in the promotion criteria for the tracks at your site early.

Another benefit of track switching is the *symbolic capital* that the new track title conveys to those internal and external to your institution [2]. For instance, if your professional identity is based in clinical teaching and you are striving to be a residency program director in the future, then clearly education is a strong priority for you. In preparation for the role and to build your curriculum vitae (CV), perhaps you are seeking to join an education interest group in your specialty's professional organization or national medical education accreditation association (e.g., Internal Medicine's AAIM-APDIM; ACGME RRC: Dermatology). If your previous title was *Clinical Associate Professor* and you switched tracks, obtaining a new title of *Associate Professor, Clinical Educator*, the modifier placement and new title will reflect your new professional identity and strongly suggest to others in the scholarly community your dedicated role to teaching. Conversely, placement of modifiers in professorial titles (e.g., clinical associate professor vs. associate professor, clinical) alters the meaning of the title. Acquiring a new title may be associated with a perceived stigma related to the modifiers [14, 23]. Finally, depending on the new roles, clinical and university affiliation legal agreements, employers, and compensation model details, one last aspect to consider is to what extent the track switch potentially impacts compensation.

An important reminder from Todisco et al. [29] is to know that,

> Occasionally, an individual may not meet the expectations of a given track. It is the responsibility of the division chair/chief in concert with the faculty member to help redirect the individual's career and, in essence, consider changing tracks. Many successful academicians have changed tracks and have had extremely successful and satisfying careers in a track different from the one originally selected. Such processes should not be viewed as failures but rather a better realignment of talents and interests. [28]

Overall, a broad cascade of events will occur when realigning your track trajectory, as captured in Fig. 4.3. As such, it is critical to research and engage with your trusted advisors to determine the optimal strategies when preparing for a track switch.

## *What Is the Review and Approval Process?*

As noted in the opening of the chapter, switching tracks is uncommon, and if it does occur for a faculty member, the occurrence will likely happen only once at their institution. There is no academic literature that is publicly available that suggests that LHS+ faculty frequently switch tracks as a result of being misplaced or needing to recalibrate their goals to the most appropriate track. Perhaps, because of its rarity, there is little effort to openly report the frequency with which faculty members switch tracks. Despite its rarity, several discussions, reviews, and approvals at multiple levels of the institution must occur before the track switch is complete. Therefore, there is much to expect.

Policies impacting academic tracks, academic reviews, and academic promotions are set by multiple entities. Depending on the type of institution (e.g., private, public, or stand-alone hospital), the entities traditionally included in policy creation and revision tend to be the state board of regents if within public

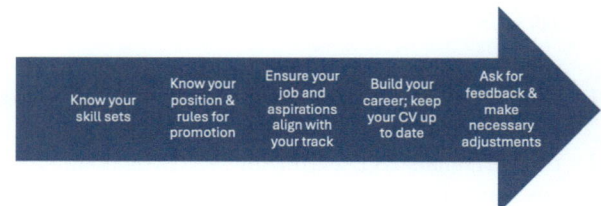

**Fig. 4.3** Career development and track trajectory

Graphic created by J.P. Sanchez MD, MPH

university systems. Within the broader academic setting, and depending on the faculty bylaws, the provost/chancellor, faculty affairs offices, and the department or division leaders are involved in enforcing and adhering to policies at each level. This includes initial appointments and track switching. The detailed operationalization of the track switching will vary widely by institution, with likely no sites being identical.

Generally, the notion of track switching is discussed at the time of one's mid-cycle reviews or annual performance reviews. Requests to switch are largely honored if both the faculty member and their immediate leader (e.g., division chief; department chair) see a need to address a significant change in professional responsibilities. Contingent upon institutional policies, the track-switching process is usually facilitated, supported, and approved by the division chief/department chair. Some sites may require additional approvals by the Office of Faculty Affairs, the department promotion and tenure committee, and/or the dean. It is important to note that for those seeking a switch on or off of the tenure-eligible/tenure track, requests are often elevated to the board of regents and high-level finance offices, depending on the case.

Overall, how does the track-switching process look different for LHS+? It is not clearly understood or documented to date. However, the process of switching should not look different than any other faculty member, but possibly due to the lack of mentorship or quality discussions with one's department chair, alignment with goals and track descriptions may not have happened accurately upon hiring or entry into the academy. Do not let that happen to you. The best practice is to stay informed and ask questions!

## Reflection Exercise

### Are You on the Appropriate Track?

In your e-journal, answer the following questions to ensure you have reviewed your institution's promotion guidelines by track, and to examine if your interests and DOE align with your current track.

### Materials Needed

1. Your school of medicine's promotion and tenure guidelines in their entirety (i.e., research, education, clinical, tenure-eligible/tenure).
2. Your personalized DOE document. If you do not have one, create one with your supervisor immediately.
3. Your CV.

Do you know what academic track you are on?

> If yes, what is the exact title?
> If no, review your hiring documents or contact your faculty affairs liaison and write the title on your CV immediately.
> Then review the track description in you.

Do you have a clear understanding of other tracks available at your institution?

> If yes, good for you! You should consider a formal role in the leadership of faculty.
> If not, budget time on your calendar to review all the tracks.

Do you perceive that the track aligns well with your current role(s) and DOE?

> Might another track be a better fit for your promotion plans?

Who played a role in determining your track with you? List them.

> Are they fully aware of your career goals and where you spend most of your time?
> Do they also serve as a mentor, coach, advisor, or sponsor for you?
> List at least one more person you would ideally like to discuss your promotion plan with. Include them in your "panel of mentors" as referenced in the chapter.

Do you think you are on track for a timely promotion at your institution?

> If yes, how do you know this based on the information you read in this chapter?
> If no, what is your plan in the next 3 months to recalibrate your aspirations and timeline?

## Skills Exercise

Brief skills exercise in the discernment of fit and alignment. Consider the following faculty scenario. A possible response is provided for you. However, review the response and rationale after you have pondered how *you* would respond and why.

Prompt: Is it appropriate for the faculty member, or would you advise Dr. DaSilva to switch tracks if you were the division chief?

*Hypothetical Scenario*: Dr. DaSilva's career track profile.

1. Currently on a nontenure *clinical educator* track. His promotion criteria emphasize the expectation of educational scholarship.
2. He is also the service line director for Medicine-ICU.
3. His division's needs in pulmonary/critical care have changed, wherein the academic division is shrinking. Clinical productivity expectations are not decreasing, so additional consult service and shifts have been added to his schedule for the last two consecutive years. He is almost at 85% clinical time on his DOE. This

is a stark difference from his 50% clinical time allocation at the time of initial appointment.
4. It has been 7 years, and he cannot gain footing on meeting the traditional scholarly requirements for the track, but given clinical exposure and contributions to new clinical protocols, and thriving with new demands, he would be excelling in another track called the nontenure *clinical series* track.
5. At his annual review, he is strongly considering switching to a clinical *series* track that emphasizes patient care/clinical excellence.

*Response and rationale:* In this case, it is appropriate for the faculty member to switch tracks to the clinical series. As division chief, you could validate and accept Dr. DaSilva's desire to make a track switch that emphasizes clinical excellence. There are five reasons to support the realignment to the clinical series track.

The very first indicator of alignment is reviewing a faculty member's DOE to see how their time distribution has shifted. You see that almost midway through his initial appointment, he has less and less time for a focus on education and more time for clinical work (50–85%).

Upon reviewing his CV and educator's portfolio, you notice there is little evidence of productivity for the last 7 years as a clinical educator. This means you see a lack of original curricula for new elective rotations for the fellows and internal medicine residents, less than seven peer-reviewed original research publications focused on medical education, educational leadership, best practices for teaching, less-than-stellar teaching evaluations in the didactic setting, and no committee service locally or nationally supporting the learner population.

Instead, you notice that the CV and clinical portfolio has multiple peer-reviewed case reports, a handful of middle-author clinical abstracts as part of team science, above average participation in internal Patient Safety/Quality Improvement (PSQI) initiatives, better scores on bedside teaching evaluations, national presentations on clinical guidelines, and substantial hospital committee service that adds to his ICU administrative responsibilities. This is confirmation that he is thriving in this mission area.

Additionally, you consider his upcoming growth and professorial promotion when thinking about the context of his switch. Your institution values time in rank as a promotable criterion after the 6-year mark. This means Dr. DaSilva could have a fair chance at a successful professorial promotion by meeting this one (of many) criterion in either track.

There would be no change to his compensation model, given that his DOE would not change for less time in the clinical setting.

All signs point to—switch!

## Conclusion

Not unlike the previous chapter, titled "Making a Decision About an Academic Faculty Track," track switching requires you to engage in continuous and deep introspection about your strengths and where your time is being allocated to meet the various missions and your passions. There are three core messages from this chapter. First, recall that the most common contextual factors that influence a faculty member's decision to switch tracks include (a) professional identity aligning with your roles, expectations, and time allocated; (b) quality and substance of engaging with colleagues and advisors; and (c) clarity on the collective needs of your department as they relate to your role on the team. Exploring, reflecting, and openly discussing these factors will greatly assist you with rationalizing and determining the appropriateness of your academic track and whether a switch is a beneficial and logical move in your career. Next, know the risks and benefits of making the switch. The idea of symbolic capital can impact perceptions both negatively and positively. Understand what the new track conveys within your local site, nationally, and within your specialty. It will give rise to either a perceived stigma or a feeling of inferiority when compared to other tracks or will lead to true alignment with your professional identity after a much-needed recalibration. The discussion to better understand what the new titling and promotion criteria are is best kept as a highly intentional discussion point when engaging advisors and supervisors. Deep contemplation, alerting important members within your professional network, and gaining support ahead of time from the entity that determines your workload distribution should make for a well-planned, positive, and timely submission experience. Finally, carefully review the written (and ask about the unwritten) general administrative process of requesting a track switch at your site. Remember, all sites have a different process, so follow the directions exactly. Like promotion dossiers, depending on the track switch type, such requests might require meticulous review and deliberation at various committees and levels, while other sites have a simplified process of approval by one's department chair. Minimize delays and frustration by doing your homework and learning the rules of the game. This chapter builds on the LHS+ faculty development work of Soto and Moreno [30], wherein they lay the groundwork for socialization, culturally relevant mentoring, and academic writing expectations to optimize the success of current LHS+ faculty. Additional research on the frequency of track switching and experiences of the process as it plays out for LHS+ is needed to understand how a team of mentors and sponsors can best serve their career advancement.

## Additional Resources

The following books are recommended to aid you in reflecting on your professional identity and your academic track:

1. Brod, H., & Skarupski, K. (2024). *The Insider's Pocket Guide to Navigating a Faculty Career in Academic Medicine.* Springer.
2. Roberts, L. W. (Ed.). (2019). *Roberts Academic Medicine Handbook: A Guide to Achievement and Fulfillment for Academic Faculty.* Springer Nature.
3. Lane, P. H. (2015). *The Promotion Game: Your Guide to Success in the Academic Medical Center.* BookBaby.

## Personal Narrative

### Guadalupe Federico-Martinez, PhD

As a nonphysician Latina faculty member, I started my professional journey and found a home in academic medicine over a decade ago. While serving as a graduate medical education residency manager, I was also working on my doctoral studies in higher education. The study of higher education is about investigating how certain sectors within university systems operate.

My home clinical department of internal medicine valued studying the social science aspect of medical education and the social construct that is academic medicine. Given my studies at the time, physician-educators and senior leaders in the department were interested in using educational theory and investigatory approaches common to the sociology of education to better understand the needs of trainees, faculty, and administrators learning and working within. It was made explicitly clear to me that leadership saw the potential benefits of having a relatively "nontraditional" faculty member in a clinical department, being a different lens toward understanding organizational culture, and the training and socialization of physicians we groom to work inside and outside of academic medicine. I think I was very fortunate to have forward-thinking leaders who took a risk, invested resources, understood the value of education specialists, and trusted in my developing expertise. Family, these leaders, colleagues, former professors, mentors, sponsors, and role models in my life merged to form a constellation of support. Some of these actors shared similar backgrounds with me, while most of them, however, shared very little in common with me in terms of upbringing, educational pathway, and demographics. It is not lost on me that we, particularly those underrepresented in medicine and leadership, need to surround ourselves with experts and people who think and look different than ourselves. My trusted group of advisers functioned as my "cabinet," if you will, for mentorship and talking out options.

Upon diving into educational research projects and managing the education department, progressive leadership opportunities present themselves. I assisted physician-faculty members with their educational research ideas, teaching techniques, and making sense of career progression at the institution. My current position still includes identifying as a faculty member. Until recently, I also served in two administrative roles: one at the local level within my institution, and another at the national level for the AAMC. At my institution, I served as the assistant of faculty affairs and career development, and for the AAMC, I served 1 year as the national chair-elect of the Group on Faculty Affairs. It pains me to say that we are still experiencing "first Latina" moments in 2024; however, I was the first Latina to serve in both roles. I found these opportunities intimidating at first, but upon long and hard reflection, they aligned with my strength: advocacy. I had to muzzle the inner critic and listen to what others saw in me and believe in my decisions. This has taken me years of practice to manage and is a continued effort.

Most recently, I made the scariest decision of my life, as I am the breadwinner of my family and have responsibilities to my son and husband. This decision included my accepting the inner call to challenge myself more and risk evolving. I decided to get additional training in coaching and counseling so I can operate within what social posts are now calling "privademics." I saw an opportunity to transition from academic leadership to business leadership. I wanted to address a gap in availability and services that I often criticized institutions for: lack of mentorship and individualized faculty development. I pulled the trigger on my vision. I retained a volunteer faculty, switched tracks from *educator scholar* to *professor of practitioner*, and started my own career coaching and consulting company for physicians. I find deep satisfaction serving as the founder and CEO of my own space within the academic career development stratosphere. I very much enjoy CV reviews and strategizing with faculty, of all walks, about their career (and life) planning and progression. The switch was rather easy in terms of processes. My Faculty Affairs Vice Dean and I deduced that the switch best aligned with my new career direction and goals. The rebalancing affords me to still achieve promotion to full professor, but on a different set of criteria.

I hope that this chapter provides overt and clear guidance on the topic of whether to switch academic tracks or not. The terms, information, and reflection exercises were intentionally crafted to serve as prompts for your career planning time, to formulate relevant questions when you meet with your chair/supervisor and "cabinet," and finally, to help you weigh the pros and cons of switching academic tracks. If you are thinking to yourself, "Over the last couple of years, I've really grown and gravitated towards a different direction in medicine than I didn't start out with when I signed on. Where I spend my time and want to spend my time are now in opposing directions, but I like it. Maybe this is who I am right now? So, is staying on my current path still the optimal track for me to get promoted? Should I even care about getting promoted?" Then, this chapter is for you!

# References

1. Holden M, Buck E, Clark M, Szauter K, Trumble J. Professional identity formation in medical education: the convergence of multiple domains. In: HEC forum, vol. 24, No. 4. Springer Netherlands; 2012, December. p. 245–55.

2. Bourdieu P, Wacquant L. Symbolic capital and social classes. J Class Sociol. 2013;13(2):292–302.
3. Mason MA. Is tenure a trap for women. The Chronicle of Higher Education; 2009. p. 4.
4. Bunton SA, Corrice A. Trends in tenure for clinical MD faculty in US medical schools: a 25-year review. Anal Brief. 2010;9(9):1–2.
5. Mallon WT, Cox N. Promotion and tenure policies and practices at US medical schools: is tenure irrelevant or more relevant than ever? Acad Med. 2024;10:1097. https://doi.org/10.1097/ACM.0000000000005689.
6. Kelly BT, McCann KI. Women faculty of color: stories behind the statistics. Urban Rev. 2014;46(4):681–702.
7. Tierney WG, Rhoads RA. Enhancing promotion, tenure and beyond: faculty socialization as a cultural process. ASHE-ERIC higher education report No. 6. The George Washington University, One Dupont Circle, Suite 630, Washington, DC 20036-1183; 1993.
8. Huston TA. Race and gender bias in higher education: could faculty course evaluations impede further progress toward parity. Seattle J Soc Just. 2005;4:591.
9. Sotto-Santiago S. 'Am I really good enough?': Black and Latinx experiences with faculty development. To Improve Acad. 2020;39(2) https://doi.org/10.3998/tia.17063888.0039.205.
10. Sánchez JP. Succeeding in academic medicine: a roadmap for diverse medical students and residents. Springer; 2020.
11. Sánchez JP, Brutus N. Health professions and academia: how to begin your career. Springer; 2022.
12. Whittaker JA, Montgomery BL, Acosta VGM. Retention of underrepresented minority faculty: strategic initiatives for institutional value proposition based on perspectives from a range of academic institutions. J Undergrad Neurosci Educ. 2015;13(3):A136.
13. Kelley WN, Stross JK. Faculty tracks and academic success. Ann Intern Med. 1992;116(8):654–9.
14. Fang D, Moy E, Colburn L, Hurley J. Racial and ethnic disparities in faculty promotion in academic medicine. JAMA. 2000;284(9):1085–92.
15. Howell LP, Chen CY, Joad JP, Green R, Callahan EJ, Bonham AC. Issues and challenges of non-tenure-track research faculty: the UC Davis School of Medicine experience. Acad Med. 2010;85(6):1041–7.
16. Ayyala MS, Skarupski K, Bodurtha JN, González-Fernández M, Ishii LE, Fivush B, Levine RB. Mentorship is not enough: exploring sponsorship and its role in career advancement in academic medicine. Acad Med. 2019;94(1):94–100.
17. Collins RT, Sanford R. The importance of formalized, lifelong physician career development: making the case for a paradigm shift. Acad Med. 2021;96(10):1383–8.
18. Hunt RJ, Gray CF. Faculty appointment policies and tracks in US dental schools with clinical or research emphases. J Dent Educ. 2002;66(9):1038–43.
19. Wieder R, Carson JL, Strom BL. Restructuring of academic tracks to create successful career paths for the faculty of Rutgers biomedical and health sciences. J Healthc Leadersh. 2020;12:103.
20. Singh U, Boxer LM. How to build the foundation for a successful career in academia. In: Roberts LW, editor. Roberts academic medicine handbook: a guide to achievement and fulfillment for academic faculty. 2nd ed. Springer; 2019. p. 9–16.
21. Roberts LW. How to prepare and strategize for academic promotion. In: Roberts LW, editor. Roberts academic medicine handbook: a guide to achievement and fulfillment for academic faculty. 2nd ed. Springer; 2019. p. 461–78.
22. Ibarra H. Provisional selves: experimenting with image and identity in professional adaptation. Adm Sci Q. 1999;44(4):764–91.
23. Beasley BW, Wright SM. Looking forward to promotion. J Gen Intern Med. 2003;18(9):705–10.
24. Lane PH. The promotion game: your guide to success in the academic medical center. BookBaby; 2015.

25. Beech BM, Calles-Escandon J, Hairston KG, Langdon MSE, Latham-Sadler BA, Bell RA. Mentoring programs for underrepresented minority faculty in academic medical centers: a systematic review of the literature. Acad Med. 2013;88(4):541–9.
26. Sambunjak D, Straus SE, Marusic A. A systematic review of qualitative research on the meaning and characteristics of mentoring in academic medicine. J Gen Intern Med. 2010;25(1):72–8.
27. Cree-Green M, Carreau AM, Davis SM, Frohnert BI, Kaar JL, Ma NS, Nokoff NJ, Reusch JEB, Simon SL, Nadeau KJ. Peer mentoring for professional and personal growth in academic medicine. J Investig Med. 2020;68(6):1128–34.
28. Xierali IM, Nivet MA, Syed ZA, Shakil A, Schneider FD. Recent trends in faculty promotion in US medical schools: implications for recruitment, retention, and diversity and inclusion. Acad Med. 2021;96(10):1441–8.
29. Todisco A, Souza RF, Gores GJ. Trains, tracks, and promotion in an academic medical center. Gastroenterology. 2011;141(5):1545–8.
30. Sotto-Santiago S, Moreno F. LHS+ Faculty Development and Advancement. InLatino, Hispanic, or of Spanish Origin+ Identified Student Leaders in Medicine: Recognizing More Than 50 years of Presence, Activism, and Leadership 2023;(pp. 209-219). Cham: Springer Nature Switzerland.

**Open Access** This chapter is licensed under the terms of the Creative Commons Attribution 4.0 International License (http://creativecommons.org/licenses/by/4.0/), which permits use, sharing, adaptation, distribution and reproduction in any medium or format, as long as you give appropriate credit to the original author(s) and the source, provide a link to the Creative Commons license and indicate if changes were made.

The images or other third party material in this chapter are included in the chapter's Creative Commons license, unless indicated otherwise in a credit line to the material. If material is not included in the chapter's Creative Commons license and your intended use is not permitted by statutory regulation or exceeds the permitted use, you will need to obtain permission directly from the copyright holder.

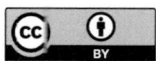

# Chapter 5
# Optimizing Your Portfolio and Executive Presence in the Recruitment Process: Perspectives from the Search Firm

Julia Omotade, David Acosta, and Philip Jaeger

> **Learning Objectives**
> - Describe the role of a search firm in the recruitment process of an academic executive.
> - List tips on how to navigate and optimize your role as a candidate during the recruitment and selection phase.
> - Outline steps to facilitate a fair and inclusive search process.

## Introduction

There is a good chance that you will interact with a search consultant in some capacity throughout the span of your professional career. Whether for a job opportunity or by serving as a member of a search committee, recruitments led by retained executive search firms are a fixture in healthcare. At the same time, academic medicine recognizes the value and importance of having a diverse healthcare and scientific research workforce to improve the health of all Americans, including those from marginalized communities like Latina/o/x/e, Hispanic, or of Spanish origin+ (LHS+) communities. The confluence of these two trends position recruitments as natural mechanisms to expand the number of faculty from historically underrepresented groups. In this chapter, we will explore how candidates—especially LHS+ faculty—can effectively work with search consultants to position themselves for their next leadership role. In addition, we will outline best practices for serving on

---

J. Omotade (✉) · D. Acosta
Association of American Medical Colleges, Washington, DC, USA

P. Jaeger
Spencer Stuart, Washington, DC, USA

search committees where those bodies evolve their practices and processes to mitigate implicit bias and engage in respectful discourse.

Search consultants can serve as valuable thought partners in a leadership transition. They simultaneously support and assist search committee members and the candidates themselves, helping both parties navigate the recruitment and selection process. Search consultants are also stewards of equity, responsible for mapping and executing a fair and inclusive search process—providing insight on best practices to attract diverse pools of talent and coaching a search committee on mitigating the role of unconscious bias.

## Working with a Search Firm as a Candidate

If it has not happened already, your phone will ring or an email will land in your inbox asking you to consider a job opportunity, and there is a good chance it will come from a search consultant. A skilled search consultant can assist in preparing you and optimizing your portfolio to maximize your competitiveness. Below are tips on how to navigate and optimize your role as a candidate during the recruitment and selection phase of the role:

*Explore*: When a recruiter calls, hear them out. Often, it is a matter of just starting to explore opportunities and seeing what is out there. Ask questions about the organization—its aspirations, financial health, faculty demographics (including LHS+), and leadership—and the authority and resources for the role to succeed. The consultant will also want to learn about you, so be prepared to share your work experiences and aspirations.

*Set your expectations*: It is rare for a first-time candidate to end up in the job. Writing cover letters, interviewing, and positioning your experience with the needs of an organization take practice. Give yourself grace through this process and be realistic with your expectations.

*Preliminary match*: The search consultant will cross-reference what they learn about you with some of the potential opportunities they are aware of (even ones that you may have not considered yourself). Ask for honest feedback from the search consultant in terms of where your goals, aspirations, and prior work experiences might or might not match.

*Timing is everything*: Despite an uncertain economic outlook, we see major healthcare, academic medical, and research organizations continue to recruit for their most important positions. If search firms know that you are looking and open for a new role, expect that you may still receive recruiting calls.

*Take the calls*: If the opportunity to have a conversation with a recruiter arises, have it—even if the job opportunity does not ignite you. Consider it a learning opportunity as it will no doubt enhance your skills at asking the right questions and building a relationship with a recruiter.

*Invest the time*: It is a learned skill to be interviewed—one that is often underestimated. At the same time, proactively ask for feedback and observations from the consultant. For example, you might say, "*I felt like I did not have a great response on working with trainees. What do you think about how I should think about my answer in the future?"*

*Consultant as a coach*: Remember, in many ways, a consultant is a coach that helps you reflect on your experience and improve in discrete ways.

## Having the "Uncomfortable" Conversations

The unhappy reality is there are some (understandably) jaded LHS+ candidates who have been a part of, or know of, a search process in which they felt tokenized. When we pitch a position to a LHS+ candidate, consultants often encounter skepticism and the question, "Am I only in the search because I am a *[insert racial/ethnic/gender identifier]*"—or—"Is this a real search?" You are well within your rights to probe here, and your questions should be met by thoughtful rationale for why you are competitive in the pool. Despite feelings of discomfort that you may have around this topic, we advise that you have this discussion—it may well show that you are not a good fit or that you are a better fit than you both thought. The point is to engage in these conversations with an open mind and have your antennae up for the best intentions. We urge you to ask the recruiter and search committee about an organization's track record not just of recruiting, but of enabling the success of LHS+ leaders. Request to speak with LHS+ leaders in the organization, which the search consultant can help facilitate. Search committees and their consultants must be forthright enough to have these sophisticated conversations to build trust because without those, institutions may recruit underrepresented candidates into the pool but ultimately fail at *sustaining* diversity.

## Working with a Search Firm as a Committee Member

A fair and inclusive process takes continuous effort. A few words from a chief diversity and inclusion officer at the launch or running an implicit bias module are important, but they are merely steps at the start of a long journey. Search committee chairs and their consultants must ensure the practice of civility and professionalism. This includes being aware of common cognitive errors and calling them in. The best search consultants are aware of certain cognitive errors encountered and practiced by search committee members, e.g., cronyism, cloning, and elitism [1]. The committee chair and consultant then work with search committee members to shape a culture of respect in the committee and create the conditions where all committee members have a voice. Here are some additional tips to consider.

### Speak Up! Your Voice on the Committee Is Key

At the start, deliberate work goes into planning a fair process. This includes ensuring search committee members possess a range of backgrounds, points of view, roles in the organization, and developing a process that allows for sufficient time to recruit and interview candidates. The search can only be as diverse as what you recruit for so search committee members, and their consultants need to ensure that the defined roles are free of any bias in the position profile and, ideally, are scoped as broadly as possible to enable candidates with valid, transferrable skills to compete. If you read biased language in the position profile or have concerns about the process, speak up early and address it with the search committee chair.

**Be a Gate Opener**
Most search consultants understand that search committee members are ideally positioned to identify and recruit diverse candidates they may know in their network. Think of your role on the search committee as a "gate opener" and not "gate keeper." In coordination with the search committee chair and consultants, leverage the relationships and the trust that you have built over time with your own networks of established and rising leaders and faculty. Networks in Historical Black Colleges and Universities, Minority-Serving Institutions, Hispanic-Serving Institutions, and Hispanic Centers of Excellence are often overlooked and not even considered—and sometimes avoided intentionally. If you can open these networks, you will strengthen the search.

**Call in the Insidious, Innocuous Slights**
Every search will have moments that test the committee's ability to put bias aside and act inclusively. As search consultants we have witnessed insensitive, sometimes hurtful comments, as well as illegal comments regarding race, ethnicity, gender, and age. Some examples of actual statements that have been made include:

> That's not where the best people train.
> Well, we're at the short list and we need a diversity candidate.
> She's very talented for a woman candidate.
> They're too old.
> He's very talented for a Latino candidate.
> We do want a diverse candidate, but we also want the best and the brightest.

These comments are far too common. The search committee chair, in partnership with the search consultant and possibly with an equity advocate, have the responsibility to serve as "guardrails" [2]—that is, to keep search committee members "centered on the path of good intentions and steering them back on course if they veer." They should set expectations for committee members to engage in these moments by respectfully "calling in" questionable behavior or word-choice. You should feel empowered to respond to these comments as well.

When it comes to equity and fairness, we all have an obligation to sustain these ongoing conversations, not just rely on transient training at the launch of the search.

# Summary

In this chapter, we hope that you found tangible, relatable insights on the best mechanisms for navigating your way through the search process—both as a candidate and as a committee member. We recognize that candidates who have been historically excluded and underrepresented in their field encounter unique experiences, perspectives, and barriers. As you reflect on future opportunities, we urge you to allow your intuition and instincts to be part of the conversation. With practice, having honest (and sometimes difficult or uncomfortable conversations) will empower you to foster the trust, openness, and inclusion that is crucial to a fair and equitable search process.

## References

1. Moody J. Faculty diversity: removing the barriers. New York: Routledge Publishing; 2012.
2. Cahn PS, Gona CM, Naidoo K, Truong KA. Disrupting bias without trainings: the effect of equity advocates on faculty search committees. Innov High Educ. 2022;47:253–72.

**Open Access** This chapter is licensed under the terms of the Creative Commons Attribution 4.0 International License (http://creativecommons.org/licenses/by/4.0/), which permits use, sharing, adaptation, distribution and reproduction in any medium or format, as long as you give appropriate credit to the original author(s) and the source, provide a link to the Creative Commons license and indicate if changes were made.

The images or other third party material in this chapter are included in the chapter's Creative Commons license, unless indicated otherwise in a credit line to the material. If material is not included in the chapter's Creative Commons license and your intended use is not permitted by statutory regulation or exceeds the permitted use, you will need to obtain permission directly from the copyright holder.

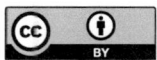

# Chapter 6
# Optimizing CV and Portfolio for Promotion Purposes

Lisa Moreno-Walton, Juliana Jaramillo, and Leon S. Sanders III

> **Learning Objectives**
> - List components of a high-quality CV and academic portfolio.
> - Describe best practices to achieve promotion in a timely fashion.
> - Explain how to highlight LHS+-specific contributions for promotional purposes.

## The High-Quality CV

Less than 5% of full professors in the mainland United States (USA) claim LHS+ identity [1]. Based on this statistic, it would appear that achieving promotion for an LHS+ academic is difficult. The contents of this chapter are your blueprint for efficiently achieving successful promotion in your academic career as an LHS+ faculty member. Fang et al. (2010) observed, while studying full-time US medical school faculty who became assistant professors between 1980 and 1989, that by 1997, 46% of White assistant professors had been promoted, while 30% of underrepresented minorities and 43% of other Hispanic assistant professors had been promoted [2]. Furthermore, by 1997, 50% of White associate professors had been promoted, while 36% of underrepresented minorities and 43% of other Hispanic associate professors had been promoted [2]. Nunez-Smith et al. reported similarly that from 1983

L. Moreno-Walton (✉)
University of South Alabama School of Medicine, Mobile, AL, USA

J. Jaramillo
Brody School of Medicine, Greenville, NC, USA

L. S. Sanders III
Department of Internal Medicine, Tulane University School of Medicine, New Orleans, LA, USA

© The Author(s) 2026
J. P. Sánchez et al. (eds.), *Advancing Latino, Hispanic, or of Spanish Origin+ Leadership in Academic Medicine*,
https://doi.org/10.1007/978-3-032-07570-3_6

through 2000 at US academic medical centers, the median institution-specific rates for White, Hispanic, and Black faculty were respectively 30.2%, 23.5%, and 18.8% from assistant to associate professor and 31.5%, 25.0%, and 16.7% from associate to full professor [3]. These racial/ethnic disparities remained consistent whether the individuals were tenured or nontenured faculty and among those who received or did not receive National Institutes of Health (NIH) research awards [2]. Despite adjusting for cohort, sex, tenure status, degree, department, medical school type, and receipt of NIH awards, underrepresented minority faculty were consistently less likely to be promoted when compared to their White faculty counterparts for associate and full professorship [2].

Consequently, it must be stressed that your CV often creates your first impression for employers/senior academic leaders when applying for initial appointment or subsequent promotion. It is both diagnostic and therapeutic, diagnostic, by helping a reviewer see how your activities fulfill expectations for employment (e.g., experience in teaching certain concepts) or promotion (e.g., number of publications), and therapeutic, by helping you illustrate work that is personally and professionally fulfilling in a standard manner. This document, when maintained in a consistent and scholarly manner, can elevate your career prospects or if neglected can leave you stagnating in the same position for many years. For this reason, your CV must match up with the format that is established by the university or medical school to which you are applying or employed [4]. You can find this resource by asking colleagues who have already been promoted or speaking to your department head. Whether or not you like the format is inconsequential, and even if you must rewrite your entire CV from another university format, you must do so. You want to remove as many roadblocks to the consideration of your CV as possible, and this is an easy hurdle to clear.

Another easy and impactful step is to speak with a faculty affairs representative or colleagues who have been promoted to the rank you aspire to during the most recent promotion cycle. Ask colleagues to share their CV that they submitted when successfully promoted. Ideally, at least one of these colleagues is within your department; however, CVs from other departments are also valuable examples. This allows you to see the most advantageous ways to set up your CV within the given format and how someone who attained the rank you aspire to emphasizes their various accomplishments, accolades, and vocational highlights to acquire the position you desire [5]. Next, schedule a meeting with one of these individuals to get advice about the process and how they succeeded. Preferably, this meeting is in person; however, a virtual meeting is acceptable. This is a critical process and should not be undertaken over texts or phone calls. This process should begin at least 1 year and, if possible, 2 years before you are ready to present your academic promotion portfolio. The person you ask should be someone who holds your desired rank and is prominent in the university. You want them to review your CV WITH YOU! The same stated rules apply; in-person or a virtual meeting is preferred. Both meeting formats allow quick edits to be displayed virtually and more rapid CV preparation. If your department has an editor, another option to consider is to seek assistance with grammar, syntax, and writing style. If not, have someone who is not a physician review your CV and portfolio, not only for grammar, syntax, and style but also for clarity in writing. It is important that you convey the information accurately. This is especially critical if English is not your first language.

To further optimize your CV and portfolio, determine who is currently on the promotion and tenure (P&T) committee. Your advisor, mentor, sponsor, or another ally can speak to a committee member if permitted by your university or medical school system. The phrase, "It is who you know, not necessarily what you know," is one of the unspoken and socially understood truths of academic advancement. If it is permitted, ask someone on the current P&T committee to review your CV and portfolio. Again, it is best if they can do this with you, in person, or virtually. If this is not permitted, try to find someone who has just rotated off the committee to review your CV and portfolio. Before making this ask, it is critical that you review the policies and procedures at your medical school and that you do not violate them. Your reputation is your most valuable asset in academia, and you want to ensure that you are putting your best foot forward, so be fully aware of all policies and procedures and act accordingly.

Keeping your CV updated is critical! Documenting your important work is a practical way to help combat minority taxation and impostor syndrome and build diversity capital [6], from the discussion groups you led in the LHS+ community on health to educational workshops you devised and led for colleagues and medical students, as well as diversity, equity, and inclusion workshops you designed and facilitated. As you document what you have done and compare your contributions to the requirements for promotion, it is a valuable way to diagnose gaps for promotion potential. It is best if you update your CV after each presentation, but barring that, make monthly updates. An alternative approach is maintaining an electronic calendar, which you fill with all of your presentations and CV citable events. Having an electronic calendar will allow you to set a day each month for this task to be completed and look at the variety of events you participated in that month at a glance. Put line items in the categories in which they belong according to your institution's standards. For example, if a particular event you participated in was a volunteer opportunity, it should be listed in that category. Again, use the format of your institution to guide the placement of these items in your electronic calendar and then on your CV.

Most importantly, do not duplicate items in your CV by putting the same item more than once. This creates the appearance of "padding" your CV. As stated previously, your reputation is your greatest asset in academia, and you besmirch it if you inappropriately double post.

Remember to document everything that you have done. If, for example, you participated in a fund-raising opportunity for an event 1 year and then the following year at the same event, you chaired a committee, it would be prudent to list both of these events and distinguish your change in role from year to year. Alternatively, you can list this event twice (with a different date) and in a different category, as your role in the event has changed from year to year. This, in fact, shows the graduation of responsibility and professional growth that a promotion committee wants to see.

## The High-Quality Academic Portfolio

The majority of universities require an academic portfolio for promotion. There are different types including teaching portfolios, research portfolios, and clinical portfolios [7]. It is your responsibility to determine which you are being asked to create and update for promotion [8]. Incidentally, there will often be differences based on the particular track in which you seek promotion, such as the research, clinical, teaching, and tenure tracks [9–11]. However, most of the same rules for creating your CV will apply to your academic portfolio [12]. Remember to conform to the format used by your institution. Ask to peruse the portfolios of recently promoted people to the rank you seek. In this case, it is more advantageous to consider portfolios that resulted in the promotion of individuals within your department or within a similar department. For example, if you are a general surgeon, you may want to look at portfolios that resulted in the promotion of a vascular surgeon or a cardiothoracic surgeon. If you are in a specialty that is equally office-based and operating room-based, such as obstetrics and gynecology, ophthalmology, or urology, seek colleagues with similar practices. The same applies to office- and consultation-based practices, such as infectious disease and palliative care, and specialties without patient contact, such as general radiology and surgical pathology. By choosing portfolios similar to or in your specialty, you will obtain important information about what is highlighted and presented by the highest-performing and selected candidates. Finally, the advice from the CV section applies here: ask someone who holds your desired rank and is prominent in the university to review your portfolio with you; schedule a meeting with someone who was promoted to the rank you seek during the most recent promotion cycle; find out if your department has an "editor"; keep your portfolio up-to-date (which can often be more work than keeping your CV updated); and understand that your portfolio will duplicate some aspects of your CV, which is acceptable [13].

## Pursue and Achieve Promotion

One aspect of academia that is often misunderstood and understated by people of color is attaining the recognition they deserve. This means that you *must* get credit for everything that you do, participate in, and receive rewards for, and for all accolades you attain. You must learn how to maximize every facet of your body of work. This means that you are going to take the audacious approach of being your own cheerleader and salesperson, for the simple reason that you ARE the largest and best marketer of yourself. One means of doing this is convincing your Chair that your promotion benefits him/her. You want to emphasize that a Chair with a large number of upper-level faculty is a successful Chair and will have a reputation for being a great mentor; furthermore, embracing diversity will enhance the Chair's reputation.

Have a plan—break it down by year and check it every 6 months. You must plan ahead for your promotional advancement instead of leaving it to the last minute. Read your institution's promotions and policy guidelines and make certain that you have the latest and most up-to-date version, as, throughout the year, there may be periodic updates. Take note of the time frame as well; do you have enough time to complete your promotion packet, or do you need to wait for the next opportunity? What are things that can "stop your clock" in an "up or out" policy institution, either planned or unplanned? This refers to times when you will need to step away from your institutional responsibilities and/or your work on your promotional packet. For example, childbirth, a sabbatical, the death of a parent/child/partner or other loved one, a serious illness, or needing to take on the role of caregiver to an ill parent or child. Who is in control of this "stopped clock"? It is critical that you communicate with these individuals as promptly as possible if you have or anticipate a life event that will impact your career. This is often difficult if you are in mourning or caring for a dying loved one; however, this *must* be done.

In most cases, you will be expected to have a regional reputation for promotion to assistant professor, have attained national prominence for promotion to associate, and have finally attained international prominence for promotion to professor. For this reason, people must know who you are. Ways to accomplish this include volunteering around the institution, participating in the committees that members of the promotion and tenure committee are on, and getting involved in regional, national, and international organizations. This means not just being a member, but someone who is pushing and facilitating the goals and purpose of the committee or organization. Join committees and task forces—many of these groups will increase your number of publications, and most importantly, many of these groups are led by people in your specialty in the highest upper echelons. Remember that publications are still the currency of academia, regardless of track. The more you have in high-impact journals, the better, and the deeper your relationship with those most reputable members of your specialty and the easier and faster your promotion will occur. Be bold in introducing yourself to people with power. Most professors with national renown enjoy the opportunity to mentor the next rising stars in their specialty. Remember that busy people are happy to have you do the first draft or the outline for them to edit, which can lead to your name being listed as a contributor for a given publication or even in the list of authors.

Furthermore, remember these social rules: it's always "no" until it is "yes," and if you do not ask, you will not receive. Just because one expert in your field denies you an opportunity does not mean that the next one will have the same response. You are your best ally and cheerleader in this regard, and it behooves you to continue to ask for exactly what you want rather than waiting and expecting it to be handed to you. Just being in the room with colleagues of an elevated station can provide untold career opportunities. Finally, before you begin to prepare your promotion packet, you should create a list of your letter writers at least 18 months in advance—the full number and two "alternates." Cultivate a deeper relationship with each of them over the subsequent 6 months. Twelve months ahead of your deadline, announce that you will be asking them for a letter. Give your letter writers at least

2 months' notice that your institution will be asking them to referee your promotion packet. Offer to draft the letter, or at a minimum, bullet points of the highlights of your career that match the promotion criteria. You must make it easy for others to help you instead of miring them in wasted time trying to figure out exactly how they can assist you.

## Maximizing Research Activities

Have you advised or mentored a junior colleague in the course of conducting research? If so, it is important that you highlight this in your CV as your advising or mentoring experience speaks volumes about your dedication to helping others attain their goals. Make sure to submit abstracts to regional, national, and international venues. This allows you to expand the reach of your research and the network of individuals who know about your work. Present your research to a diverse range of audiences in locales all over the nation and the world.

Are you developing scholarly products—poster or oral presentations and publication for each of your research projects? All research projects can and should be turned into abstracts for presentation at conferences. It is most critical that you turn abstracts into manuscripts as often as possible, a common problem for many. Ensure that you are presenting this research either via a poster or an oral presentation. The more of these presentations, the better for your academic prestige, and the more widespread your name will be in academic circles. This can be dubbed "the trifecta publication plan": you complete a study, present the research at a conference, and publish the abstract, and finally, you write and publish a manuscript on this same study. This optimizes and synergizes your research activities in a way that will yield multiple CV entries and expand your network opportunities exponentially.

## Maximizing Day-to-Day Operational Work

Titles matter! Ask the person who assigned you a task if you can have a title to go along with the job you are completing. Make sure to list this title and activity on your CV. Remember that every task mandates a task force! Request that the leader who assigns you a task that requires you to recruit, consult with, or work with others allows you to call the team a task force, and then list this on your CV. Even something as seemingly small as a social event, like residency graduation party planning, can become a committee or task force activity. For example, with our local Latino Medical Students Association (LMSA) chapter, we wanted to focus on fundraising for our group as well as highlight the organization. We developed an annual local gala during Hispanic Heritage Month which required extensive planning, marketing/promotion, and collaboration with local community groups to aid in participation, sponsorship, and donation of goods. We had to operationalize the development and execution of the event. This was a large project, and we did assign roles and titles for each person who worked on part of the event. These various activities require time and energy in bringing them to fruition, and consequently, you deserve recognition, which is reflected in its inclusion on your CV.

## Highlighting LHS+-Related Contributions

Diversity, equity, and inclusion (DEI) has been a mission area for many academic health centers. Historically, before the 2025 White House Administration's Executive Order, many departments wanted to prove they were champions in DEI-related areas. Since the order, some higher education institutions and departments within medical schools may have experienced a chilling effect that could potentially reverse course on this commitment and visibility [14, 15]. Nonetheless, as part of your legacy and advocacy practices as a faculty member, you must do your best to remind and focus your Chair and Dean on the importance of promoting scholarly activities that promote safe and quality educational environments and clinical care for LHS+-identified individuals and providing an equivalent chance for all faculty to be promoted to the rank of full professor. Strive to communicate and illustrate how LHS+-related scholarly activities will attract like-minded individuals to join the department and the institution, which will raise the success and profile of the institution as a whole.

As you consider your day-to-day activities, there are numerous possibilities to engage in LHS+-related, promotion worthy, activities. Advising or mentoring students of LHS+ lived experiences to achieve academic success, such as matriculating to medical school or graduating medical school summa cum laude, qualifies as a significant contribution. Other significant contributions might include providing a grand rounds presentation or returning to your residency program or medical school to provide presentations related to DEI. You might also consider delivering a diabetes workshop in Spanish to a primarily Spanish-speaking audience or organizing a fundraiser for DACA students or organizing a medical Spanish class. Think of the times when you were the only Spanish-speaking member of the medical team, and the entire patient list admitted that day was Spanish-speaking, and your presence contributed to their feeling of well-being, respect, and consideration.

Don't forget social media! If your presentation includes a recorded or live component, share the link with your Chair and Dean so they can hear exactly what you said! You want to highlight the various activities you are involved with and make known if you are receiving an award or recognition. If you have and utilize social media accounts (e.g., YouTube, TikTok, Instagram) and do not mind putting yourself out there for professional purposes, you could consider doing some short videos highlighting disease prevention, proper diet and nutrition, resources for the community on tobacco cessation, etc. Remember that you are a leader and a specialist in your field and that with this highly respected position comes a high level of social responsibility, so give your utmost back to the community when and wherever possible.

Also, include on your CV any LHS+-related professional development activities undertaken to be up-to-date on best or promising practices in caring for LHS+ community members. For example, the LMSA Instruction, Support, Training, and Orientation Session for Advisors (LISTOS), a program for medical school faculty and staff to be better prepared in supporting the success of medical students with LHS+ lived experiences [16]. The NHMA Advancing Physician Leaders Fellowship, formerly the Leadership Fellowship Program, was launched in 1999 to support Hispanic physicians in health policy and academia [17]. It aims to enhance leadership skills and increase representation in governmental, academic, and institutional executive roles. By equipping physicians with essential skills and resources, the fellowship empowers them to become impactful leaders to drive meaningful change in the Hispanic community and promote health equity for all Americans. Remember that not just anybody can do the work that YOU are doing, and you must highlight this fact [18].

Proper formatting matters! On your CV, LHS+-related activities should be incorporated under their respective headings. Have you participated in or led a committee, or been invited to participate as a speaker or panelist related to LHS+ topics? Are you an active member of the Latino Medical Student Association, National Hispanic Medical Association, or another LHS+ focused organization? These all need to be included and demonstrate your own diversity in activities. For example, if you are a member of LMSA, this can be listed where you have all the organizations you are a member of under "Affiliations." If you have participated in national or regional LMSA conferences as a speaker or panelist, be sure to include this under "Invited Presentations." Depending on your particular institution, they will require a certain number of invited presentations that are not at your institution which are required to be either regional or national.

## Example

### Invited Presentations

| October 2019 | LMSA 6th Annual Policy Summit at the AAMC, Washington DC Speaker & Physician Panelist at Health Policy & Community: Current State of Affairs |
|---|---|

A heading on service leadership activities should be included as well, where you can add additional LHS+-related activities. Generally, there is an aspect of service that is required to be included in your portfolio for promotion. If you have any peer-reviewed publications or abstracts related to LHS+, ensure you are placing those under the respective research headings. It can be overwhelming to consider creating a CV. It is not something that can be accomplished overnight. Everyone's CV is going to look a little different and can have variations on certain section headings depending on what you have accomplished so far. This does require some reflection on what activities you have undertaken. While compiling your portfolio, take time to reflect on what drives you and what you wish to highlight about your journey. Do you have a particular niche? What would your professional mission statement be? Taking some time to reflect on these points can help determine the best aspects to highlight. You can try the following exercises to help get you started.

## Skills Exercise: Initial Approach to CV

It is likely from past residency, fellowship, or graduate school applications that you already have a basic CV. You can look at your institution's Office of Faculty Affairs and Career Development website for the required format. Each school has its unique style and requirements. The AAMC also offers a generic template that you can get started with at *Create My CV template webpage*—https://www.aamc.org/professional-development/affinity-groups/gfa/faculty-vitae/preparing-your-curriculum-vitae (Table 6.1).

We hope this helps you to take inventory and visualize what activities you have participated in and organize your timeline for future plans and compare to the institutional criteria for promotion.

## Reflection Exercise: CV Themes

Read through your CV and make a note of themes in another document. Themes that emerge should reflect either your passions, opportunities, or both (Table 6.2).

**Table 6.1** CV template exercise

| CV template headings utilized | Exercise |
|---|---|
| Your institution ___ AAMC ___ | Write a list of the various activities you have participated in according to the multiple headings. Include everything for now, and you can go back to review if it truly fits in that area |

**Table 6.2** Approach to group CV activities into themes

| |
|---|
| *Reflection prompts after noting your themes:* |
| Have most of your presentations and publications dealt with a particular theme or topic (e.g., social determinants of health)? |
| What theme seems to occur almost as often? (i.e., Do you work within a predominantly LHS+ community and often present in Spanish?) |
| *Tips after noting themes:* |
| Highlight these in your cover letters, letters of intent, or promotion candidate statements |
| Highlight them when you market yourself |
| Moving forward, focus on developing the areas that might be lean based on promotion criteria, but where your interest or passion lie, so that you can grow into a content expert in those focused areas |

## Conclusion

Currently LHS+ academic physicians are not well represented in the ranks of associate or full professor in comparison with other major groups. Various factors may have contributed to this, and with less LHS+ individuals within these ranks, it may be harder to seek advice from other LHS+ within the rank you desire. Our hope is to change this moving forward and have provided a framework to provide guidance on how to develop your CV and portfolio for advancement. As in all science, the steps of the appointment and promotion processes must be delineated, precisely planned, meticulously executed, well organized, and concisely presented in the required format. Hard work alone will not ensure success. Appropriate advising and mentorship, early planning, and detail-oriented preparation are essential. We hope you took away three key points from this chapter: (a) preparation is imperative for career planning and progression in academic medicine, (b) make day-to-day activities count for something that you can legitimately add to your CV for promotion, and (c) ensure that leaders at your institution know that the promotion of people of LHS+ lived experiences is in everyone's best interest.

## Personal Narratives

**Lisa Moreno-Walton, MD, MS, MSCR, FAAEM, MAAEM, FACEP, FIFEM**
I was born in New York City. My family was not college-educated, but placed a high priority on education as the way to achieve success, respect, and financial security. During college, I was advised that I would not be able to succeed in medical school because I was a mother. I pursued a Master's Degree in Social Work and became a psychiatric social worker. I attribute the courage to pursue my dream of becoming a physician to the encouragement of my daughter and the mentorship of a psychiatrist in charge of the Inpatient Child Psychiatry Unit where I worked, the first example of the value of good mentorship in my career. I attended the Albert Einstein College of Medicine in my home borough of the Bronx, where I was active in the Boricua Health Organization and the Latino Medical Student Association (LMSA), and I credit my survival through the rigors of medical school and motherhood to the relationships fostered in these organizations. My involvement in LMSA helped me to find support and fellowship that is essential to professional development in what can sometimes be an unwelcoming or even hostile environment. LMSA also provided those lines on my CV that illustrated my professional service. My fluency in LHS+ culture and the Spanish language significantly increased my patient satisfaction and patient compliance outcomes. My supervisors and hospital leaders valued this tremendously. I was attentive to updating my CV once a month to include the training I did for my department, the hospital, and the medical school. I have maintained the habit of updating my CV monthly, ensuring that I do not overlook any activities that should be part of my CV. I also mark every invited lecture or manuscript submission

on my electronic calendar to minimize the chance of forgetting something that should be included. I am sometimes asked why, as a Professor with Tenure, a rank above which there is no promotion, do I continue to update my CV with such rigor. For faculty at the highest academic level, Deans want to see that Professors are mentoring others and enhancing the reputation of the university in the larger academic community. Keeping your CV and your teaching portfolio current make it easy to complete your annual faculty review forms and to document your worth to the university, especially for those faculty not bringing in grant funding. My own research has focused almost entirely on elucidating health disparities and exploring methods of amelioration. In this way, I was able to serve my community, educate my peers, and have a significant number of presentations and publications on my CV. Community engagement and my ability to move comfortably within the patient community and to be embraced by our patient population were the most critical factors in the success of my HIV testing program. This program resulted in significant grant funding, presentations, and publications. Mine was the first ED-based opt-out HIV testing program in the nation and was used as a prototype by the Centers for Disease Control and Prevention [19]. Most importantly, it reduced the incidence of HIV in the community by half [20].

Once in practice, I set a goal of becoming a full professor within 10 years of completing my Emergency Medicine Residency at the Montefiore-Jacobi Emergency Medicine Residency Program in the Bronx. I achieved that goal at the Louisiana State University Health Sciences Center in New Orleans. My career has focused on promoting diversity, equity, and inclusion in medicine; research in infectious diseases; and the development of emergency medicine internationally. A current CV and teaching portfolio have been instrumental in curating focused letters of intent for my roles in national organizations such as the American Academy of Emergency Medicine, where I was elected the first female President, and the National Hispanic Medical Association, on whose Board of Directors I currently serve. I continue to commit my career to the goal of increasing the number of high-quality underrepresented minorities in the physician workforce, both in the USA and internationally, and the elimination of disparate health outcomes globally. I, like many other faculty, have been promoted to full professor in part based on LHS+-related activities that have been personally fulfilling and that have yielded better outcomes for the LHS+ diaspora.

**Juliana Jaramillo, MD**
I was born in Massachusetts and moved often during my childhood, living in Bogota, Colombia, as well as Guayama, Puerto Rico. Eventually we settled back in New York where I spent most of my upbringing. I am of Colombian, Puerto Rican, and Dominican heritage. I had said I would be a doctor since I was 5 years old. This was not an easy journey but I was dedicated. As frequently described by others of similar background, I experienced various microaggressions including being told I should consider something else as I likely would not be a doctor. I did use this as fuel to keep going because I was determined to pursue this as a career. It had always been instilled in me that I needed to work twice as hard and prove my worth and I did. I

went to college with an academic scholarship and ultimately graduated from SUNY Downstate Medical School. I fell in love with Emergency Medicine and truly felt that was my calling. I completed my Emergency Medicine Residency training at SUNY Downstate Kings County where I gained an amazing family and had incredible training. I decided I truly loved Pediatric Emergency Medicine as well and decided to then pursue additional training. I completed a fellowship in Pediatric Emergency Medicine at Atrium Health/Carolinas Medical Center in Charlotte, North Carolina, where I had great exposure and awesome training to learn to deal with sick children with some amazing colleagues. Currently, I am an Assistant Clinical Professor at East Carolina University (ECU) in Emergency Medicine/Pediatric Emergency Medicine, as well as the Director of Off-Service Residents during their emergency medicine rotation. In my role, I participate in educating emergency medicine residents as well as other learners in the space. I serve as the Latino Medical Student Association (LMSA) Faculty Advisor for the Brody School of Medicine as well as for the Southeast region. I am very passionate about Hispanic populations, specifically mentoring and providing support to future physicians. To continue that mission, I have also been very involved with the National Hispanic Medical Association (NHMA), where I previously served as the Chair of Council of Residents and Fellows (COR) followed by the Chair of the Council of Young Physicians (CYP), and presently sit on the board of directors for the organization. I recently completed the American Academy of Pediatrics Women's Wellness through Equity and Leadership program (WEL), where I help support others now by participating as a steering committee member through NHMA. I am very grateful for all the support and mentorship I have had along the way through all these organizations and programs. I became involved with the planning of this chapter at a perfect time as I am also in the midst of organizing a portfolio with the aim to go up for academic promotion in the near future. This chapter has a lot of helpful information that I have counseled by other associate or professor rank colleagues.

**Leon Sanders III, MD, MS, MS**
I had a passion for research and science at a very young age. At the tender age of 6, I set curing AIDS as my life goal. To that end, I pursued a career as a scientist with my very first research presentations beginning in my sophomore year of college at the University of Pittsburgh. While there, due to my love of Japanese culture, I pursued a Bachelor of Arts in Japanese culture and Language and attended the Temple University Tokyo branch in Tokyo, Japan, during my junior year. I continued conducting scientific research throughout my undergraduate tenure, culminating in my first, first author publication with Dr. Yenamula Reddy at Grambling State University. It was there during my summer break that I devised a neural network program capable of diagnosing blood clot disorders with >93% accuracy. I then attended Louisiana Tech University, where I earned a Masters in Biology studying the effects of microtubule poisons on glioblastoma multiforme. To pursue a PhD, I attended the University of Minnesota, where my research focused on the effects of an unknown human factor on HSV-1 replication and protein expression. It was during my second year of doctoral studies that I faced the racism endemic in academic research and

was prevented from earning my PhD. I earned my second Master's at the University of Minnesota in Cancer Biology, Immunology, and Microbiology, and with my dreams of being a scientist unperturbed, I worked in a small biotech company, Vergent Biosciences. There I became the lab manager, lead tester, and manufacturer of all products and learned how to interact with customers. I desired to earn a terminal degree, and with the help and support of my parents, I took the MCAT and was accepted into medical school at Louisiana State University, New Orleans. I earned my medical doctorate in 5 years after both of my parents passed away from cancer during my first years of medical school. My goal is now set on eradicating cancer. I applied and was accepted into the STARR program at Tulane University. This program offers me the unique opportunity to pursue a career as a physician-scientist during 4 years of Internal Medicine residency. On the day of my medical school graduation, I was contacted by the Journal of Virology informing me that my research at the University of Minnesota, which once had been called a "fishing expedition" and a "waste of time," was being published as the premier article in the #1 journal for virologists. I am currently focused on research looking at the connection between COVID-19 and malignancy at Tulane University.

**Acknowledgments** We would like to acknowledge Angela Velez, MD, for her insightful review and critiques of our chapter.

# References

1. American Association for Medical Colleges AAMC Table 15: U.S. medical school faculty by gender, race/ethnicity, rank, and tenure status. 2021. https://www.aamc.org/media/9746/download. Accessed 11 Nov 2024.
2. Fang D, Moy E, Colburn L, Hurley J. Racial and ethnic disparities in faculty promotion in academic medicine. JAMA. 2000;284(9):1085–92. https://doi.org/10.1001/jama.284.9.1085.
3. Nunez-Smith M, Ciarleglio M, Sandoval-Schaefer T, Elumn J, Castillo-Page L, Peduzzi P. Institutional variation in the promotion of racial/ethnic minority faculty at US medical schools. Am J Public Health. 2012;102(5):852–8.
4. Anita N, Erin L, Indra K. Writing an effective curriculum vitae: a module for teaching and grading student CVs. MedEdPORTAL. 2023;6:8101. https://doi.org/10.15766/mep_2374-8265.8101.
5. Gottlieb M, Promes SB, Coates WC. A guide to creating a high-quality curriculum vitae. AEM Educ Train. 2021;5(4):e10717. https://doi.org/10.1002/aet2.10717.
6. Sánchez JP, Ellis D, Plaza V, Velez A, Rodriguez J, Duque Lasio L, Quintero-Rivera F. Addressing the minority tax by building diversity capital: a case based discussion. Accepted to MedEdPORTAL.
7. Callahan EJ, Banks M, Medina J, Disbrow K, Soto-Greene M, Sánchez JP. Providing diverse trainees an early and transparent introduction to academic appointment and promotion processes. MedEdPORTAL. 2017;13:10661. https://doi.org/10.15766/mep_2374-8265.10661.
8. Andre K, Heartfield M, Cusack L. What do I have and what do I need? In: Portfolios for health professionals. 3rd ed. Chatswood: Elsevier Australia; 2017. p. 59.
9. Baldwin C, Chandran L, Gusic M. Guidelines for evaluating the educational performance of medical school faculty: priming a national conversation. Teach Learn Med. 2011;23(3):285–97. https://doi.org/10.1080/10401334.2011.586936.

10. Chandran L, Gusic M, Baldwin C, et al. Evaluating the performance of medical educators: a novel analysis tool to demonstrate the quality and impact of educational activities. Acad Med. 2009;84(1). https://journals.lww.com/academicmedicine/Fulltext/2009/01000/Evaluating_the_Performance_of_Medical_Educators__A.22.aspx
11. Gusic ME, Baldwin CD, Chandran L, et al. Evaluating educators using a novel toolbox: applying rigorous criteria flexibly across institutions. Acad Med. 2014;89(7). https://journals.lww.com/academicmedicine/Fulltext/2014/07000/Evaluating_Educators_Using_a_Novel_Toolbox_.19.aspx
12. Hong DZ, Lim AJS, Tan R, et al. A systematic scoping review on portfolios of medical educators. J Med Educat Curri Develop. 2021;8:23821205211000356. https://doi.org/10.1177/23821205211000356.
13. Kuhn GJ. Faculty development: the educator's portfolio: its preparation, uses, and value in academic medicine. Acad Emerg Med. 2004;11(3):307–11. https://doi.org/10.1111/j.1553-2712.2004.tb02217.x.
14. Blake J. Trump takes aim at DEI in higher ed. inside higher ed. 2025, January 23. https://www.insidehighered.com/news/government/politics-elections/2025/01/23/how-trumps-order-targeting-dei-could-affect-higher-ed. Accessed 20 Mar 2025.
15. Sciacca A. Amid plummeting diversity at medical schools, a warning of DEI crackdown's 'chilling effect'. California Healthline. 2025, March 19. https://californiahealthline.org/news/article/dei-crackdown-trump-diversity-medical-schools-universities-enrollment/. Accessed 20 Mar 2025.
16. LMSA Instruction, Support, Training & Orientation Session for Advisors (LISTOS). https://fpac.lmsa.net/center/listos/. Accessed 5 July 2025.
17. NHMA Advancing Physician Leaders Fellowship. https://www.nhmaphysicianleaders.org. Accessed 5 July 2025.
18. Lin PS, Kennette LN. Creating an inclusive community for BIPOC faculty: women of color in academia. SN Soc Sci. 2022;2(11):246. https://doi.org/10.1007/s43545-022-00555-w.
19. Lin X, Dietz PM, Rodriguez V, Lester D, Hernandez P, Moreno-Walton L, Johnson G, et al. Routine HIV screening in two health care settings—New York City and New Orleans, 2011–2013. Morb Mortal Wkly Rep. 2014;63(25):537–41.
20. Moreno-Walton L, Simmers EM, Rhodes S, DeBlieux PMC. Assessing the need for acute HIV testing in the emergency department. EC Emerg Med Crit Care. 2021;5(4):S63.

**Open Access** This chapter is licensed under the terms of the Creative Commons Attribution 4.0 International License (http://creativecommons.org/licenses/by/4.0/), which permits use, sharing, adaptation, distribution and reproduction in any medium or format, as long as you give appropriate credit to the original author(s) and the source, provide a link to the Creative Commons license and indicate if changes were made.

The images or other third party material in this chapter are included in the chapter's Creative Commons license, unless indicated otherwise in a credit line to the material. If material is not included in the chapter's Creative Commons license and your intended use is not permitted by statutory regulation or exceeds the permitted use, you will need to obtain permission directly from the copyright holder.

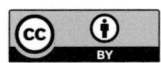

# Chapter 7
# A National Perspective on LHS+ Leadership in US Medical Schools

David Acosta, Joel Dickerman, and David J. Skorton

> **Learning Objectives**
> - Describe the rationale for enhancing LHS+ leadership in academic medicine.
> - Analyze the present landscape of LHS+ representation in leadership positions in the academy.
> - Explore the importance of LHS+ identity and the power of LHS+ leadership.
> - Identify executive leadership and system-based inhibitors and effective practices for executive leadership.
> - Explore where academic medicine needs to go.

## Introduction

This chapter will explore national perspectives on Latina/o/x/e, Hispanic, or of Spanish+ (LHS+) leadership in US medical education, focusing on medical schools, colleges of osteopathic medicine, and graduate medical education programs. Leadership from these organizations will provide updates on the current landscape and highlight opportunities for advancing LHS+ faculty in leadership roles. We will first examine the rationale for enhancing LHS+ representation in leadership, the barriers hindering their progress, and the existing disparities in academic medicine.

---

D. Acosta (✉) · D. J. Skorton
Association of American Medical Colleges, Washington, DC, USA

J. Dickerman
Rocky Vista University, Englewood, CO, USA

Although LHS+ individuals make up nearly 18% of the US population, they face significant health disparities, including higher rates of obesity and mortality from chronic diseases compared to non-Hispanic whites. Cultural and language barriers, limited access to care, and a lack of health insurance contribute to these disparities, compounded by the underrepresentation of LHS+ physicians in the workforce. For example, LHS+ students comprised only 7.9% of first-year osteopathic medical students (in comparison with 12.7% of first-year allopathic medical students) in 2021, a figure that remains well below their national demographic representation.

This chapter will also examine efforts to address these issues, such as initiatives led by the American Osteopathic Association and the American Association of Colleges of Osteopathic Medicine to increase LHS+ representation among students and faculty. Programs like the COMPASS mentorship initiative and the pipeline programs at various osteopathic schools have made strides in promoting diversity and cultural competence. Additionally, the National Board of Osteopathic Medical Examiners has adopted principles to enhance diversity, equity, and inclusion in examinations.

By identifying challenges and highlighting ongoing initiatives, this chapter aims to present strategies for fostering LHS+ leadership at individual, institutional, and national levels, ultimately promoting greater diversity and equity in academic medicine.

## Rationale for Enhancing the LHS+ Representation in Leadership Positions in Academic Medicine

There are many justifications for enhancing the LHS+ representation in leadership positions in academic medicine. This section will highlight a few of the rationales that are creating the sense of urgency: (1) the changing demographics of the US population; (2) the health injustices unveiled by the COVID-19 pandemic that devastated the LHS+ communities; and (3) the invisibility of LHS+ leaders in the academy and for the future. Each will be discussed in some detail.

### *Changing Demographics of the US LHS+ Population in the Immediate Future*

Data from 2019 cite that the LHS+ population represented 18% of the US population estimated at 60.6 million [1]. Translated this means that one in six people in the USA today are Latino and four in five Latinos living in the USA (80%) are US citizens [2]. Figure 7.1 depicts the projections of the LHS+ population growth, e.g., 81.2 million by 2035 (or 1 in 4), 99.8 million by 2050. However, we are reminded that in the pediatric population, LHS+ are already the majority. For example, in

# 7 A National Perspective on LHS+ Leadership in US Medical Schools

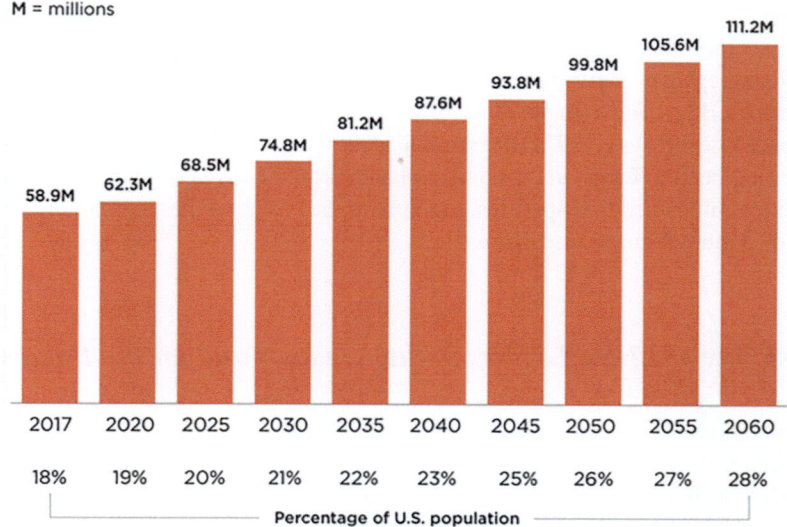

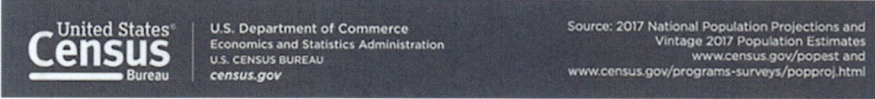

**Fig. 7.1** Hispanic population to reach 111 million by 2060. Projected Hispanic population 2020 to 2060, United State Census Bureau [1]

2020, one in four children enrolled in US K-12 public schools are LHS+ in comparison with one in six students enrolled in US colleges and universities [3].

Figure 7.1 also reminds us that the LHS+ population is clearly a heterogenous group and not a homogenous group [4]. Each LHS+ group has their own unique set of traditions, cultural norms, and beliefs as well as their own unique set of issues and challenges they face—a gentle reminder that not all Hispanics/Latinx people should be categorized into one box, and each should be respected for their own identities.

Despite these population numbers, LHS+ faculty only account for 5.5% of all full-time (FT) allopathic medical school faculty [5]. Given what the immediate future holds for the demographic changes in the USA that are coming at a rapid pace, it would behoove all leadership in the academy to have LHS+ leaders and faculty at the table to better prepare our institutions for the immediate future.

## Health Injustices Unveiled by the COVID-19 Pandemic That Devastated the LHS+ Communities

LHS+ faculty bring a different perspective to the table than our non-LHS+ colleagues cannot and will not bring. The health injustices inflicted upon the LHS+ communities by the pandemic were made visible (Fig. 7.2). Data revealed in comparison with non-Hispanic Whites, LHS+ suffered 1.9 times the number of cases, 2.8 times the number of hospitalizations, and 2.3 times the number of deaths [6]. This data begs the question, "Would these injustices have been as prevalent if we had more LHS+ leaders in positions of power and decision-making that could have influenced health systems?" From the impact of the pandemic, we learned that there is a strong need to focus, understand, and address the LHS+ community issues and health inequities/health disparities, to improve the health of these communities and provide a more focused research agenda.

## Invisibility of LHS+ Leaders in the Academy and for the Future

If you randomly chose several academic medical institutions in the USA and reviewed their websites (specifically looked at the faces in the photos provided), one would immediately note the lack of LHS+ student, resident, and faculty faces. This is exactly what aspiring LHS+ students, residents, and early career and mid-career faculty see when they visit the websites of our US medical schools, teaching hospitals, and research centers. You will also see stark absence and lack of LHS+ representation in all leadership positions in the academy. And despite the number of us that are LHS+ and in leadership positions, we are invisible to society and to other leaders in power and decision-making positions at all levels in our academic medical institutions. One is compelled to ask, "Is this invisibility intentional?" To answer that question, let's turn to the data regarding the race, ethnicity, and gender of faculty and leaders in the academy. And here lies one of the many problems. That is, we do not have sufficient data in our academy that is needed to accurately identify how many LHS+ faculty are in leadership positions. When examining the present status of US allopathic medical schools and teaching hospitals:

- Good data exists for medical students.
- Some data exists for residents, faculty, faculty ranking, department chairs, and deans.

**Fig. 7.2** COVID-19 cases, hospitalizations, and deaths by race/ethnicity—July 21, 2016 [6]

| Rate ratios compared to White, Non-Hispanic persons | American Indian or Alaska Native, Non-Hispanic persons | Asian, Non-Hispanic persons | Black or African American, Non-Hispanic persons | Hispanic or Latino persons |
|---|---|---|---|---|
| Cases[1] | 1.7x | 0.7x | 1.1x | 1.9x |
| Hospitalization[2] | 3.4x | 1.0x | 2.8x | 2.8x |
| Death[3] | 2.4x | 1.0x | 2.0x | 2.3x |

- Little to no data exists for fellows, part-time faculty, non-ladder faculty, volunteer faculty, center directors, residency program directors, DIOs, department vice chairs, departmental division chiefs, vice deans, senior associate deans, and associate/assistant deans:
  - Many of our community volunteer faculty are people of color and are the predominant source of mentors, role models, and teachers for our learners (medical students, residents), yet they are not included in the data collection. Therefore, we do not have an accurate picture of the true diversity of all faculty that our learners are exposed to and have experiences with.

In addition, the data for race/ethnicity is not disaggregated for specific population groups, e.g., the AAMC data category for African American/Black was subcategorized for the first time in 2016: US-born African Americans, Caribbean African American, Africans, and Other. Before 2016, the AAMC only had aggregate data for all URM and non-URM population groups.

## Data for LHS+ Faculty and Leaders in US Medical Schools

### Faculty in US Medical Schools

A recent review by Xierali and colleagues looked at the trend of full-time (FT) faculty (both clinical and basic sciences) by race, ethnicity, and gender over the last 40 years in US medical schools [7]. Overall, we see a familiar trend that mirrors what we see in the applicant/matriculant data for medical school—namely, a flat slope of the curve for all URMs in comparison with non-URM men and non-URM women faculty. Overall, the total FT faculty in US medical schools increased by over 3.5-fold from 49,909 in 1979 to 175,326 in 2018. Clinical sciences FT faculty increased 4-fold and basic sciences FT faculty increased 1.8-fold. The proportion of representation grew more among non-URM FT faculty, especially for non-URM women FT faculty, compared with FT URM faculty. The greatest rise for FT URM faculty occurred among LHS+ faculty, e.g., from a total of 1243 (2.9%) in 1979 to 9720 (5.5%) in 2018. In 2018, LHS+ FT faculty made up 5.6% of total FT faculty in clinical sciences, and 4.4% of the FT faculty in basic sciences.

The most recent data for FT faculty in US medical schools is depicted in Fig. 7.3. In 2020 the total number of FT faculty was 184,682—21.1% were FT professors (39,001), 20.4% were FT associate professors (37,781), 47.0% were FT assistant professors (86,458), and 11.6% were at other ranks (21,442) [8]. In 2020, the total number of LHS+ FT faculty at all ranks was 5391—2.5% were FT professors (vs. 75.6% non-Hispanic (NH) Whites), 3.1% were FT associate professors (vs. 65.6 NH Whites), and 3.6% were FT assistant professors (vs. 58.2% NH Whites).

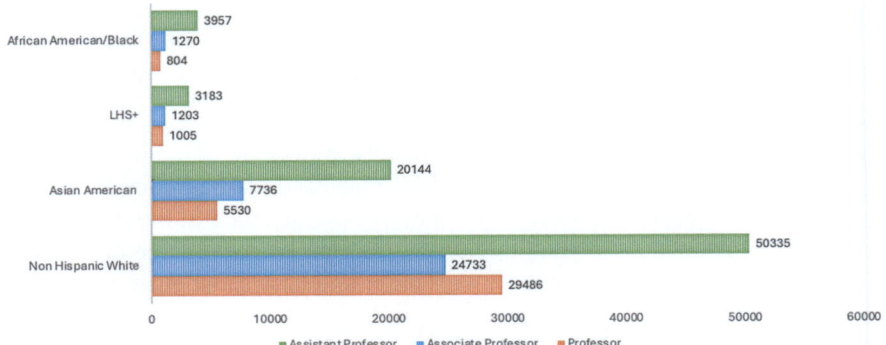

**Fig. 7.3** US medical school faculty by rank (full-time) and race/ethnicity, 2020 [8]

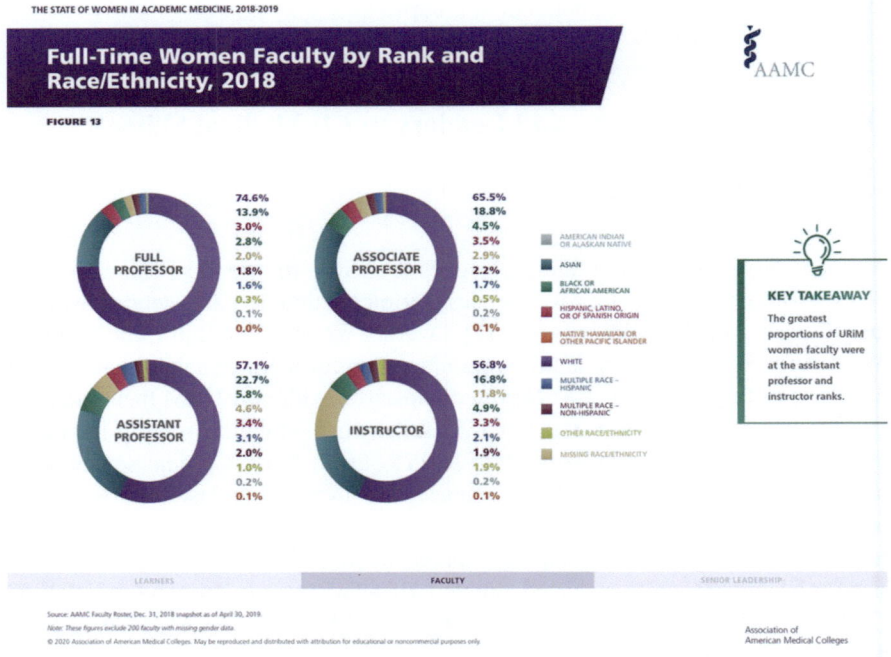

**Fig. 7.4** FT women faculty in US medical schools by rank, race, and ethnicity, 2018 [9]

Figure 7.4 illustrates the trend for FT women faculty by rank, race, and ethnicity in 2018 [9]. Women represented 41% of all FT faculty in US medical schools and a higher percentage of NH White women were at the full professor rank (75%), associate professor rank (65.5%), and assistant professor rank (57.1%) by significant margins in comparison with LHS+ FT women faculty, e.g., 3.0% FT professors, 3.5% FT associate professors, and 3.4% FT assistant professors. Also of note is that the majority of all URM FT women faculty were at the assistant professor and instructor rank in comparison with NH White and Asian American FT women faculty.

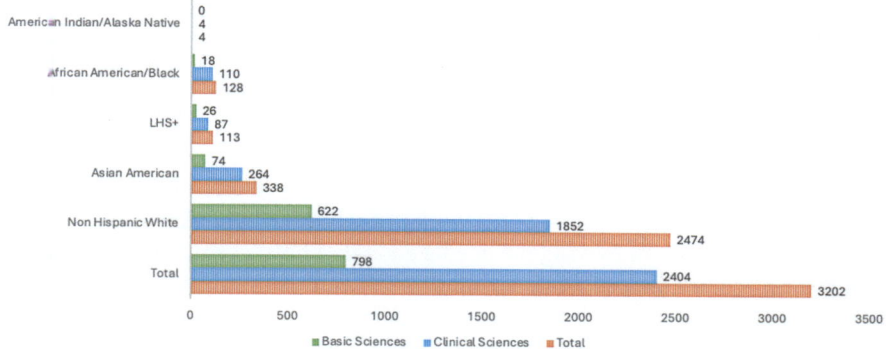

**Fig. 7.5** Department chairs in US medical schools by race/ethnicity, 2020 [10]

## Department Chairs in US Medical Schools

In 2020 there were a total of 3202 department chairs (both basic science and clinical sciences). The large majority were in the clinical sciences (2404, or 75% of total department chairs vs. 798 basic science department chairs, or 24.9% of the total). Figure 7.5 shows that the largest number of department chairs were NH White (77.2%), e.g., the majority were men in both the basic sciences and clinical sciences. LHS+ department chairs made up 3.5% of all chairs—3.2% basic science chairs (highest in biochemistry, microbiology, physiology) and 3.6% clinical science chairs (highest in surgery, pediatrics, OB/Gyn, psychiatry, family medicine, and internal medicine) [10].

## Medical School Deans in US Medical Schools

In 2018 there were a total of 151 deans (both full-time and interim) in US medical schools. URM Deans made up 11.2% and LHS+ Deans made up 3.3% (almost all were from Puerto Rico medical schools). In comparison 82.8% were NH White, 7.9% were African American/Black, and 2.6% were Asian American. There were no Deans that were American Indian/Alaskan Native, Native Hawaiian, or Pacific Islander [11].

## Challenges Facing LHS+ Faculty

> We know Latinos are racialized in this country when the most successful members of the Latino community, those who have 'done everything right,' regularly experience discrimination…this paradoxically demonstrates how deep racism and discrimination run in America. [12] Maria Chavez, PhD, Associate Professor, Political Science, Pacific Lutheran University and author of Everyday Injustice: Latino Professionals and Racism

> No Latino in America, whether a citizen or a professional, can truly escape the consequences of racialization that brand him or her as foreign, unwelcomed, and unwanted. Latinos are not allowed to assimilate…No amount of assimilation efforts on the part of Latinos can compete with the structural barriers and cultural constructions of what it means to be an American…. [12] Dean Kevin Johnson, Dean, School of Law, University of California Davis School of Law and author

This paradoxically demonstrates how deep racism and discrimination run in the academy. After 20 years of doing DEI work to enhance the diversity of the healthcare workforce, and not moving the needle enough, I have come to the conclusion that our next generation of work for moving forward is to dismantle the system-based problems (the inhibitors), and dismantle the white social frame that is embedded within academic medicine as these continue to challenge our well-intentioned efforts in diversifying the workforce and excludes more and more LHS+ faculty from entering leadership positions within the academy. As this quote so aptly states,

> The system isn't broken. It's working exactly as designed. Michael Arceneaux

We can no longer afford not to address this system problem and the consequences of LHS+ being racialized. It's time to disrupt it! This concept of racialization challenges our LHS+ identities. It's time we stand together to realize and understand the power of and the role of our LHS+ identity. This is in alignment with the following quote:

> I treasure who I am, I treasure who my parents were, my culture, my language, and I don't have to give any of that up in order to succeed. Indeed, if I keep all those things, it will make me more successful in practical terms as well as in self-fulfilling terms. Latinos have a unique contribution to make to America. We can't do that if we give up our cultural core – that which makes us who we are. Raul Yzaguirre, Past president and CEO of the National Council of La Raza and past U.S. ambassador of the Dominican Republic

## What Does the Key and Executive Leadership Need to Know?

It can start with helping our leaders within the academy understand the unique and different challenges that LHS+ faculty face that other non-URMs do not (Fig. 7.6). There is now ample evidence that these challenges exist in our academy and in our workplace environments that have been deemed invisible by many. We are at a critical point where our leadership needs to be consciously aware, recognize, and understand the manifestations of what a toxic learning and workplace environments are for LHS+ faculty (as depicted on the right-hand side of Fig. 7.6). Leaders that belong to the major dominant group in the academy have asked for the data and the evidence for the challenges and barriers that inhibit LHS+ faculty from advancement and it has been delivered. But this evidence is still invisible to our executive and key leadership. This invisibility is a manifestation of privilege that brings forward two defense mechanisms commonly used by the major dominant group—the luxury of ignorance, e.g., "I didn't know about these challenges," and the luxury of

**Challenges Faced by Graduate & Medical Students, Residents and Faculty from HEUGS***

Odom KL et al, Acad Med 2007; Dyrbye LN et al, Mayo Clin Proceedings, 2006; COGME, 2006; Osseo-Asare A et al, JAMA Network Open, 2018; Smith WA et al, J Negro Ed, 2011; Smith WA et al, Int J Qual Studies in Ed, 2016; Misra J et al, Sociological Forum, 2012; Pololi L et al, J Gen Intern Med, 2010; Rodriguez JE, Campbell KM, Fam Med, 2014; Boulton C, Howard J Communications, 2016; Cyrus KD, JAMA 2017; Shayne J, Inside Higher Ed, 2017; NASEM, 2019

| | |
|---|---|
| • Lack of exposure to BIPOC faculty, scientists, health care providers<br>• Lack of BIPOC faculty, scientists, health care provider role models & mentors<br>• Difficulties in acculturation to culture of medicine & science<br>• Expectation to assimilate<br>• Undesirable geographic distance of school from student's home and community | • Daily microaggressions<br>• Stereotype threat<br>• Imposter syndrome<br>• Racial biases, prejudice, discrimination<br>• Racial battle fatigue<br>• Identity interference<br>• Code switching<br>• Minority tax<br>• Mistreatment<br>• Sexual/gender harassment<br>• Isolation/marginalization |

**Fig. 7.6** Challenges faced by graduate and medical students, residents, and faculty from historically excluded and underrepresented groups in STEMM (HEUGS)

denial, e.g., "Do these challenges really happen? It's hard to believe that they exist in our institution?" [13].

Cultural/climate assessments can help to inform the leadership what the lived experiences are for our LHS+ faculty and should be regularly performed to inform them. There is a need for a call to action for the tenured LHS+ faculty (who are protected) and LHS+ faculty in key leadership positions to assist in teaching the top leadership what they need to know, e.g., identifying the systems-based inhibitors to success that are unique to LHS+ faculty.

## *Exercise: Questions for Self-Reflection*

So, what are the most effective practices to address and mitigate these challenges?

It must start with self-reflection. The following set of questions are for our LHS+ readers to contemplate and reflect on, and perhaps, are questions that you should discuss with your LHS+ faculty mentors as well. The questions will require a lot of self-reflection and truth-telling so be sure to allot the time necessary to pause and do some mindfulness thinking. As you answer these questions for yourself, consider documenting your thoughts so you can refer back to them in the future:

Question 1: What holds LHS+ faculty back?
Question 2: What holds you back?

Question 3: What holds key and executive leaders at your institution back?
Question 4: Do you see yourself in a leadership position?
Question 5: Do you possess a "leadership identity"?
Question 6: Do the key and executive leaders at your institution see you in a leadership role?
Question 7: Does your cultural identity contribute to the leadership attributes needed?
Question 8: Do you see your cultural identity as an asset? Or as a detriment?
Question 9: Is the key and executive leadership at your institution aware of your cultural identity? If so, what do they understand about it? Do they respect it? If not, why not?
Question 10: If the key and executive leadership were sensitized to how you felt about how important your cultural identity was to you, would things change?

After you have completed answering these questions for yourself, it might be helpful to reflect on the same questions with a group of LHS+ faculty at your institution. Sharing insights and perspectives through guided, facilitated, interactive dialogue might be beneficial. The outcome might lead to collective action strategies that your key and executive leadership might be willing to discuss.

## The Power and the Role of Cultural Identity

We contend that we have a systems problem in academic medicine. We exist in an educational system, an academy, which has a social frame embedded throughout that does not recognize or value other cultural identities outside of whiteness. As Joseph Feagin has demonstrated in his research, "Latinos have been racialized as non-white and thus experience discrimination in countless ways" [14, 15]. To dismantle this social frame and disrupt the system, Feagin suggests we consider offering a counter-frame to deconstruct the racialization of LHS+ people. We exist in a system with a hierarchy that expects LHS+ faculty (and other URM faculty) to assimilate to this social frame. As long as you do, you will be promoted, and you will thrive. If you don't, you will be marked (and sometimes targeted) as a "difficult faculty member." But as demonstrated in the quote by Raul Yzaguirre, most Latinos have preserved their cultural identity by being "culturally adaptive." The question is, "Is the key and executive leadership aware of cultural identity? Do they understand and respect cultural identity? If they don't, what holds them back? But there's a belief that one should not challenge the status quo because it's too risky for one's career in the academy. Does this belief hold you back? Does this hold any LHS+ faculty back at your institution? Are you allowed to see yourself in a leadership position? Are you allowed to have a leadership identity? If so, how does that connect with your LHS+ identity? How does a leadership identity connect with the other multiple identities that make up who you truly are? Have you been taught or ever told that your LHS+ identity is an asset? How many times have you heard that focusing on your cultural identity interferes with the science identity [16], and therefore you should only focus on your science identity and assimilate to the culture of science and medicine and minimize your cultural identity if you want to succeed? Do you buy-in to that opinion?" The real question is: "What system-based issues need to be addressed and changed in academic medicine and how can Latinos collectively contribute to changing the dysfunctional system?" Perhaps it can start with helping our leaders understand the unique value and assets that LHS+ faculty bring to the table and that LHS+ leadership styles are influenced by that cultural identity [17–19].

## The Power of LHS+ Leadership

Research by Juana Bordas [17] contends that Latinos are programmed differently when it comes to leadership styles. Her research has discovered that Latinos lead in different ways than the major dominant group leads who are more hierarchical, e.g., more self-centric, self-serving, more power oriented. This is opposite of Latino leadership style that is more egalitarian, e.g., more community-centric, culturally based, focused on collective stewardship, and more "we"-oriented than "I"-oriented. This is illustrated by the ten principles of Latino leadership in Fig. 7.7 [18]. For example, *personalismo* means valuing that everyone has inherent worth, is interconnected, and is faithful to the communities they came from. *La cultura* refers to keeping a "cultural balance" in strategic thinking and problem solving. LHS+ leaders are "culturally based" and maintain a "we" orientation. *De colores* refers to the importance of inclusiveness which is recognized as a critical component for leadership given the heterogeneity of the LHS+ population. *Juntos* refers to collective stewardship where a community of leaders sharing responsibility and capacity is the norm. *Si se puede* emphasizes the role of social activism and coalition building which are

| | | | |
|---|---|---|---|
| Personalismo | -Everyone has inherent worth, value<br>-Never forget where you came from<br>-Interconnectedness | Juntos | -Collective stewardship<br>-Community of leaders sharing responsibility & capacity<br>-Working *paso a paso* |
| Consciencia | -In-depth reflection, self-exam<br>-Know your cultural assets<br>-Personal intention<br>-Listen to inner voice | Adelante | -Global vision & immigrant spirit (bring initiative, hard work, optimism, faith)<br>-Be cultural adaptive |
| Destino | -Life path, purpose, heart's desire<br>-Alignment, sense of direction<br>-Vision<br>-Open the door when ops knock | Si Se Puede | -Social activism; coalition bldg.<br>-Perseverance, commitment<br>-Be cultural broker, build partnerships |
| La Cultura | -Culturally based leadership → keep 'cultural balance' in strategic thinking & problem solving<br>-"We" orientation<br>-*Simpatico, respeto* | Gozar la Vida | -Communicate with *carisma, cariño, corazón*<br>-Speak the "people's language"<br>-"Stir the *salsa* & *gusto*" into leadership |
| De Colores | -Heterogeneity, inclusiveness<br>-Practice "*bienvenido*"<br>-Create allies | Fe y Esperanza | -Have faith & courage to be bold, to inspire & motivate<br>-Show gratitude, humility |

**Fig. 7.7** Ten Latino leadership principles [18]

| Four Dimensions of Transformational Leadership | Latino Leadership Principles |
| --- | --- |
| 1. Individual considerationa | Personalismo and destino |
| 2. Inspirational motivation | Fe y Esperanza and goza de vida |
| 3. Idealized influence | La cultura and juntos |
| 4. Intellectual stimulation | Si se puede and la cultura |

**Fig. 7.8** The Alignment of the Four Dimensions of Transformational Leadership with the Latino Leadership Principles [19]

believed to be keys to success. LHS+ leaders are cultural brokers, are relationship-centered, and recognize the benefits of building partnerships through trust. As LHS+ leaders I contend that we need to return to these Latino roots and draw from these leadership principles. Why? Because many of these principles are connected to the four dimensions of transformative leadership (Fig. 7.8) that is needed today to solve systems-based problems and find systems-based solutions.

Transformational leaders work with their people to implement change. They guide the change through inspiration and motivation. They are role models, and their followers emulate their action. They inspire by motivating others to perform beyond expectations [20]. This is what Latinos bring to the leadership table, and that's exactly what our key and executive leadership in our institutions need to know. Many of the principles of Latino leadership cited in Fig. 7.7 are in alignment with the four dimensions of transformational leadership in Fig. 7.8. For example:

*Individual consideration* is the extent to which a leader attends to each follower's needs. This aligns with features of *personalismo* and *destino* (alignment with heart's desire and sense of direction).
*Inspirational motivation* is the degree to which a leader articulates an appealing vision that inspires and motivates. This aligns with *fe y esperanza* (having the faith and courage to be bold, take risks, and driven by hope) and *gozar la vida* (knowing when to "stir the salsa").
*Idealized influence* describes leaders that are role models who engage in high standards of ethical behavior. This aligns with *la cultura* and *juntos*.
*Intellectual stimulation* is the extent to which leaders challenge assumptions, take risks, and solicit ideas from followers. This aligns with *si se puede* and *la cultura*.

# Leadership and Advancement Opportunities for Advancement for LHS+ Faculty

## What Are Some Things That Can Be Addressed Now?

1. Increase the visibility of LHS+ leaders by identifying them and describing the impact they have made in academic medicine and society.

2. Create and disseminate a new adage for our leadership, e.g., "If they (the key and executive leadership) see it, they will believe it" that translates to "Latinos can be leaders"!
3. Change the narrative. There is a sense of urgency to address another crisis—the shortage of LHS+ leadership. Given what the future will bring, academic medicine must be prepared to deal with the societal changes that will impact healthcare.
4. Disseminate information to all of the LHS+ faculty about the many leadership development opportunities that exist. At a recent LIDEReS conference, less than one-quarter of the faculty attending were aware of the programs listed in Fig. 7.9 [21].

## *What Are Some Things That Can Be Addressed in the Near Future?*

AAMC should take another look at each of their leadership programs and consider adding pathways or tracks that specifically target the unique challenges that face LHS+ faculty. It is true that these types of leadership development programs exist elsewhere, e.g., NHMA and others, but the numbers enrolled in those programs are small, and they need to expand their capacity to enhance their impact.

Secondly, this work cannot be the responsibility of one association alone. There needs to be an effort to stop working in siloes and think of more creative ways to bring associations and other industries to the table (key stakeholders like hospital associations, health insurance companies) to invest and contribute to these efforts with the hopes of creating a substantial pool of LHS+ healthcare executives.

Organized medicine needs to engage in this effort and should be encouraged to collectively and collaboratively accelerate the creation of new leadership academies that specifically target LHS+ faculty within their specialties and subspecialties, e.g., LHS+ members who are aspiring to become our next generation of leaders in academic medicine. Every organization and academic society needs their fair share of LHS+ leadership they can leverage to position themselves better for the future.

Perhaps developing an agreed-upon faculty development framework based on best practices from lessons learned from AAMC, LMSA LISTOS and LIDEReS, NHMA programs, and others will provide the nidus specialty/subspecialty societies need to start up their own programs.

Partnering with other organizations/associations that are already focusing on LHS+ faculty. For example, the National Association of Latino Healthcare Executives (NALHE)—a national organization led by LHS+ executive leaders of US hospitals and healthcare organizations with expertise in healthcare policy and practice. Their goal is to create a future workforce of highly talented LHS+ healthcare executives who can meet the challenge of delivering and

| | |
|---|---|
| **AAMC Minority Faculty Leadership Development Seminars for Early-Career Faculty**<br>For URM faculty at the assistant professor level, build foundational leadership skills and explore paths to leadership in academic medicine and science. | **AAMC Grant Writer's Coaching Group for NIH Awards**<br>For faculty who are actively working on a NIH Career Development (K or R) proposal, writing successful grants. |
| **AAMC Minority Faculty Leadership Development Seminars for Mid-Career Faculty**<br>For URM faculty at the associate professor level, build foundational leadership skills and explore paths to leadership in academic medicine and science. | **AAMC Career Development Program for MOSAIC Scholars**<br>For cohorts of NIH-awarded K99/R00 scholars, facilitating the transition of promising postdoctoral researchers from diverse backgrounds into independent faculty careers. |
| **University of Pittsburgh TRANSFORM Faculty Development Initiative for Mid-Career Faculty**<br>For all faculty at the associate professor level, a one-year longitudinal faculty development experience following participation in the AAMC mid-career faculty development seminar that will build upon the foundational leadership skills learned and further explore paths to leadership in academic medicine and science. | **AAMC Healthcare Executive Diversity and Inclusion Certificate Program**<br>For new and aspiring CDOs and assistant/associate deans of DEI, develop and enhance the competencies needed to meet the administrative demands associated with this role. |
| **AAMC Early-Career Women Faculty Leadership Development Seminar**<br>For women faculty at the assistant professor level, build foundational leadership skills and explore paths to leadership in academic medicine and science. | **AAMC Chief Medical Officers Leadership Academy**<br>For new and aspiring CMOs, develop and enhance the competencies needed to meet both the clinical and business demands associated with the role. |
| **AAMC Mid-Career Women Faculty Leadership Development Seminar**<br>For women faculty at the associate professor level, build foundational leadership skills and explore paths to leadership in academic medicine and science. | **AAMC Organizational Leadership in Academic Medicine for new Associate Deans and Department Chairs**<br>For new associate deans and department chairs, develop and enhance the essential leadership and management skills needed to support your institutions' mission and goals. |
| | **AAMC Leadership Education and Development Certificate Program**<br>For emerging leaders in medical education, gain a foundation in leadership theory and applied practice to advance your career. |

**Fig. 7.9** AAMC leadership development programs [20]

improving healthcare in diverse communities and promote health equity. It may be a prime time to convene a summit that brings all partners together, including organizations like the National Association of Diversity Officers in Higher Education and other associations of higher education, to formulate best approaches moving forward.

## Summary

This chapter focuses on the urgency we are facing with the lack of LHS+ leadership in academic medicine, and how the academy can best create and promote the development and advancement of LHS+ leaders at the individual, group, institutional, and organized medicine levels. Let's review.

### *Individual Level*

The work starts with our own self-reflection efforts…not only contemplating the answers to the questions presented above but also transforming those responses into action. LHS+ faculty should review the *10 Latino Leadership Principles* presented and ask themselves, "Which ones resonate with my leadership identity? Which principles are assets that I as an LHS+ faculty bring to the table? How can I move from a habit of assimilation (the path of least resistance) to acculturation and maintain my cultural identity? What needs to be in place for me to do that?"

### *Group Level*

LHS+ faculty collectively need to learn how to practice *juntos* and move beyond working independently of one another in siloes. The same questions answered at the individual level should be addressed as a group transforming reactions and responses to action. The power of many will make a better impact as opposed to attempting to do this alone. The group should address how best to reach out to LHS+ members in specialty/subspecialty societies and recruit them to participate in these efforts. At the same time, the group should create a mechanism that enhances the engagement with LHS+ community-based physicians who are in leadership positions in medicine and healthcare, e.g., those that are chief medical officers, medical society leaders, and state medical association leaders.

LHS+ faculty need to realize the collective power of their LHS+ identity and of their own LHS+ leadership style. The group should ask, "How can LHS+ faculty collectively create a mechanism that enhances the engagement of successful mid-career and senior LHS+ faculty that don't attend the types of meetings like

LIDEReS?" "How can they be leveraged in this quest to move the needle forward?" As a reminder the data reveals that there are over 5300 LHS+ FT faculty across all US medical schools and teaching hospitals—are they all involved in this quest? If not, is there a reason they are not engaged? LHS+ faculty need to consider these questions as these seasoned LHS+ faculty could serve as significant assets to the group by providing career and leadership consultations, mentorship, and sponsorship.

## *Institutional Level*

Where can organizations like the AAMC help? AAMC could help with changing the narrative and leverage the influence of the AAMC Board, the Council of Deans, the Council of Teaching Hospitals, and the Council of Faculty and Academic Societies, to help educate and influence academic medicine and its key and executive leadership that make the decisions at our academic medical institutions. AAMC could assist in reaching out to other boards of nationally recognized associations they have relationships with, e.g., NHMA, AMA, AHA, NBME, ABMS, CMSS, ACGME, AACOM, and other specialty societies. AAMC affinity groups could assist in these efforts as well, e.g., GDI, GFA, CFAS, GREAT, and GRAND—all could have a role in crafting a new narrative and disseminating the message of the need to focus on the development of more LHS+ leadership. AAMC could enhance their efforts further to disaggregate the data by LHS+ subgroups and complete data collection in those areas where we don't have sufficient data that has been mentioned above.

Organized medicine should consider amplifying the development of leadership academies themselves that specifically target LHS+ faculty aspiring to become our next generation of leaders in academic medicine. Identifying a best practices framework for leadership development that could be replicated is doable. This includes encouraging AAMC that has a number of leadership development venues to consider re-envisioning their programs to include pathways/tracks that specifically target LHS+ unique needs.

Lastly, the voice of LHS+ faculty and leaders needs to be "louder" and be present in places where policy decisions are being made, e.g., LHS+ faculty need to step up and volunteer to serve on association boards, e.g., AAMC, ABMS, ACGME, AACOM, CMSS, AMA, AOA, and more.

The effort will take a village...but a new order of things can be achievable.

> There is nothing more difficult to take in hand, more perilous to conduct, or more uncertain in its success, than to take the lead in the introduction of a new order of things. Niccolo Machiavelli

## Personal Narratives

### David A. Acosta, MD, FAAFP

As I reflect on my journey as faculty, having been at two different academic medical institutions (the University of Washington School of Medicine [UWSOM] and the University of California Davis Health [UCDH]) in two different states [Washington, California] (both with anti-affirmative action laws in place), there were some experiences that I had that were similar to other LHS+ faculty in academia, and some that were very different.

I can totally relate to the invisibility of LHS+ leadership during my entire academic career. One would assume that being a primary care faculty would have increased my exposure to faculty and leaders that looked like me…but this was certainly not the case at the UWSOM where I initially served as the associate dean for multicultural affairs and then later the inaugural chief diversity and inclusion officer (CDIO). I continued to be one of the only faculty members in my department who was Latino…or at least I could count the number of LHS+ faculty in the entire medical campus on one hand. Most of the LHS+ people that were visible to me were essential workers who, as expected, were not in leadership positions. Nonetheless, they played a significant role in my career. They were part of my community at the hospital. I felt that they were my *familia* away from my own personal *familia*. They were the reason I thrived at both of these institutions, and I will forever be grateful for the gift they provided me. It was their unconditional support and their shared stories that kept me afloat, and their constant reminder of never forgetting where I came from. They reminded me of and kept me in check with my cultural identity and the attributes I gained from my *familia* and my *communidad* (*personalismo, simpatia, respeto, familia, juntos*). They reminded me of the power I had because of my position as a physician and as an executive who had the privilege to sit at the table where decisions were made. I was their voice. This was the driver that kept me on the path toward sustaining my path as an LHS+ leader. As my father's voice inside my head would tell me, "…you have to be at the table to make change happen—but make sure you are not on the menu." As CDIO at the UWSOM, I anticipated that I would finally be at the C-suite table with the other chiefs and VPs…but that never came to fruition. The dean deliberately excluded me from his cabinet meetings. When I finally mustered up the courage to ask him why he excluded me, he simply told me, "…there was no reason for you to be there." I felt invisible. I felt powerless.

This all changed for me when I transitioned to UCDH as their inaugural chief diversity and inclusion officer and associate vice chancellor for equity, diversity, and inclusion. It was the first time in my career that I encountered a number of LHS+ faculty (in both primary care and non-primary care specialties), and LHS+ faculty in leadership positions, e.g., division chiefs, vice chairs, assistant deans, and executive directors. It made sense given the demographics of Sacramento, CA. In addition, the surrounding community had a large LHS+ community that were engaged with the health system and its leaders. I felt welcomed in this new community, and similarly, I brought their voices (the LHS+ faculty, staff, students, and the LHS+ community) to the dean's cabinet. It is true that I was the only Latino serving on the dean's cabinet. However, I had the good fortunate of having a dean that was a strong ally who understood the value of diversity, equity, and inclusion, who recognized the inequities impacting LHS+ faculty and students, and the healthcare inequities that burdened the surrounding LHS+ community we served. We formed the inaugural Dean's Standing Advisory Committee for HEUGS [5]. Faculty that reported directly to the dean and the CDIO to assist with faculty development, advancement, and recruitment, and resolve faculty issues. My experiences at UCDH reaffirmed for me that leadership, intentionality (investment), and accountability do matter, and can lead to enhancing LHS+ leadership. *Si se puede!*

## David J. Skorton, MD—President and CEO of the Association of American Medical Colleges (AAMC) Personal Reflection and Anecdote of the Association of American Medical Colleges' Perspectives on Hispanic/Latinx and Leadership

What I have to share comes from my position leading the AAMC and from my career-long experiences in higher education. I have been blessed with a variety of leadership positions in higher education and related areas, and I learned from each one of them. And since diversity, equity, and inclusion have long been a very high priority in every one of these positions, I have spent much time observing and learning from the mistakes that I and others have made.

Unfortunately, the data shows that the academic establishment in this country has failed to move the needle forward very much with medical school enrollment of students from groups underrepresented in medicine (race, ethnicity, rural, disabled, and others). This is true over my career—close to a half a century—and with some groups in many areas, we have barely moved the needle at all. I want to share what I have learned.

When it comes to inclusion, I believe the first responsibility of leadership is to cultivate the ability to see all groups as capable of taking on leadership responsibilities, including those of different ethnicities, races, ages, backgrounds, perspectives, life experiences, and more. I heard the term "executive leadership" used and I am going to expand that to say leadership at any level. I say this because if leaders do not see a broader range of individuals as capable of taking on additional leadership responsibilities, then diversification and advancement will not occur—no matter how many programs we try.

In the case of LHS+ colleagues, there is an additional, critical learning that those leaders who are not a part of the LHS+ community must undertake to understand the tremendous breadth and variety within the LHS+ community. I want to ask you to bear with me as I tell you a bit about my personal history.

I am a second-generation American. My family came over from Russia; my dad came over during the influenza pandemic about a hundred years ago when he was 9 years old. Their ship was diverted to Cuba. My dad lived there for about 3 years, and to the day he passed away (may he rest in peace) over 40 years ago, he spoke English, Russian, a little bit of Yiddish, and Spanish with a Cuban idiom. In our home, when I was a child, he taught me a little Spanish and spoke it at home. More importantly, he drove home the lesson for me—and this is over 40 years ago, so he did not use the term "LHS+," but the meaning remains—that there is incredible diversity within the LHS+ community worldwide.

To paraphrase a late colleague of mine in higher education discussing another vibrant, diverse community, the LHS+ community is a "mosaic not a monolith." Many leaders do not understand the incredible richness and variety within the LHS+ community. They tend to miss the possibilities of ways that individuals, including LHS+ colleagues, can contribute in as many different ways as there are backgrounds. All leaders must learn and internalize this truth.

The next thing that I've learned is that leaders must be intentional and deliberate in working to diversify our institutions, from the brand-new student all the way to the top leadership positions. That's easy enough to say; it sounds like rhetoric. What would actually motivate this kind of intentionality? What will finally break the log jam to make our intentions effective?

As leaders, our intentions are a critical first step, but good intentions are not enough. The second, critical step is the willingness to be humble, learn, and ask others for continued learning, no matter the heights the leader may have reached. It is very possible for a leader of any background to start to believe that because they have reached a certain level and title, that they have a firm grasp of all things that fall under the rubric of what they are leading. But it is important to understand that we all have more to learn in this regard. I repeat it is a rare week that I do not learn something from colleagues based on data or other elements to further inform my own thinking.

But the most important step for leaders is the acceptance of accountability. If there is no personal accountability to make a difference, there is a very small probability that a difference will actually occur. I believe very strongly that in any organization, the governance process should hold top leadership accountable for two aspects of inclusion at our institutions.

The first is for the institution to be inclusive of individuals from a broad variety of backgrounds in all its different divisions, areas, and categories. The second is the climate of the institution. In my experience, no matter how effectively we recruit a broad composition of individuals in a student body or workforce, if the climate of the institution is not such that it feels safe and the person feels likely to succeed, they will not succeed or will not stay at the institution. It is important that boards hold leaders accountable for both the composition and climate of the institution.

But that is not enough. An accountable leader should, in turn, hold the next level of leaders accountable. And they should hold the next level of leaders accountable, and so on throughout the entire organization. If leaders within an organization hold one another accountable, and if the accountability is real accountability (and shows up, e.g., in annual evaluations), then there is a better chance that the organization can make progress.

We are practicing this at the AAMC, although most certainly we are a work in progress. When I first joined the organization, I asked for the board of directors to hold me accountable for the composition and climate of the AAMC in my annual evaluation. I have also assigned that accountability to every one of the chiefs who make up our leadership team. In addition, I expect each of the chiefs to hold me accountable for an improved composition and climate across the organization. We have adopted this approach as a leadership executive body.

Another extremely important avenue is the concept of shared governance. Top leaders—no matter whether they have held their positions for 6 months or 6 years or more—need to continue to learn by listening to input garnered directly from students, faculty, staff, and other leaders. Hopefully, your institution already has some ready and effective mechanisms for such "shared governance" through, for example, a faculty senate, an assembly, or other means. If so, take advantage of it. Make it as effective as it can be. Participate even though it takes more time.

What if not? What if there is no organized, formal shared governance system, or no effective one? Then get one started or make suggestions to those at the very top of the organization that this be done. I feel very strongly about the need to lead by listening.

And finally, I have a message for leaders throughout higher education. I am asking you, as fellow leaders, get to know your LHS+ colleagues more directly. If you have not had the privilege and joy of working with them, I encourage you to do so as soon as possible, and I imagine you will learn something that will enrich your life and your organization.

# References

1. 2017 national population projections and vintage 2017 population estimates. www.census.gov/popest; www.census.gov/programs-surveys/popproj.html. Accessed 16 Sept 2025.
2. Pew Research Center. Key facts about U.S. Latinos for national Hispanic heritage month. 2021, September 9. Accessed at https://www.pewresearch.org/fact-tank/2021/09/09/key-facts-about-u-s-latinos-for-national-hispanic-heritage-month/#:~:text=Four%2Din%2Dfive%20Latinos%20are,who%20have%20become%20naturalized%20citizens on 07/26/2022.
3. U.S. Department of Education. White House initiative on advancing educational equity, excellence, and economic opportunity for Hispanics. 2022. Accessed at https://sites.ed.gov/hispanic-initiative/2021/10/recognizing-2021-hispanic-national-blue-ribbon-schools/ on 08/01/2022.
4. Moslimani M, Hugo Lopez M, Noe-Bustamante L. 11 facts about Hispanics origin groups in the U.S. Hispanic Pew Research Center. https://pewrsr.ch/44dSIIZ. Accessed 15 Oct 2025.
5. Guevara JP, Wad R, Aysola J. Racial and ethnic diversity at medical schools—why aren't we there yet? NEJM. 2021;385(19):1732–4.
6. Centers for Disease Control and Prevention. Risk for COVID-19 infection, hospitalizations and death by race/ethnicity. 2021, July 21. Accessed at https://www.cdc.gov/coronavirus/2019-ncov/covid-data/investigations-discovery/hospitalization-death-by-race-ethnicity.html on 02/22/2022.
7. Xierali IM, Nivet MA, Rayburn WF. Full-time faculty in clinical and basic science departments by sex and underrepresented in medicine status: a 40-year review. Acad Med. 2021;96(4):568–75.
8. AAMC. Faculty Roster, medical school faculty by rank, race/ethnicity. 2020. Accessed at https://www.aamc.org/media/8906/download?attachment on 02/22/2022.
9. AAMC. Full-time women faculty by rank and race/ethnicity, 2018. State of women in academic medicine. 2020. Accessed at https://www.aamc.org/data-reports/data/2018-2019-state-women-academic-medicine-exploring-pathways-equity on 02/22/2022.

10. AAMC. Faculty Roster: U.S. medical school faculty, Table C: Department Chairs by Department, Gender, and Race/Ethnicity. 2021. Accessed at https://www.aamc.org/media/9871/download?attachment on 02/22/2022.
11. AAMC. Faculty Roster: U.S. medical school faculty, U.S. medical school deans by dean type, and race/ethnicity (URiM vs. non-URiM). 2019. Accessed at https://www.aamc.org/data-reports/faculty-institutions/interactive-data/us-medical-school-deans-trends-type-and-race-ethnicity on 08/01/2022.
12. Chavez M. Everyday injustice: Latino professionals and racism. Lanham: Rowman & Littlefield Publishers, Inc; 2011.
13. Howard GR. We can't teach what we don't know: white teachers, multiracial schools. 3rd ed. New York: Teachers College Press; 2016.
14. Feagin JR. The white racial frame: centuries of racial framing and counter-framing. 3rd ed. New York: Routledge; 2020.
15. Chun EB, Feagin JR. Rethinking diversity frameworks in higher education. New York: Routledge; 2020.
16. National Academy of Science, Engineering, and Medicine. The science of effective mentorship in STEMM. In: Chapter 3: "mentoring underrepresented students in STEMM: why do identities matter?". Washington, DC: The National Academies Press; 2019. p. 51–73.
17. Bordas J. Salsa, soul, and spirit: leadership for a multicultural age. San Francisco: Berrett-Koehler Publishers, Inc; 2012.
18. Bordas J. The power of Latino leadership: culture, inclusion, and contribution. San Francisco: Berrett-Koehler Publishers, Inc; 2013.
19. Rodriguez R, Tapia AT. Autentico: the definitive guide to Latino career success. 2nd ed. San Francisco: Berrett-Koehler Publishers, Inc; 2021.
20. Bass BM, Riggio RE. Transformational leadership. 2nd ed. Taylor and Francis. Access at https://wwwperlego.com/book/1546534/transformational-leadership-pdf on 02/22/2022.
21. AAMC. Leadership development. 2022. Accessed at https://www.aamc.org/career-development/leadership-development

**Open Access** This chapter is licensed under the terms of the Creative Commons Attribution 4.0 International License (http://creativecommons.org/licenses/by/4.0/), which permits use, sharing, adaptation, distribution and reproduction in any medium or format, as long as you give appropriate credit to the original author(s) and the source, provide a link to the Creative Commons license and indicate if changes were made.

The images or other third party material in this chapter are included in the chapter's Creative Commons license, unless indicated otherwise in a credit line to the material. If material is not included in the chapter's Creative Commons license and your intended use is not permitted by statutory regulation or exceeds the permitted use, you will need to obtain permission directly from the copyright holder.

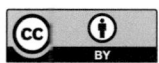

# Chapter 8
# Succeeding Along the Clinical Track from Assistant to Full Professor

Leon McDougle, Jeannette E. South-Paul, John Paul Sánchez, and A. Orlando Ortiz

---

**Learning Objectives**
- Justify the concept of promotion along the clinical track to current and future LHS+ medical school faculty
- Appraise the promotions process, step by step
- Differentiate the requirements for promotion in the clinical track
- Construct an organized promotion strategy for LHS+ faculty on the clinical track

---

## What Does It Mean to Be on the Clinical Pathway?

Several pathways or *tracks* for faculty professional advancement are available at medical school–affiliated academic medical centers [1]. Traditionally, these have consisted of clinical, research, and educator tracks. Over time, some of these tracks have become hybridized to address faculty interests and institutional missions [2]. Indeed,

---

L. McDougle (✉)
The Ohio State University Wexner Medical Center, Columbus, OH, USA

J. E. South-Paul
Meharry Medical College, Nashville, TN, USA

J. P. Sánchez
Latino Medical Student Association Inc., Chicago, IL, USA

Building the Next Generation of Academic Physicians Inc., Rye Brook, NY, USA
e-mail: exec.director@lmsa.net

A. O. Ortiz
Albert Einstein College of Medicine, Bronx, NY, USA

new tracks such as public health tracks have been implemented, and more will follow, to address the evolving roles of these institutions. The clinical track is designed for clinical faculty who invest the majority of their time in providing patient care, supervising and instructing trainees, and fulfilling all clinical mandates for their respective departments. A faculty member who chooses this pathway for advancement at their institution (i.e., promotion) provides full-time or nearly full-time clinical service. Promotion along the academic continuum, from assistant to associate to full professor, is determined by the fulfillment of specific institution-determined metrics and criteria, the majority of which are clinically driven. Clinical work includes direct patient care (i.e., number of patients seen per week in outpatient, inpatient, and community spaces; diagnostic/consultative service; hospital committees; clinical administration (i.e., service/division chief and clinical director). These are predicated on the faculty member achieving one or more areas of distinction, including clinical, research, education, or institutional/community service.

Medical schools may offer clinician educator, clinician scholar, or clinician investigator pathways where additional full-time-equivalent (FTE) effort is protected for education, scholarly, or research activities, respectively [3]. However, inadequate progress toward research and scholarship goals may often lead to loss of the protected time. Regardless of whether there is or is not protected time available, clinical track faculty can, with appropriate guidance, support, and mentorship, plan and get promoted [4].

To gain a better perspective on why we need more LHS+ academically oriented clinical faculty, an understanding of recent performance benchmarks provides an objective framework with which to monitor future progress and develop creative interventions based upon diversity, equity, and inclusion (DEI) initiatives. Overall, how have LHS+ faculty fared so far in the medical school promotions process (Table 8.1)?

Imagine if there were a 10% increase in promotion from assistant to associate professor based on the 2024 data [5]. What would be the result of this change? About 10% of the 7257 assistant professors equals 726 additional associate professors and 726 fewer assistant professors. Add those 726 individuals to the existing complement of 2597 associate professors: 2597 + 726 = 3323 and the total number of all associate professors, 43,981 + 726 = 44,707. The incremental percentage of LHS+ associate professors would increase from 5.7% (Table 8.1) to 3323/44,707 = 7.4%. Using a similar approach, with simple assumptions, a 20% increment in promotion rate would result in 8.9% LHS+ associate professors. By comparison, in 2024, 63% of associate professors were White, 22% were Asian, and 3.7% were African American or Black [5]. These data come as no surprise to LHS+ faculty. When they go to work, the noticeable dearth of colleagues with a similar background is the rule. Whether they are the person preselected or called to see a Spanish-speaking patient or to attend a community event in a Latino neighborhood, the LHS+ faculty member often understands that they will be a solo act. Such are the potential challenges and barriers to academic promotion for LHS+ faculty. A paucity of mentors and role models, a taxing number of LHS+ responsibilities, and an imbalance of clinical demands overshadow and outweigh any time or energy

**Table 8.1** LHS+ medical school faculty by rank

| Year | Race ethnicity | Professor | Associate professor | Assistant professor | Instructor | Total |
|---|---|---|---|---|---|---|
| 2022 | Hispanic, Latino, Spanish Origin | 1091 | 1244 | 3595 | 731 | 6661 |
| | Multirace/ethnicity Hispanic | 694 | 982 | 2717 | 338 | 4731 |
| | Subtotal LHS+ | 1785 (4.4%) | 2226 (5.5%) | 6312 (6.9%) | 1069 (6.3%) | 11,392 (6.0%) |
| | All Faculty | 40,224 | 40,181 | 91,951 | 17,063 | 189,419 |
| 2023 | Hispanic, Latino, Spanish Origin | 1146 | 1252 | 3966 | 796 | 7160 |
| | Multirace/ethnicity Hispanic | 737 | 1158 | 2842 | 382 | 5119 |
| | Subtotal LHS+ | 1883 (4.5%) | 2410 (5.7%) | 6808 (7.1%) | 1178 (6.9%) | 12,279 (6.2%) |
| | All Faculty | 41,490 | 42,051 | 95,953 | 17,185 | 196,679 |
| 2024 | Hispanic, Latino, Spanish Origin | 1180 | 1313 | 4242 | 800 | 7535 |
| | Multirace/ethnicity Hispanic | 849 | 1284 | 3015 | 353 | 5501 |
| | Subtotal LHS+ | 2029 (4.7%) | 2597 (5.9%) | 7257 (7.1%) | 1153 (6.6%) | 13,036 |
| | All Faculty | 42,900 | 43,981 | 101,824 | 17,396 | 206,101 |

Modified from AAMC Faculty Roster [5]

allotment for professional development [6]. This is what makes promotion a prize worth striving for, as it is a critical step toward rebalancing the academic scorecard and creating tomorrow's mentors and leaders within the LHS+ academic community.

## How Should LHS+ Faculty Navigate the Journey from Assistant to Full Professor on the Clinical Pathway?

All journeys commence with a decision to make a move. This requires resolve on the part of the faculty member, and that resolve can be fostered by self-reflection. Thought should be given to the basis or rationale for embarking on this journey, for pursuing this clinical pathway. There are many reasons why an LHS+ faculty member should consider academic promotion. These extend beyond the financial incentives that go hand in hand with advancement. Academic promotion represents the achievement of a formal milestone in your career trajectory. It is a direct recognition and validation of your clinical contributions. Advancing along the clinical pathway is one manifestation of professional growth. Career-building opportunities will present themselves with a greater frequency as the faculty member is promoted. This, in turn, expands the faculty member's scholarly network and provides more opportunities for academic and professional collaboration. It is known that a faculty member's clinical reputation is monitored by numerous entities, including colleagues, referral sources, insurers, patients and patient groups, and various medical societies. The direct and indirect implications of an academic promotion in the clinical track for clinical practice growth are extremely positive. Whether it is associate professor or professor, tenure or nontenure, the personal advantages or gains that are associated with promotion also include recognition of a faculty member's scholarly and intellectual pursuits, a source of pride and honor with the creation of a potential legacy, and upgraded status in the academic medical center as well as in the home community. LHS+ faculty members serve as role models and are potential mentors for up-and-coming LHS+ medical students. Last, a faculty member considering promotion should be aware that they can use the promotion guidelines process to align their professional activities with their institution's missions. This will allow the faculty member to have a smoother journey along their clinical track as they will likely encounter support and other opportunities because of this team approach. Typically, promotion guidelines can be found on the website of your Office of Faculty Affairs or the Office of Career Development. Examples include Office of Faculty Development, Albert Einstein College of Medicine (https://einsteinmed.edu/administration/faculty-development); Office of Faculty Development, the Ohio State University, College of Medicine (https://medicine.osu.edu/departments/homes/faculty-development); and Office of Faculty Affairs and Development, Meharry Medical College, School of Medicine (https://home.mmc.edu/about/administration/administrative-offices-divisions/faculty-affairs-development/).

Early-career faculty need to be knowledgeable about their institutional promotion requirements for their respective pathway, for example, clinical faculty [7]. An awareness of the most common requirements enables the faculty member to better understand the progression from assistant to associate to full professor [8]. This allows the faculty member to focus and better coordinate their activities as they formulate their strategic plan for promotion and develop their academic portfolio (Tables 8.2 and 8.3). The institution-dependent promotion guidelines for a clinical faculty track will usually be available online on the institution's intranet. Interested faculty members can also obtain an up-to-date copy of these guidelines from their chair or division chief or from the institutional office that oversees faculty development and promotion. Be aware that, as previously stated, your institution may use the title of "clinical track," "clinical educator," "clinical scholar," or "clinical investigator," or other terms based upon that institution's policies and missions. An underlying theme that tends to be consistent across institutions is the type of recognition that a faculty member must achieve to be promoted. At the clinical instructor or assistant professor level, the recognition is considered local, within the academic medical center where the faculty member practices. To be considered for promotion from clinical assistant professor to clinical associate professor that faculty member must achieve regional and national recognition. National and international recognition are requirements for promotion from clinical associate to clinical professor. While at first glance this may seem vague and daunting, the institution promotion guidelines will outline the specific criteria that are demonstrative of these types of recognition.

**Table 8.2** Generic example of guidelines for promotion in the clinical educator track

| Required activity | Evidence | Your checklist |
|---|---|---|
| *Clinical* | 1. Directs a clinical service recognized as excellent | |
| | 2. Regional/national (associate professor) or national/international (professor) recognition | |
| | Must include at least two of the following: | |
| | Invited presentations | |
| | Ability to draw clinical trainees | |
| | Journal reviewer | |
| | Journal editorial board member | |
| | Chapter or review article author | |
| | 3. Clinical scholarship | |
| | Peer-reviewed publications | |
| | Research grants | |
| | Involvement in clinical research protocols | |
| *Teaching* | | |
| Clinical | 1. Clinical teaching with distinction (as attending, director of service, CME educational workshop …) | |
| | Frequency/duration | |
| | Independent assessment of teaching performance from department, residency program(s), numerical score ranking your teaching performance as compared to that of your colleagues | |
| OR | Trainee (resident, fellow) testimonials | |
| Medical school | 2. Medical school teaching with distinction (lecturer, course leader, preceptor) | |
| | Description of teaching commitment (content, hours, number and level of students, number of sessions) | |
| | Testimonials from students and course leaders | |
| | Independent assessment of teaching from medical school | |
| | 3. Program director and/or development of courses | |
| | 4. Teaching awards | |
| | 5. Invited lectures at the regional or national level | |
| | 6. Educational scholarship related to teaching assessment and/or education programming | |
| | Publications related to pedagogy or educational programming | |
| | Participation in educational research protocols | |
| | Invited presentations of educational approaches at national meetings | |
| | Education grants | |

**Table 8.3** Additional promotion guidelines for a clinical educator track

| Other activities | Evidence | Your checklist |
|---|---|---|
| Research | Publications | |
| | Grant support | |
| | Recognition: Invited presentations, editorial boards | |
| Service | Administrative: Program director, committee participation in the hospital and/or medical school | |
| | Organization and operation of a service | |
| | Mentorship: Students, junior faculty | |
| | Awards: Hospital or community service | |
| Other | Evidence of prior rank at another institution | |

## How Is the Promotion Process Along the Clinical Track Initiated?

There are essentially three ways of initiating the promotion process. First, if you are employed at a medical center that is affiliated with a medical school and if you are involved in teaching medical students, then it is likely that you will have already received a faculty appointment, as either a clinical instructor or assistant professor, at the start of your employment. To ensure accountability for educational quality, the Liaison Committee for Medical Education (LCME) requires that faculty members involved in medical student teaching hold academic appointments at the medical school. Similarly, if you are involved in resident or fellow education, then the Accreditation Council for Graduate Medical Education (ACGME) will also require an academic appointment at the medical school. The second way is to be identified as a viable candidate for promotion by either your division chief or your department chair. Alternatively, the chair of your clinical department's promotion committee, if one is in place, can also nominate you and discuss it with your department/division leaders. The third way to be considered for academic promotion is to self-identify and to express your interest and inquire, with your chair or division chief, if the timing is right and if you are ready for promotion. Carefully read and assimilate the guidelines for your institution's clinical track. This is where the support of your department chair, division chief, or department promotion committee chair and your mentors will prove most helpful. It is paramount that early-career or junior faculty, with assistance from their department chair/division chief, identify faculty who have been promoted on their clinical pathway to provide mentorship [9].

Once the promotion process is initiated, it must be monitored. Keep in mind that each institution has specific timelines that are strictly observed for the timely and thorough review of a candidate's proposed promotion. All documents must be provided by the institution-specific deadlines as promotion and tenure (P&T) committees meet at only specific times each year. It is both the candidate's and the department chair's responsibility to ensure prompt submission of all components of the promotion packet. P&T committees will not review incomplete packets and will defer the submission until the next promotion cycle, which may be a year later.

## Creating Your Promotion Packet

Once you understand the requirements for promotion, the so-called rules of the game, then you can participate with a strategic focus (Tables 8.2 and 8.3). This will enable you to efficiently create a "promotion packet" that supports your application for promotion (Table 8.4). This will also facilitate and assist you with collecting, organizing, and categorizing your documentation. In building one's dossier for promotion, frequent recordkeeping is important. Consideration should be given to labeling file folders with categories that count toward promotion, for example, teaching evaluations, clinical excellence, and service, including advising. Regarding advising, it is important to record the person's name, year of training, institution, date, and amount of time spent. For more formal mentoring activities, it is beneficial to track and document the career outcomes of the mentees (i.e., acceptance to college or graduate school; accepted poster presentations). Most institutions have an office of faculty affairs and a website that has standard templates (e.g., CV, dossier) to record and track productivity and contributions [10, 11]. It is critical to regularly accumulate, save, and store all your documents. In addition to cloud-based storage, consider backing up your precious documentation on additional drives and external drives. Difficult-to-replicate hard-copy documents should be scanned and stored as soft copies. All these supporting documents, including an updated copy of your curriculum vitae (CV), a copy of your academic portfolio, and a list of your referees (individuals who will be writing your letters of support), will comprise your promotion packet (Table 8.4). Store the documents in your main "Promotion" folder in their respective categories. Again, do this regularly (biweekly, monthly, or quarterly), and do not wait until the last minute before dossier submission.

Table 8.4 Promotion packet contents

| Document | Comments |
| --- | --- |
| Curriculum vitae | Use institutional template |
| Academic or teaching portfolio | A concisely written summary of your clinical, educational, and scholarly accomplishments. This should complement and not duplicate your CV |
| Academic portfolio appendix | Includes a few documents that demonstrate your best work |
| Referee list | Individuals who will write letters of recommendation supporting your promotion |
| | Includes chair's letter<br>Faculty: Internal and external<br>Suggested by you, your chair, or division chief |
| | Prior learners: Medical students, residents, fellows, or other trainees |
| Supporting documents | Includes any item that attests to your clinical and scholarly pursuits at a local, regional, national, or international level |

Do you consider your promotion packet as your personal marketing packet? You should! It will be reviewed, analyzed, and critiqued at several levels and by multiple key individuals. Your department chair will need it to write a letter supporting your promotion. Your department promotions committee, if active, will review it for completeness and determine if the criteria for promotion are satisfied before forwarding the packet to the medical school promotion and tenure committee. Your referees, or letter-writers, will also need to review your packet so that they can write more relevant and stronger letters endorsing your promotion.

## Your Curriculum Vitae

In preparing your curriculum vitae (CV), make sure that you strictly adhere to your institution's required template. Be a perfectionist with respect to format, content, grammar, and spelling. Publications and other citations should be cited properly and retrievable by a reviewer. Check any hyperlinks to make sure they are active and access the correct document. While you should include works in progress, consider excluding submissions that have been sitting in limbo for a few years. The latter creates an unfavorable impression. List accomplishments in chronological or reverse chronological order as per the template requirements at your institution. Most importantly, get into the habit of updating your CV quarterly; do this more frequently if you are involved in many clinical, educational, scholarly, administrative, or community activities. An intelligent and creative strategy that is key to your success is to be able to transform any of your professional activities into clinical, educational, scholarly, or service contributions. Make sure that your department chair or chief of service reviews your initial CV draft to confirm that you are using the correct format and to make sure that you are including and properly categorizing all your clinical, scholarly, research, and service activities. A properly drafted CV will also assist you in crafting your academic portfolio.

## The Academic, Educational, or Teaching Portfolio

The academic or clinical and/or teaching portfolio is a collection and summary of your educational activities and accomplishments [12]. Most importantly, it is your assessment of your activity. It differs from a CV, which shows your activity in quantity and in chronological order, in that it shows quantity, quality, and the impact of your work as it relates to the missions of the medical school. This portfolio combines with your CV to provide a complete overview of your clinical and academic productivity. It is your supporting evidence in the faculty promotion process and should "speak" on your behalf during the evaluation process. It should create a clear and accurate description of you as a clinician, scholar, and educator. The creation of this portfolio is simultaneously a proactive, prospective, and retrospective activity

[13]. You should begin accumulating and filing documented evidence of your professional, educational, scholarly, and service work from your first day as a faculty member.

A critical step in the preparation of your academic portfolio is to familiarize yourself with the guidelines for promotion in the clinical pathway that is available at your institution and plan the portfolio to show that you fulfill the criteria for promotion (Tables 8.2 and 8.3). Think broadly as to what is considered clinical service, teaching, scholarly work, and institutional and community service. Transform all your activities into scholarly, educational, or service contributions! Ask yourself or your mentor or chair if the activity, project, or product has a specific value that pertains to one or more of your professional pursuits. This will enable you to create a portfolio that complements your CV. You are marketing yourself to the promotions committee, make sure to present your materials in an organized and concise fashion that follows the recommended guidelines. This will make your application for promotion more attractive as it will enable the committee members to fairly and efficiently assess the quality and quantity of your work in your quest for promotion.

## How Should the Academic Portfolio Be Organized?

This will be a highly structured and concise document that, for example, may consist of a 10–15-page double-spaced document in 12-point font. The document should be clear and succinct. It should address the requirements for promotion (Refer to: Personal Narrative for A.O. Ortiz). Use narrative for important achievements and use tables and grids for lists. Discuss your philosophy of education and how it relates to the mission(s) of the academic medical center and medical school. State your specific goals when teaching and comment on your unique strengths as a clinical educator. Discuss your didactic and bedside teaching methods and how you assess the success of your interventions. It is a medical school, so do outline your contributions to the medical school curriculum, your teaching responsibilities, educational projects, and your activities as a faculty advisor and mentor. Do include any regional, national, or international educational programs that you contribute to. Participate in local or society education committees and document your input and responsibilities. Include any original work in these educational endeavors, especially educational materials that have been shared or disseminated. All your administrative and clinical coordination activities are worthy of mention. Most academic medical centers have or support faculty development programs. It is prudent to participate in and document the educational workshops and courses that you have attended. Save all those certificates, acknowledgment letters, awards, and thank you notes as proof of local, regional, national, and/or international recognition of the importance and impact of your professional work [3]. Once this document is organized, prepared, and written, do proofread it. Some medical schools allow you to include an academic portfolio appendix. Some examples of supporting documents include recent publications, links to recorded presentations interviews, or educational media, and clinical service or teaching or community service awards. To reflect clinical excellence, you can consider summarizing dimensions of your contribution to the clinical mission with redacted referral communication examples; short narratives about second opinions solicited; Patient Safety/Quality Improvement (PS/QI) outcomes; clinical awards from your clinical site; acceptance letters as a fellow (e.g., Fellow of the American College of Surgeons FACS); patient volume or throughput; new service lines, clinics, or programs you started; and patient education materials developed. This appendix allows you to include representative samples or documents that show your best work. Important materials should also be summarized in the body of your portfolio.

You should have your chair, section chief, and mentor(s) review your academic portfolio prior to its submission. They can help make any modifications or suggest potential additions that you may have overlooked. Moreover, it will help your chair and your referees write your letters of support.

## Letters of Recommendation

A preset number of individuals or referees, depending on your medical school's promotion guidelines, will be writing letters of recommendation on your behalf to support your academic promotion. In general, this consists of a small number of internal and external faculty (from other institutions) who possess the academic rank that you aspire to. Furthermore, these may include faculty that are suggested by you or your chair. External referees are important because they are perceived as less biased and can stipulate that you would be a successful candidate if you applied for that same promotion at their institution. External referees can also attest to the impact of your work outside of your institution. The solicitations for these letters usually occur through the department chair or a designee as per the medical school's promotion process. Each referee is confidentially contacted regarding your candidacy and is asked if they can write a letter of support for your promotion. A specific deadline for the letter of recommendation is also provided. So, the two main reasons a referee might refuse to write a letter are: (1) They do not believe that you fulfill the criteria for promotion to the proposed rank; (2) they have conflicting obligations and would not be able to meet the deadline. If the referee agrees to write a letter of support, then they are provided with a copy of your CV, a copy of your academic portfolio, and a copy of the institution's guidelines specific to the rank and category of interest. This is why a CV and academic portfolio are so critical to your promotion, as it is your way of indirectly providing supporting information, as to the depth and breadth of your clinical contributions, to your referees. In turn, the referees can validate the scope of your regional, national, and international reach. They can also use key achievements in your packet, in the composition of their letter, as evidence of excellence in the clinical, educational, research, or service arenas. Your department chair will also write a letter of support on your behalf. This letter also carries considerable weight as the department chair is in the best position to assess your achievements and contributions to the department, hospital(s), medical school, and community. This should be an enthusiastic letter that makes a strong case for your promotion. It therefore mandates that you meet with the department chair before they write the letter so that you can update the chair as to all your contributions as you review your up-to-date CV and your academic portfolio. The letters of support are forwarded directly to the dean's office, the office of academic appointments, or the promotions committee, according to the medical school's specific protocol.

## The Review Process

The clinical track promotions application, review, and decision processes vary for each medical school. A useful exercise is to look up and save a copy of the faculty promotion process for your respective medical school (e.g., Faculty Affairs—UMass Chan Medical School) [14]. The following is a general overview that will provide you with some familiarity with these processes, which will in turn assist you with your preparation and expectations. The promotion packet is first reviewed within your department by the department promotion committee and/or by your chair for both completeness and to ascertain that the criteria for promotion are being met by the candidate. This committee may or may not write a letter of endorsement that is included with the promotion packet, but, at a minimum, the committee will endorse your application. Your chair will also write a letter to support your promotion, and that letter will be included with your packet. The packet is then forwarded to the medical school. Your promotion packet is carefully reviewed at the medical school office of faculty affairs, or equivalent, to ascertain completeness prior to forwarding it to the promotions and tenure (P&T) committee. This assessment consists of determining if there is sufficient supporting documentation with which to make a fair determination of the candidate's status for promotion. The P&T committee usually adheres to a calendar schedule for their meetings to efficiently evaluate candidates for promotions at specific time intervals at your institution. Occasionally, under special circumstances, an ad hoc P&T meeting may take place to address a pressing promotion issue. The P&T committee reviews the promotion packet and discusses and decides as to whether the candidate merits promotion. The committee members will follow the medical school's criteria for promotion in the clinical track. They will assess your level of recognition based on the proposed promotion rank and will address all major clinical track parameters that are demonstrative of clinical excellence. Your additional documents and contributions to the medical school, hospital, and community will also be evaluated by the committee. These deliberations are confidential. In certain instances, the P&T committee may request additional information from you via your chair, from your chair, from a referee, or may wish to solicit the input of an additional referee.

**Table 8.5** Some common reasons for not being promoted in the clinical track

| |
|---|
| 1. Application package was incomplete or poorly organized. |
| 2. Key elements for review were not submitted in a timely fashion. |
| 3. Candidate was not proposed in the correct track/pathway. |
| 4. Candidate's reputation (regional/national, national/international) was insufficiently documented. |
| 5. Significant accomplishments were excluded from the CV and/or academic portfolio. |
| 6. Appropriate referees were not selected. |
| 7. Specific promotion packet materials needed to be revised or added. |
| 8. Evidence of independent scholarship was lacking. |
| 9. Promotion proposal was premature. |

## The Decision Process

Once the P&T committee reviews and discusses your request for promotion, if they feel there is sufficient documentation with which to decide, then they take a vote and make a recommendation. In general, if the criteria for promotion are met, then a favorable recommendation is likely. Once the P&T committee approves your faculty promotion in the clinical track, their recommendation is forwarded to the executive medical council and dean's office for review. The executive medical council and dean accept the recommendation of the P&T committee. The dean drafts and signs your promotion letter. Alternatively, the dean may approve the promotion and await the approval of the provost and/or chancellor prior to signing your promotion letter.

If the P&T committee decides not to approve your promotion, then they will discuss the situation and reasons for rejection with your chair. Your chair will discuss the P&T committee's decision with you. The reason(s) for the committee's decision are often valid, and you should look at this as an opportunity to remediate and strengthen your application for the next application cycle or as per the recommendations of the P&T committee that have been discussed between you and your chair (Table 8.5). Approach the decision as a temporary situation and respond with a growth mindset. Discuss with your division chief, chair, and/or mentors what you can do in the next year or two to increase your likelihood of being promoted.

## Corrective or Proactive Protocol Seen Through an LHS+ Lens

Identify any real or potential weaknesses or deficiencies in your quest for promotion. Get in the habit of touching base with your mentors, identifying new mentors, and discussing your career plans with these mentors, as well as your division chief and chair. You should set aside time each year to reflect on your clinical, teaching, research, and service activities [4]. Your mentors can help guide you on potential activities that can augment your presence in these mission-based categories. This may be an opportunity to create and deploy an innovative clinical program that increases the presence of your medical school and/or institution in an LHS+ community (e.g., a syphilis control intervention targeting black and Hispanic men who have sex with men) [15]. Develop educational programs directed to medical students that focus on LHS+ patients and track the outcomes for these programs from both a medical student (course evaluations and reviews) and a patient perspective (patient satisfaction surveys, compliance indicators) (e.g., using Promotores Programs to Improve Latino Health Outcomes: Implementation Challenges for Community-based Nonprofit Organizations) [16]. Create lectures and symposia that focus on LHS+ healthcare issues (e.g., Diseases Transmitted by Arthropods: Module to Train Medical Providers in English and Spanish) [17]. Present these talks locally, regionally, nationally, and/or internationally as you develop your expertise on these topics. Identify research topics and questions that pertain to your LHS+ patients, with respect to your specialty, and create research projects designed to address those research questions. This will often require collaboration with your colleagues within your department and from other departments and from community leaders. A collaborative mindset will catalyze your professional growth and your scholarly productivity. Volunteering to be a journal manuscript reviewer in your specialty and hosting journal clubs are keyways to get you to think of important clinical research questions. Attend your specialty's regional and national conferences [18]; some may even be LHS+ specific, such as the Latino Surgical Society [19]. This will introduce you to the "how" of presentation delivery, whether didactic or research related. It will also stimulate ideas for future projects. Submit abstracts for scientific presentations or exhibits or case presentations to your specialty's regional and national meetings. Once you start presenting at these meetings, you will understand the process, and with each iteration, the preparation and submission become second nature. But in the beginning, your advisors, mentors, and colleagues will guide and help you. Over time, you will appreciate that abstracts become presentations and presentations can become publications.

It cannot be stated enough, the LHS+ patient–clinical care field needs scholarly contributions. Get involved. You may need to increase your organizational and institutional involvement, for example, in DEI activities, so that you enhance your service commitment and become a known entity in your medical school. Volunteer for your specialty society committees and work your way up to become part of their leadership team [18]. This will enhance your professional network and create opportunities for collaboration [8]. Plan for your professional future and use the promotion guidelines as a strategic planning tool. Document your work prospectively and keep it organized, according to your medical school's template, so that you can find it and track your accomplishments. It is critical that you get into the habit of obtaining and saving learner (medical student, trainee) evaluations related to any of your lectures, presentations, or educational workshops. Proactively monitor your progress and follow up on any outstanding items. Never make assumptions about the status of any document or process as it relates to your promotion and professional growth. Therefore, develop and maintain an inquisitive mindset.

## Challenges for LHS+ Faculty in Career Tracks

### Diversity Tax

Clinical faculty who are from historically minoritized groups will soon discover the diversity tax that they will be asked to pay [5]. Consider the tax as an opportunity to strategically build diversity capital and influence across the campus and community to advance academic promotion and community health [20]. Please review your department's appointment, promotion, and tenure document to determine how best to document these activities that advance the mission, vision, and values of the institution. At most medical schools, there is an inherent mismatch between the percentage of learners as compared to faculty who are from historically minoritized groups. This imbalance may result in those faculty being potentially overextended by learners requesting advice and mentorship. This may include serving as an advocate for learners experiencing academic or learning environment difficulties thought to be related to bias, racism, and ethnic discrimination. Consider identifying and collaborating with other faculty to assist in sharing the responsibility for responding to these students' needs—both in and outside of your department or institution [21]. In addition to the diversity tax paid in support of learners, clinical associate professors may also be asked to advise or mentor early-career faculty from historically minoritized groups who also outnumber clinical associate professors (Table 8.1). Serving on multiple medical school and clinical department committees that benefit from diverse perspectives can also delay or derail promotion. The average time for promotion from clinical assistant professor to clinical associate professor is typically 6 years [1]. Prior to becoming over-committed to paying diversity tax, consultation with faculty mentors and discussion with the medical school's diversity, equity, inclusion, and accessibility (DEIA) or academic affairs leadership for guidance is strongly encouraged [22]. In the absence of DEIA Offices, individuals should reach out to SOM or institutional Offices for Faculty Affairs or Career Advancement.

### Patient Satisfaction

Clinical faculty who are from historically minoritized groups are more likely to receive lower patient satisfaction scores related to bias [23]. This may negatively impact clinical performance evaluations, access to financial incentives, and perceptions of clinical excellence. If such a differential policy or practice exists within the clinical department, consideration should be given to proposing an alternative promising practice that averages patient satisfaction scores across all clinicians at the practice site. For LHS+ faculty, the addition of a clinic day for Spanish-speaking patients, combined with a Spanish language patient experience survey, may help to level the playing field. This may be a more realistic goal in areas where the demographics support this type of initiative.

## Institutional Culture

Institutional climate and isolation may form barriers to career advancement. Leadership commitment to initiatives that advance anti-LHS+ discrimination, anti-racism, diversity, equity, inclusion, accessibility, and belonging is key to optimizing the work and learning environment. In addition to implicit bias awareness and mitigation, priorities should include allyship and bystander training and behavior so that persons from historically minoritized\groups are not the sole voices in response to microaggressions. Observing unsolicited support from colleagues in response to microaggressions helps to develop a sense of belonging [24–26]. Developing relationships with affinity group members may require outreach beyond one's department. Joining an employee resource group or affinity group network may also promote well-being and decrease isolation. Consideration should be given to becoming active members of local, regional, or national professional organizations (i.e. Association of American Indian Physicians; Faculty Physician Advisory Council, Latino Medical Student Association; National Medical Association; National Hispanic Medical Association; and National Council of Asian Pacific Islander Physicians). Advancing to leadership positions in such organizations may be looked upon favorably by promotion committees [18, 27].

## Case Discussion

*Scenario 1* After completing the academic track within her residency program, where she obtained a master of public health degree in clinical translational science, Mary Martinez, MD, MPH, (pronouns, she/her/ella) joined the University of High Aspirations faculty as an assistant professor on the clinical scholar pathway with 20% protected time. Dr. Martinez is a first-generation college graduate and committed to improving the health of Spanish-speaking communities. During her recruitment, the Department Chair applauded Dr. Martinez for serving as chief resident and obtaining the MPH from the prestigious institution. Upon arrival at the University of High Aspirations, Dr. Martinez is greeted warmly by numerous constituents, including learners, faculty, and community members. Before long, Dr. Martinez had agreed to serve as advisor for a first-generation student affinity group and joined the medical school admissions committee. In addition to being invited to after-work-hours recruitment dinners, she routinely receives requests to speak at community events by the Spanish-speaking community. Most recently, Dr. Martinez has been asked to serve on the Department's Diversity Committee. During her fourth-year review, the Department Chair voiced serious reservations about her continuation on the clinical scholar pathway: "Your clinical research and scholarship are inadequate. How can I continue to justify your being away from the clinic? We're short staffed and our department can benefit from reallocation of your 20% FTE to patient care."

- How should Dr. Mary Martinez respond to the chair's threat to remove the Clinical Scholar pathway protected time?
  Dr. Martinez should ask for further information on what constitutes adequacy in clinical research and scholarship. Dr. Martinez should also prepare to explain how her activities are helping the department meet the school's and institution's mission and accreditation standards. Dr. Martinez should ask for guidance and support to adequately meet metrics tied to clinical research and scholarship.
- What should have been done to optimize the likelihood of career advancement at the time of employment?
- Initial steps to be taken to increase Dr. Martinez's likelihood of career advancement include:

  1. Assign her an associate professor faculty member who can serve as a role model or advisor and guide Mary with first-hand knowledge and skills on how to achieve promotion to associate professor. Also, asking Mary if she would prefer an identity-congruent advisor or offering her a nonidentity- and identity-congruent advisor to discuss personal, professional, and cultural issues.
  2. Discussing and documenting how Mary's personal and professional interests and activities align with departmental and institutional mission and goals.
  3. Help her consider an academic niche in LHS+ health equity, whereby her LHS+ related activities are framed as deliverables and outcomes aligned with promotion criteria.
  4. Provide biannual check-ins with Mary to review her activities and help her document outcomes of value for promotion.

- What other resources are available to Dr. Martinez?
  Dr. Martinez should consider a number of resources in her department or institution or external institutions to help her achieve promotion. Her department may have a vice chair of faculty development or chair of faculty development who can provide guidance. On the school or institutional level, there may be a career development advisor or office that can provide support. Externally, there are a number of specialty- or identity-based organizations that can provide professional advancement workshops, seminars, or programs. For example, the LMSA Faculty Physician Advisory Council offers LIDEReS—LHS+ Identity Development, Empowerment and Resources Seminar; this two-day seminar is for residents, fellows, faculty, and staff from across the United States. The seminar provides participants with inspirational and practical guidance and tools for pursuing career advancement in academic medicine, such as progressing from assistant to full professor with tenure and from assistant dean to dean of the medical school. The seminar helps participants develop key professional competencies that build self-efficacy, communication skills, and leadership while expanding their network of colleagues, role models, advisors, and champions. (https://fpac.lmsa.net/center/lideres/. Accessed on June 7, 2025.)

**Scenario 2** Dr. Dakota Alverez (pronouns, they/them) completed the surgical residency at the University of High Aspirations and immediately agreed to join the faculty after an offer was extended by the department chair. Within the employment agreement, 90% of Dr. Alvarez's FTE was devoted to surgical practice. The demand for surgical services outpaced the supply of surgeons, and Dr. Alvarez was a welcome addition to the department, especially because of ability to communicate directly with Spanish-speaking patients. Dr. Alvarez decided to become a surgeon while in elementary school and loved the complexity and volume of surgical cases at the University of High Aspirations. During faculty orientation, Dr. Alvarez was given a PDF version of the department's appointment, promotion, and tenure document that was subsequently saved within their computer server.

Six years have flown by, and Dr. Alvarez is considering going up for promotion after noticing that colleagues with similar time in rank had been promoted to Clinical Associate Professor. Upon retrieving data for inclusion within the dossier, Dr. Alvarez discovers that their aggregate patient satisfaction scores were below the department mean; therefore, limiting the amount of annual clinical performance bonus payment. Dr. Alvarez also has concerns about how service in support of diversity, equity, and inclusion did not appear to be a value-added criterion for promotion. Dr. Alvarez had informally mentored and advised many medical students and residents from historically marginalized and minoritized groups throughout the 6 years as faculty. In addition, the high clinical load has limited Dr. Alvarez's ability to publish peer-reviewed journal articles or book chapters. Therefore, Dr. Alvarez decides to forgo promotion and to be content with the rank of clinical assistant professor.

- What are your thoughts about Dr. Alvarez's decision to forgo submitting a dossier for promotion consideration to clinical associate professor?
  Six years is the typical length of time taken before being promoted to associate professor. Dr. Alvarez should be encouraged to meet with the chair or departmental designee of faculty affairs or career development and discuss the portfolio and opportunity to pursue promotion at this moment or during a subsequent year. During this meeting, Dr. Alvarez should be prepared to describe contributions (i.e., education, service, research) and explain the circumstances in which deliverables were achieved (i.e., "The demand for surgical services outpaced the supply of surgeons and Dr. Alvarez was a welcome addition to the department."). Dr. Alvarez can also describe how uniquely congruent care was provided by communicating directly with patients in Spanish and addressing nuanced cultural issues for LHS+ patients, which offers a unique skill set.
- How should Dr. Alvarez address the lower patient satisfaction scores?
  Dr. Alvarez should explore with the chair or vice chair of clinical affairs the factors contributing to lower patient satisfaction scores. Some of these factors may be systemic and out of the oversight of Dr. Alvarez, such as wait time for procedures and systemic bias by other clinical team members. Other factors, such as communication and follow-up, may be more feasible for Dr. Alvarez to improve.

Dr. Alvarez should determine an action plan with the departmental leaders to improve her patient satisfaction scores.
- What can Dr. Alvarez do to meet the criteria for promotion to clinical associate professor?

Dr. Alvarez should review the criteria for promotion, especially teaching, research, and service criteria. They should inquire how diversity-, equity-, and inclusion-related activities are considered or calculated in the promotion process, because DEI-related activities did not appear to be a value-added criterion for promotion. Dr. Alvarez should also explore how to better document advising or mentorship of medical students and residents from historically marginalized and minoritized groups, which fulfills SOM requirements. Given she is 90% clinical time and has assumed a greater number of patients, she should inquire with departmental leadership how to properly document this level of clinical contributions. It is important for Dr. Alvarez to routinely meet her departmental leadership, potentially on a biannual basis, to receive ongoing advising on how to achieve successful promotion in the near future.

## Summary

A case has been made for LHS+ faculty to proactively and strategically participate in the promotion process at their respective medical schools. There are many reasons that favor this academic pursuit beyond monetary remuneration, such as the multiplier effect of incremental scholarly opportunities. Each LHS+ faculty promotion honors the legacy of previous LHS+ leading faculty who endured much more to open doors on our behalf. Embracing this legacy of mentorship and excellence is key to accelerating the pace of career advancement of students, trainees, and early-career faculty. The power of promotion motivates and inspires and has the potential to favorably impact the quantity and quality of LHS+ clinical faculty. An improved understanding of the promotion pathway using a step-by-step approach shows that academic promotion is a realistic and achievable objective. By learning how to translate many of their current clinical, educational, and service activities into the language of promotion and developing a disciplined method for tracking and documenting these activities faculty are well on their way in their quest for academic promotion in the clinical track. Active service participation in the medical school and specialty societies will expand an aspiring faculty member's network and reputation. This is conducive to recognition at multiple levels, the kind of recognition that enhances the chances for promotion. By being open to professional collaboration, a faculty member can increase their scholarly and research productivity. Most importantly, LHS+ faculty should identify advisors who can help them navigate difficult situations, thereby avoiding diversity taxation without mentor representation. Savvy advisors can help LHS+ faculty convert their LHS+ "capital" and LHS+ service commitments into academic currency that will satisfy one or more of the clinical track guidelines. By charting a course for promotion and crafting a powerful promotion packet, with the help of these senior colleagues and mentors, LHS+ faculty markedly increase their chances for a favorable outcome.

## Personal Narratives

**Excerpts from My Academic Portfolio—A. Orlando Ortiz, MD, MBA, FASSR**
This is a condensed example of my teaching portfolio during my request for promotion to Professor of Clinical Radiology in 2018 at the Albert Einstein College of Medicine in New York. It provides insight into the creation of a teaching or academic portfolio. While there may be variation with respect to format and content requirements, the academic portfolio will allow you to speak to your achievements and contributions in concordance with the promotion guidelines for your specific clinical track. Take note of how this differs from the traditional CV. While only a few publications and presentations are listed here for the sake of brevity, their purpose in this case is to reinforce, with respect to excellence in the field and/or level of recognition, a specific criterion in one of the major promotion categories (clinical, teaching, research, service). As a marketing tool or an instrument of self-promotion, the prose is used to send a consistent message to the intended audience that you are motivated by a spirit of perpetual inquiry and a desire to contribute to the medical school and its missions in a meaningful way, all in keeping with the requirements of your desired academic rank. Admittedly, the messaging will be different for each candidate, but it should be consistent throughout each section of the medical school's template. This specific template consists of 7 sections.

*Teaching Portfolio: A. Orlando Ortiz, MD, MBA, FACR*
I. Philosophy of Education
   As a career academic radiologist, I see each day as an opportunity for academic improvement—at my institution, within my radiology department, and within myself. My roots as an educator, in a one-to-one format, developed during my work as a tutor while in high school. Subsequent growth of my radiology education was stimulated by my favorable experience as a chief resident teaching in a group format, while providing weekly radiology conferences to my peers. My interest in academic radiology continued to flourish as a neuroradiology fellow at the Neurological Institute at Columbia University—with active involvement in intra-departmental and multidisciplinary conferences as well as teaching radiology residents on a case-by-case basis. With these early experiences, I quickly developed an open architecture approach toward radiology education and scholarship, as learning opportunities do arise in any clinical or administrative encounter. Furthermore, these learning opportunities are continuous, fluid, and multidirectional as learning involves any person in any situation. There is a cyclical duality with the teacher as both instructor and student, as well as with students and patients serving as teachers and sources of instruction. My initial endeavors in these educational processes as a junior radiology faculty were

centered on traditional structured curriculums with formal didactic sessions as the major teaching instrument. As my career has progressed, I have had the opportunity to explore other teaching tools and learning environments from audience response systems, hands-on courses to small group interactive sessions. My involvement in faculty development programs has exposed me to new methods and tools for "getting my message across."

My interest in academic radiology to this day continues to grow. As chair of a radiology department, it has enabled me to communicate the value of our profession across the enterprise and to the public that we serve. Programmatic developments, including faculty development programs to empower and support junior faculty, research clubs, visiting professor programs, medical student clerkships in radiology subspecialties, and safety initiatives, are a natural byproduct of this interest. I would state that my most significant contribution as chairman of the department of radiology at NYU Winthrop Hospital is evidenced by the fact that 2/3's of my resident trainees have embarked on a career in academic radiology, all radiology faculty secured academic appointments, and all junior radiology faculty successfully completed a formal Winthrop faculty scholars' program. As continuous, lifelong learners, we put ourselves in a position to enhance education and positively impact the future of global healthcare.

II. Contributions to Medical School Curriculum

  A. Teaching Responsibilities

*NYU Winthrop Hospital/Stony Brook University School of Medicine (2000–2018)*

Stony Brook University and other visiting medical students:

Lecturer in medical student radiology clerkship
Co-director for medical student radiology research elective

Radiology resident education: Active contributor to the neuroradiology and interventional neuroradiology curriculum at NYU Winthrop on a broad spectrum of topics in this field, including general neuroradiology, head and neck radiology, pediatric neuroradiology, interventional neuroradiology, and spine radiology.

Diagnostic teaching at the PACS workstation: on average 5–10 h per week
Clinical instruction in my spine clinic: 1–2 h per week
Sponsor for fourth-year resident elective concentration in Spine Interventions

Radiology Residency Program Director at NYU Winthrop: 3/2006–6/2007; 1/2011–6/2013

  B. Curriculum Development

As radiology chairman, I have been involved in organizing, implementing, and continuously monitoring the focused curriculums for the medical students and for the radiology residents. This includes the addition of topics such as the business of radiology, medico-legal issues in radiology, and patient safety in radiology.

Emergency radiology for the first-year radiology resident (symposium)

I created and coordinated a one-day (7 h) educational symposium for the Winthrop first-year radiology residents on various emergency radiology topics to prepare them for the start of their radiology call. Total 16 of the radiology faculty volunteered to teach on their day off to help the residents. The feedback was so positive that in the third year of the course (2017), we also included the first-year radiology residents from Stony Brook University. On the course evaluation, which had an overall rating of 5/5 (excellent on the scale), all residents stated that they would highly recommend the course to future first-year residents. I intend to initiate this course at Jacobi Medical Center in the fall of 2018.

C. Projects for Which I Have Primary Responsibility

Spine intervention service

A major area of personal interest within radiology is diagnostic and therapeutic spine care. While the spine is an overlap structure between general radiology and various radiology subspecialties, it is also an overlooked and incompletely understood structure. I have dedicated a significant portion of my clinical, academic, and research endeavors toward improving how patients with symptomatic disorders of the spinal axis are managed. As a neurointerventionalist and clinical radiologist, I developed my own spine intervention clinic. This enabled me to combine my diagnostic and interventional core competencies as a radiologist in providing prompt and quality care to this specific patient group. For this work, I have been recognized by multiple "Best Doctor" and "Top Doctor" awards over the past two decades. I was an early adopter of this philosophy and the interventional spine clinic model within the radiology community. Moreover, I have shared this model with others at national and international meetings. In addition to providing clinical care, the model facilitates education, clinical research, and information gathering—the results of which have been shared via presentation and publication formats to advance spine care throughout the world.

D. Faculty Advisor/Mentor
E. Education Committees

Member: NYU Winthrop Graduate Medical Education Committee 7/1/2000–3/15/2018

III. Educational Scholarship

1. Co-developer and founder of *Oztech, Inc.* (1999)—an educational media company—my colleague, Dr. Gregg Zoarski, and I developed an educational CD to train other physicians on how to perform two major percutaneous image-guided spine intervention procedures: Vertebroplasty and kyphoplasty. The CD, a two-volume set, includes chapters with active links

to PowerPoint images and video clips, and was widely used by spine operators.
2. Authored textbook on how to prepare for and perform image-guided spine biopsy: **Ortiz AO**. *Image-guided Percutaneous Spine Biopsy*. New York, Springer-Verlag. 2017

IV. Contributions to Regional/National Educational Programs

**Ortiz AO.** Course director: Vertebral augmentation how-to workshop: vertebral augmentation imaging. RSNA Scientific Assembly and Annual Meeting (12/3/2015) (12/1/2016) (11/30/2017) Chicago, IL

*Invited International Scientific Presentations (past 5 years)*

**Ortiz AO.** Actualizacion: vertebroplastia y cifoplastia. Sociedad Iberolatinoamericana de Neuroradiologia Diagnostica y Terapeutica 25th Annual Meeting (6/20/2013); Panama City, Panama

**Ortiz AO**. Vertebral augmentation: Review of literature and update on trials. World Federation of Neuroradiology, XX Annual Symposium Neuroradiologicum (9/9/2014), Istanbul, Turkey

*Invited National Scientific Presentations (past 5 years)*

**Ortiz AO**, Riascos R. Spine—Maintenance of certification review. American Society of Neuroradiology Annual Meeting (5/20/2013); San Diego, CA

V. Professional Development

Faculty Skills Update: Beyond the Podium—Tips for Teaching and Testing; Radiological Society of North America workshop; 9/22/2015; 6.25 AMA PRA Category 1 Credits

VI. Administration/Clinical Coordination

Chairman: American College of Radiology subcommittee for revision of Guidelines for Computed Tomography of the Spine 2010, 2015

American Society of Spine Radiology mentor committee (2004–2010): I created the Mentor Program to encourage and support junior researchers interested in spine radiology.

American Society of Spine Radiology President (2002–2003)

American Society of Neuroradiology Gadolinium Deposition Committee (2015)

*NYU Winthrop Hospital Committees* (7/1/2000–3/15/2018)

Member: Executive Committee of the Medical Staff

Chairman—Department of Radiology; NYU Winthrop Hospital 7/1/2000–3/15/2018

Chairman—Departments of Radiology; Jacobi Medical Center (4/2/2018–)

VII. Evaluations, Honors, and Awards for Teaching

Distinguished faculty award 2005 SIR Annual Scientific Meeting Spine interventions workshop

Stony Brook University School of Medicine Contributions to Teaching: 2001, 2004.

Radiological Society of North America annual course evaluations: highly favorable (4.41–4.5/5.0), hence the annual renewal of each of the three workshops (spine biopsy, spine injections, vertebral augmentation)

Radiology resident evaluations at NYU Winthrop: "Excellent," "allows us to learn to perform basic spine injection procedures under supervision"

Medical student evaluations from Stony Brook: "lectures are tailored to our needs"; "neuroanatomy review is helpful"

Academic Certificate of Merit: Miller TS, Brook A, Georgy BA, Gangi A, **Ortiz AO**. Avoiding complications before, during, and after vertebral augmentation. RSNA 103rd Scientific Assembly and Annual Meeting (11/27–12/1/2017); Chicago, IL

Editorial Review: Editor's Recognition Award; *Journal of Women's Imaging: 2000–2004*

| Name | Year | Project | Result |
|---|---|---|---|
| College Student(s) | | | |
| S. Martinez | 2012 | Dual puncture epidural steroid injection | Publication |
| Medical Student(s) | | | |
| F. Cohen | 2017 | MRI safety | Presentation |
| Resident(s) | | | |
| J. Flug | 2013 | Economics of vertebral augmentation | Publication |
| Fellow(s) | | | |
| J. Agris | 2003 | Intravertebral pressure during vertebroplasty | Presentation |

## Leon McDougle, MD, MPH, DHL (h.c.), FAAFP

Doctor of Humane Letter (honoris causa) from Eastern Virginia Medical School, 2021, Fellow of the American Academy of Family Physicians.

Among the class of over 200 Ohio State University College of Medicine graduates, six of us were Black. My experience as a college of medicine student sparked my interest in becoming a medical school faculty member. Beyond Dr. Wilburn Weddington, who was the minority affairs associate dean, I encountered few Black faculty during preclinical courses and clinical rotations. I decided that I would pursue a pathway to become a faculty member to help become an answer the question that I asked: Where are the Black college of medicine faculty?

A family medicine research elective taught during the fourth year of medical school by Larry Gabel, PhD, helped me to establish foundational knowledge regarding review of medical literature, research terminology, and methods. This was followed by a research elective as a family medicine resident at the Naval Hospital Camp Pendleton, California with Gerald Klien, MD, an allergist who led a clinical research practice in San Diego, California. With mentoring by Dr. Klien, I conducted a national preventive medicine survey regarding instructions that emergency medicine physicians provided patients who developed Hymenoptera sting anaphylaxis. I was invited to present the findings at the Annual Conference of Allergy and Immunology in Manhattan, New York, during my third year of family medicine residency. Having an opportunity to present my research poster in New York was exciting.

Following completion of residency and encouragement by Captain Warren Jones, MD, I became a member of the National Medical Association. This enabled me to develop a national network of mentors while serving as secretary/historian, vice chair, and then chair of the Aerospace Military and Occupational Health Section. As I transitioned to leadership in the National Medical Association House of Delegates, I would gain additional academic career mentors. The National Medical Association also provided an excellent venue for me to give national presentations about my research and scholarship during the annual conventions and scientific assemblies that were helpful toward future academic medicine promotions in rank.

My first tour of duty following residency included service as the family physician member of Fleet Surgical Team Five for 2 years, and I participated in two Western Pacific (WestPac) deployments at sea with the US Marines and US Navy. Between deployments I served as faculty for the Naval Hospital Camp Pendleton Family Medicine Residency Program and later Research Coordinator after completion of 2 years of service on Fleet Surgical Team Five. I volunteered for as many training opportunities as time permitted. I completed the Medicine in the Tropics course in Puerto Rico and the Dominican Republic, the Cold Weather Medicine course 9000 feet above sea level in Bridgeport, California, and the Total Quality Leadership course among other courses.

After more than 7 years of active duty in the US Navy Reserve, where I gained proficiency in the full spectrum of Family Medicine, including obstetrics, I decided to transition to civilian practice. I was invited to interviews at about five family medicine residency programs in Ohio. My first interview was at a residency training program in my spouse's hometown, and after the department chair gave me the hard sell of needing to make a decision the same day, I accepted the offer to become a faculty member that I would soon learn was not the best decision. Within 6 months of being hired, I started looking for a new academic position. I would say, "I always wanted to obtain a Master's of Public Health degree." So, I explored family medicine departments affiliated with a school of public health. This go round, I interviewed at about five family medicine departments, and the final two programs being considered were competing for my services. The leadership, clinical, teaching, and research skills that I had acquired served me well. I selected the University of Michigan where I became a *clinical assistant professor* of family medicine and completed the 25-month On-Job-On-Campus Executive Master's of Public Health degree in Health Management and Policy. During each appointment as a faculty member, I had the good fortune to help teach and mentor Black and minoritized corpsmen, medical students and residents, some of whom I run into during national conferences. It is heartwarming and meaningful to learn about the positive influences that one can have on a learner's career.

I would then be offered an opportunity to complete a full circle and become the next assistant dean for diversity and multicultural affairs and founding associate program director for a new Urban Family Medicine Residency Program at the Ohio State University College of Medicine. I would be reunited with Dr. Larry Gabel, who, along with other professors, would provide the needed mentorship for advancement in rank.

**Jeannette E. South-Paul, MD, DHL(Hon), FAAFP**
EVP and Provost, Meharry Medical College
J. South-Paul Academic Consultants, LLC

As a child of immigrant parents from the West Indies who prioritized faith, family, and education, I recognized the importance of building networks and working hard to achieve career goals. I was fortunate to attend the University of Pittsburgh on an Army scholarship and soon realized that completing medical school would be dramatically influenced more by the discrimination I experienced as an African American woman, more so than the financial pressures I initially envisioned. Lack of mentorship at the institutional level and overt racial discrimination by faculty became rapidly apparent, so I sought support from a variety of professional sources inside the medical school and outside of medicine and joined the Student National Medical Association to help establish my community. Mentors were significant in my decision to commit to academic medicine and began with a support biochemistry professor at Pitt, Dr. Robert Glew, and an African American endocrinologist who took me under his wing on an away rotation at an Army Medical Center, James Reed, MD and ultimately came to the same med center I matched to as a founding director of a new Internal Medicine residency. My journey in Family Medicine impressed on me the importance of cross-disciplinary collaboration, community engagement, and supporting the next generation of physicians. These lessons also taught me how to manage discrimination that occurred later in my career—even in leadership positions—and the importance of integrity, commitment to the most vulnerable, quality practice, and solidifying one's personal support outside of one's local professional environment.

I served as a Medical Corps officer in the US Army, retiring in 2001 while serving as chair of family medicine at the Uniformed Services University of the Health Sciences and previously as vice president for minority affairs at the same institution. I was then recruited back to my alma mater to unify the Department of Family Medicine and became the Andrew W. Mathieson UPMC professor and chair of the Department of Family Medicine at the University of Pittsburgh School of Medicine from 2001 to 2020 (returning to Pittsburgh after 22 years in the army—although I had vowed never to return to Pittsburgh). I retired from Pitt in 2020—as the Covid pandemic began to surge—and began a consulting group to address issues of leadership and supporting those from diverse backgrounds who were in higher education and the health sciences. After more than 10 years of service as a member of the Meharry Medical College Board of Trustees, I stepped off the board to begin a new leadership role where I can work with the academic leaders of the five schools (medicine, dentistry, graduate studies, applied computational sciences, and global health). As the executive vice president and provost since December 2021—I have the opportunity to contribute to the vision of an institution branching its commitment to diversity, education, clinical care, creating new knowledge, and creating health equity for the local and global community.

I have served in leadership positions in the Society of Teachers of Family Medicine (STFM), the American Academy of Family Physicians (AAFP), the Association of American Medical Colleges (AAMC), and the Association of Departments of Family Medicine (ADFM), including serving as president of the Uniformed Services Academy of Family Physicians (USAFP) and the STFM. I am also a member of the National Academy of Medicine, the Gold Humanism Society, and the Alpha Omega Alpha Medical Honorary Society.

## References

1. Beasley BW, Simon SD, Wright SM. A time to be promoted. The prospective study of promotion in academia. J Gen Intern Med. 2006;21(2):123–9. https://doi.org/10.1111/j.1525-1497.2005.00297.x. Epub 2005 Dec 7. PMID: 16336619; PMCID: PMC1484667.
2. Coleman MM, Richard GV. Faculty career tracks at U.S. medical schools. Acad Med. 2011;86(8):932–7.
3. Collins J. Teacher or educational scholar? They aren't the same. J Am Coll Radiol. 2004;1:135–9.
4. Levine MS. Primer for clinician scholars in academic radiology. Radiology. 2004;231:622–7.
5. Faculty Roster: U.S. Medical School Faculty, Association of American Medical Colleges. https://www.aamc.org/data-reports/faculty-institutions/report/faculty-roster-us-medical-school-faculty. Accessed on 5 July 2025.
6. Rodriguez JE, Campbell KM, Pololi LH. Addressing disparities in academic medicine: what of the minority tax? BMC Med Educ. 2015;15:6.
7. Chapman T, Carrico C, Vagal AS, Paladin AM. Promotion as a clinician educator in academic radiology departments: guidelines at three major institutions. Acad Radiol. 2012;19(1):119–24.
8. Jhala K, Kim J, Chetlen A, Nickerson JP, Lewis PJ. The clinician-educator pathway in radiology: an analysis of institutional promotion criteria. J Am Coll Radiol. 2017;14(12):1588–93.
9. Lalwani N, Shanbhogue KP, Jambhekar K, Jha S, Ram R, Itri JN, Tappouni R. New job, new challenges: life after radiology training. Am J Roentgenol. 2019;212:483–9.
10. Callahan EJ, Banks M, Medina J, Disbrow K, Soto-Greene M, Sánchez JP. Providing diverse trainees an early and transparent introduction to academic appointment and promotion processes. MedEdPORTAL. 2017;13:10661. https://doi.org/10.15766/mep_2374-8265.10661.
11. Fernandez CR, Lucas R, Soto-Greene M, Sánchez JP. Introducing trainees to academic medicine career roles and responsibilities. MedEdPORTAL. 2017;13:10653. https://www.mededportal.org/doi/10.15766/mep_2374-8265.10653
12. Kuhn GJ. Faculty development: the educator's portfolio: its preparation, uses, and value in academic medicine. Acad Emerg Med. 2004;11(3):307–11.
13. Thomas JV, Sanyal R, O'Malley JP, Singh SP, Morgan DE, Canon CL. A guide to writing academic portfolios for radiologists. Acad Radiol. 2016;23(12):1595–603.
14. UMass Chan Medical School, Office of Faculty Affairs: Process FOR faculty promotion Faculty Affairs—UMass Chan Medical School. Accessed 12 Nov 2024.
15. Sánchez JP, Lowe C, Freeman M, Burton W, Sánchez NF, Beil R. A syphilis control intervention targeting black and Hispanic men who have sex with men. J Health Care Poor Underserved. 2009;20(1):194–209. https://doi.org/10.1353/hpu.0.0103. PMID: 19202257.
16. Twombly EC, Holtz KD, Stringer K. Using promotores programs to improve Latino health outcomes: implementation challenges for community-based nonprofit organizations. J Soc Serv Res. 2012;38(3):305–12. https://doi.org/10.1080/01488376.2011.633804. Epub 2012 Apr 24. PMID: 23188929; PMCID: PMC3505454.

17. Wrench A, Vélez-Figueroa AC, de Lamadrid JJRG, Pommells K, Sánchez JP. Diseases transmitted by arthropods: module to train medical providers in English and Spanish. MedEdPORTAL. 2025;21:11509. https://doi.org/10.15766/mep_2374-8265.11509.
18. Aby ES, Kriss M, Rubin DT, Pillai A. How to navigate national societal organizations for leadership development and academic promotion: a guide for trainees and young faculty. Gastroenterology. 2021;161(5):1361–5.
19. Latino Surgical Society. https://www.latinosurgicalsociety.org. Accessed on 9 June 2025.
20. Sánchez JP, Ellis D, Plaza V, Vélez A, Rodriguez J, Duque Lasio L, Quintero-Rivera F. Addressing the minority tax by building diversity capital: a case-based discussion. MedEdPORTAL. 2025;21:11536. https://doi.org/10.15766/mep_2374-8265.11536.
21. Williamson T, Goodwin CR, Ubel PA. Minority tax reform—avoiding overtaxing minorities when we need them most. N Engl J Med. 2021;384(20):1877–9.
22. Campbell KM, Rodriguez JE. Addressing the minority tax: perspectives from two diversity leaders on building minority faculty success in academic medicine. Acad Med. 2019;94:1854–7.
23. Poole KG, McDougle L. There is still bias in-patient satisfaction data. J Natl Med Assoc. 2020;112(3):242.
24. Bullock JL, O'Brien MT, Minhas PK, Fernandez A, Lupton KL, Hauer KE. No one size fits all: a qualitative study of clerkship medical students' perceptions of ideal supervisor responses to microaggressions. Acad Med. 2021;96(11S):S71–80.
25. Hill Weller LM, Tang J, Chen R, Boscardin C, Ehie O. Tools for addressing microaggressions: an interactive workshop for perioperative trainees. MedEdPORTAL. 2023;19:11360. https://doi.org/10.15766/mep_2374-8265.11360.
26. Stephens KC, Redman T, Williams R, Bandstra B, Shah R. Considering culture and conflict: a novel approach to active bystander intervention. MedEdPORTAL. 2023;19:11338. https://doi.org/10.15766/mep_2374-8265.11338.
27. Lin MP, Lall MD, Samuels-Kalow M, Das D, Linden JA, Perman S, Chang AM, Agrawal P. Impact of a women-focused professional organization on academic retention and advancement: perceptions from a qualitative study. Acad Emerg Med. 2019;26(3):303–16.

**Open Access** This chapter is licensed under the terms of the Creative Commons Attribution 4.0 International License (http://creativecommons.org/licenses/by/4.0/), which permits use, sharing, adaptation, distribution and reproduction in any medium or format, as long as you give appropriate credit to the original author(s) and the source, provide a link to the Creative Commons license and indicate if changes were made.

The images or other third party material in this chapter are included in the chapter's Creative Commons license, unless indicated otherwise in a credit line to the material. If material is not included in the chapter's Creative Commons license and your intended use is not permitted by statutory regulation or exceeds the permitted use, you will need to obtain permission directly from the copyright holder.

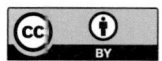

# Chapter 9
# Succeeding Along the Educator Track from Assistant to Full Professor

Alvaro Pérez Arcila and Maria Soto-Greene

> **Learning Objectives**
> - Outline expectations to move from Assistant to Full Professor.
> - Demonstrate how conducting LHS+-related work can facilitate promotion.
> - Summarize available resources to support the promotion of individuals identifying as LHS+ along the educator track.

This is an exciting time to consider being on an educator track. Medical education continues to evolve from the legacy of the two plus two preclinical to clinical education model. The accelerating pace of transformation in medical education, coupled with the expansion of new medical schools and class sizes, has intensified the demand for skilled medical educators to shape the next generation of physicians [1, 2]. Our present state invites and challenges medical schools to incorporate content, activities, and experiences for learners to prepare for patient care across multiple populations. Schools are seeking to better equip learners with the skills, knowledge, and behaviors necessary to practice in this ever-changing landscape of health systems. This change has been fueled, in part, by the American Medical Association (AMA) Accelerating Change in Medical Education initiative in response to the Lancet Commission on Education of Health Professionals for the Twenty-First Century report [1]. Equally important is the imperative to achieve a diverse workforce and inclusive learning environment as highlighted in lessons learned by the AMA Accelerating Change in Medical Education Consortium, which reaffirmed

A. P Arcila (✉)
Universidad Central del Caribe, Bayamon, Puerto Rico

M. Soto-Greene
Rutgers New Jersey Medical School (NJMS), Newark, NJ, USA

© The Author(s) 2026
J. P. Sánchez et al. (eds.), *Advancing Latino, Hispanic, or of Spanish Origin+ Leadership in Academic Medicine*, https://doi.org/10.1007/978-3-032-07570-3_9

the need for collective efforts to address recruitment and support historically marginalized groups [3]. Moreover, "A Snapshot of Medical Student Education in the United States (US) and Canada: Reports From 145 Schools," published in Academic Medicine, featured 145 out of the 171 allopathic medical schools at the time of the report. The snapshot provides key highlights into the curriculum, the overall medical education program, governance, and other new initiatives. Of particular note, this compendium does not include the type of unprecedented changes in medical education that have occurred in response to the *COVID-19* pandemic and that continue to transform how and what we teach [4]. The aforementioned changes were overlaid throughout a 25-year time span from 1980 to 2005 during a period when there was essentially no growth in the number of graduates from MD-granting schools. The decision to implement the changes was based on the initial recommendations of reports by the Council on Graduate Medical Education (COGME) that repeatedly cautioned against overproducing the number of physicians, only to later note the need for physician workforce expansion [5–7]. Subsequently, the Association for American Medical Colleges (AAMC) issued a series of workforce projections that upheld the recommendations and demonstrated the need for more physicians [2].

Educators are a subgroup of the academic medicine workforce. Carrying responsibilities and duties that support an institution's teaching mission is central to the track. Although the inclusion of Latina/o/x/e, Hispanic, or Spanish Origin+ (LHS+) professionals in the educator workforce within academic medicine has gained attention in recent years, their representation remains limited. While many medical schools and healthcare institutions have recognized the value of diversity, tangible representation of LHS+ faculty, particularly in senior academic ranks, is still disproportionately lower relative to the growth rate of the LHS+ population in the USA [8]. Several factors impact this underrepresentation. LHS+ individuals face unique challenges and facilitators in achieving inclusion and success in academic medicine, which are shaped by both systemic barriers and cultural strengths. A key challenge includes underrepresentation in faculty and leadership positions, often stemming from historical disparities in educational access, implicit biases, and limited mentorship opportunities [9]. Programs that provide early mentorship and sponsorship opportunities have proven effective in helping LHS+ faculty gain critical academic skills and create supportive professional networks. Thus, increasing their sense of belonging and career satisfaction [10].

Increased representation of LHS+ educators enhances medical education by introducing critical cultural competence and bilingual capabilities to learners, both of which strengthen patient-centered education and improve healthcare outcomes for underserved communities [10, 11]. LHS+ educators, when included in the academic workforce, are uniquely positioned to shape medical curricula by addressing health disparities, embedding cultural competence, and fostering trust within historically underserved communities [10, 11]. The inclusion of LHS+ educators within the academic workforce fosters a more supportive learning environment for LHS+ medical students and residents by providing culturally concordant role models, which can enhance students' sense of belonging, mentorship opportunities, and academic success [10, 11]. Although progress is being made, increasing LHS+ inclusion in medical education requires concerted efforts. This includes investing in mentorship programs, promoting equitable hiring and promotion practices, and ensuring accountability within diversity, equity, and inclusion (DEI) initiatives [11]. Academic institutions that intentionally cultivate inclusive environments for LHS+ educators not only advance faculty success and retention but also enhance the quality, relevance, and cultural responsiveness of medical education in an increasingly diverse society [10, 11].

## What Does an Educator Track Encompass?

An academic track description will always align with the track's promotion criteria. No matter the size of the institution, the rules for promotion along the selected track are pretty similar, varying mainly by the weight assigned to each component (teaching, research, and service) and the amount of evidence required.

Assuming that your list of professional priorities includes having the opportunity to influence the next generation and that you have decided that the best way to do this is to dedicate your time and continued professional development to teaching, then the educator track may be the best track option for you. The next step is to decide whether you want to do this as a faculty member who (a) primarily focuses on your area of clinical expertise and also teaches students or trainees or (b) is responsible for shaping what is taught, how learners learn, effective evaluation, and influencing the learning environment. The latter pathway, requiring formal expertise in educational theory and practice, remains both a critical gap and an identified strategic need in many medical schools [12].

Being on the educator track, you will be expected to spend the majority of your time teaching medical students, residents, fellows, and colleagues. Generally, promotion on this track will depend on the results of your teaching evaluations from learners across the continuum; invitations to guest lecture across your institution, regionally, nationally, and internationally; contributions to curricular development; medical education scholarship and research; committee work related to clinical teaching; and your clinical service efforts. Academic institutions have a variety of names for their faculty tracks. Some, but not all, institutions have a unique blend of titles under the educator umbrella, and it is important to be aware of the weight assigned to each mission-based component in your selected track. At Universidad Central Del Caribe, including the School of Medicine, different tracks have different weights assigned to mission-based components: (a) educator (90% teaching, 10% service), (b) researcher-educator (60% research, 30% teaching, 10% service), (c) clinical-educator (clinical 60%, teaching 30%, service 10%), and (d) educator-administrator (Administration 70%, teaching 10%, service 20%). Whereas at New Jersey Medical School of Rutgers University, for Clinician Educator/Academic Educator, Assistant Professor, "Time Allotment is up to 80% devoted to patient care and/or medical education/teaching and at least 20% for scholarly activities, including research focused in the areas of medical education (M.D. or Ph.D.)" [13]. The relevance of these two examples is to be aware of the evidence that would be required for you to be promoted at your own institution, so you can tailor your faculty development plan accordingly.

## Overview of the Missions

As an overview, each one of the missions, teaching, research, and service (both clinical and administrative), requires documented evidence to demonstrate compliance with the particular institution's requirements. This is why maintaining a regular monthly practice of updating your CV is imperative! The daily work of an educator provides opportunities to meet promotion criteria, but we need to transform the daily work into tangible evidence that can be appropriately cited (Table 9.1).

These are some examples of common activities that are part of an education or teaching portfolio. For some tracks at specific institutions, a teaching portfolio could be included as part of your promotion application or dossier package. Given this requirement, you must reframe how you think about and document your education contributions such that you can legitimately transform them into scholarly

**Table 9.1** Teaching activities

| Teaching activities that could count as evidence are: | | |
|---|---|---|
| At the hospital | At the classroom | At curriculum design and administration |
| Bedside teaching | Scheduling activities | Developing teaching materials (study guides, syllabus, assignments) and assessments (rubrics, checklists, MCQ) used by others |
| Grand rounds | Lectures | New curriculum development/renewal |
| Morbidity and mortality conference | Direct teaching activities | |
| Resident core conferences | | |
| Chief of service conferences | | |
| Journal club | | |
| Residents as teachers | | |
| Board review conferences | | |
| Simulation conferences | | |
| Biostatistics conferences | | |
| Wellness curriculum | | |
| Mentoring/tutoring | | |

**Table 9.2** Service and administrative activities

| Clinical service | Course or clerkship director | Administration |
|---|---|---|
| Direct patient care | Scheduling activities | Committee membership |
| Supervising trainees at clinical settings | Curricular tagging | Quality improvement activities |
| Mentoring community activities | Administering exams | Department director |
| | Proctoring | Program director |
| | Grading | Dean (Assistant, Associate, or Dean) |
| | Reporting | |
| | Keeping the learning management up to date | |

production. In this reframing, you want to note the various types of scholarship you are engaging, so that project offshoots become peer-reviewed publications (e.g., original articles, invited commentaries, abstracts, book chapters, monographs, patents, and in some schools, even case reports). There are several prestigious journals for educators to consider, such as Academic Medicine, MedEdPORTAL, Clinical Teacher, and Medical Education, to name a few. Other forms of service for educators to be promoted include membership and activity in national professional societies; presentations as an invited speaker; being a member of an editorial and reviewer team for journals; or being invited to review manuscripts, books, and conference submissions. We review these options in the table below (Table 9.2).

When you can document that you have become regionally, nationally, and internationally known in your field, it bodes well for promotion. The key to promotion on the educator track is to demonstrate your prestigious "reach" outside of the four walls of your institution. From a clinical standpoint, this could also mean that your "reach" leads to increased patient referrals, naming as director of a clinic or clinical service line, including patient outcomes, development and publication of clinical education materials, or leading successful quality improvement activities. This is a golden opportunity for an LHS+ faculty to highlight their efforts in addressing the Hispanic/Latino health disparities through the development, implementation, and evaluation of curriculum that reflects the Latino experiences (e.g., Taking Care of the Puerto Rican Patient: Historical Perspectives, Health Status, and Health Care Access) [14], electives in medical Spanish (e.g., Medical Spanish in US Medical Schools: a National Survey to Examine Existing Programs) [15], research in health disparities, healthcare services initiatives, and voluntary work directed to address these issues among the LHS+ communities (video tool to promote knowledge of syphilis among black and Hispanic men recruited from clinical and nonclinical settings) [16]. Be sure to include such efforts in your submission materials, CV, and portfolio.

Research activities are the most common and best understood of all missions, as traditional measures of scholarly productivity used by decanal promotion review committees include [17] (Table 9.3) the following:

**Table 9.3** Research categories

| Internal or external funding research | | | | |
|---|---|---|---|---|
| Bench research | Translational research | Clinical research | Community research | Educational research |

Even for educator tracks, the number of publications, your H-index, conference presentation of your original education research findings, and/or educational grant award funding totals from industry, state, or federal sources will be assessed and scored for promotion.

## Overview of Advancing by Rank

Most faculty begin their career at the instructor level. In most institutions, if you are a clinician, once board-certified, you can be promoted or appointed to the assistant professor rank. It should be noted that appointment as an instructor may allow for additional time to be considered for those seeking a tenure-track position. In some institutions, time to promotion to the next academic rank is delineated, and not doing so, achieving promotion within the specified number of years, may result in nonrenewal of your academic agreement. Thus, the next question to consider is whether your educator track has term limits during which advancement must be achieved.

Advancement from Assistant to Associate Professor criteria vary by institution [18]. For some faculty, they may select "areas of excellence" within several domains:

*Scholarship*, know the type of scholarship that is accepted [19], and the amount your institution requires, which is often less specific.
*Clinical excellence*, if applicable, which may include productivity.
*Teaching*, demonstrated contribution, type of education (pre-clerkship, clerkship, residency), volume and impact as noted by student/resident outcomes, awards (teaching awards, nomination), mentorship (list outcome of the relationship), and.
*Service*: State or regional reputation, including invited grand rounds, and service on committees (describe role with a level of detail, as committee members may not always know the impact).
*Other* key emerging criteria include diversity-related work and evidence of impact.

Once successful, you are considered mid-level faculty and have an incredible opportunity to have influential seats at the table that contribute to the careers of others. However, remember you have not reached the next and, in many cases, the last rung on the ladder. You need to continue to forge ahead with meeting the criteria for Full Professor, which are similarly structured to Associate Professor, with an expectation of national and/or international prominence based on the school.

## Additional Considerations That Extend Beyond the Missions

When you are developing your initial plan, take a look at the proportions of faculty members in each rank available at your institution, a wider base of instructors or assistant professors with a narrow apex, will require a very structured plan with strong support from mentors and all available resources, with close monitoring of the timely and efficient outcomes achievements. Be sure that the institutions provide a strong mentorship program and a wide range of options via the office of faculty affairs and career development, or its equivalent. In addition to the proportion, the expected time that it will take you from one rank to the following and up to the full professor is a key factor to include in your analysis when you are creating your plan.

Know that all institutions, whether at the university level or the school of medicine level, have an administrative system to support your goal to be promoted and get to the final rank of professor. Seek out support and guidance from your faculty affairs and career development office, department/hospital or school-level faculty-to-faculty mentoring program, local or abroad peers, professional associations, and your immediate supervisor (chief/chair/dean) and dotted-line supervisors (residency/fellowship director). There are even LHS+ specific faculty development programming where individuals of LHS+ lived experiences or non-LHS+ faculty engaged in LHS+-related activities can discuss unique barriers and facilitators to being promoted, such as the LHS+ Development, Identity, Empowerment, and Resources Seminar (LIDEReS) of the LMSA Faculty Physician Advisory Council [20]. You are not alone in the process. There are many resources in-house and externally that will help you navigate the academic world, but you need to start the process; your sole determination is the main fuel to move the machine. For an LHS+ faculty member or leader in any healthcare institution or teaching center, it is highly recommended to explore if these criteria are already included in their own "institution's procedures," or "review it," and propose new and expanded up-to-date best practices [21].

## Reflection and Skills Exercise

**Case Scenario**
Margarita, a South American descendant, is an internal medicine physician who began her academic career as a faculty member 10 years ago. She completed her residency program at a large academic center and started her faculty position on the nontenured academic track as an assistant professor focused on clinical scholarship. Over the decade, she developed a robust clinical program focused on the LHS+ community and has fellows from different specialty programs under her guidance. During her time as an academic faculty member, she published about three articles as a second author. She also participated as a mentor for team-based learning

activities where she developed many case scenarios and relevant assessment tools, served as the medical student director, and was an active member of the curriculum committee. She has continued at the rank of assistant professor on her current track.

At this point in her career, is she ready for academic promotion?

- As you consider this question, it is important to collect information. Review the faculty promotions manual to better understand the criteria for promotion. Margarita should speak with leadership in her department and with individuals who were recently promoted to learn more about the process and consider if she meets criteria for promotion.

What resources can she use to drive her career to pursue a promotion to associate professor?

- In addition to reviewing the faculty promotions manual, Margarita should attend faculty development sessions, often through the department or Office of Faculty Affairs and Career Development and seek out mentors who can guide her in the process of being promoted.

What would you advise her to focus on to obtain the goal of promotion?

- It is important for Margarita to consider the criteria outlined in the faculty promotions manual and appropriate outcomes. She has three articles as second author, but she should strive to be first author on a few publications. She should note the number of mentees she has and what goals she has assisted them in achieving, for example, performing well on exams, matching into preferred specialty, etc. She should collect evaluation forms from her teaching sessions that show her competence and excellence in teaching.

Taking the time to reflect on questions such as these and thinking about *your* own accomplishments are important for your growth and understanding. Seek input from your advisors and/or mentor/s may have longer-term implications in providing you with the joy and fulfillment that contributes to retention and job satisfaction.

**Skills Exercise**
CV audit with criteria comparison: As stated in the teaching mission section, updating your CV regularly is important. However, aligning your past activities and making plans to accept a project or not are equally important in order to stay focused on meeting educator promotion criteria.

*Step 1.* Pull up your institution's latest promotion criteria for educators. If you do not know where to access it, contact your department chair or faculty affairs office. Be aware that criteria and dossier requirements can be revised annually depending on your department or school of medicine.

*Step 2.* Go through your CV and highlight your teaching activities (papers, courses, service, single talks, curricular development). Note how many activities you have done during the time of your current rank *only*. On paper, do you look like someone on an educator track? Is your "area of excellence" shining through?

**Table 9.4** Sample worksheet for CV self-audit

| Teaching-related activity listed on promotion criteria | Quantity and importance | Planning: note to self |
|---|---|---|
| Formal course teaching | Note how many | How can I improve my evaluations? Should I get more involved in certain teaching activities? How do I get more involved? |
| Informal bedside teaching, M&M, clinical case conference | Scores on evaluations from trainees | How can I improve my scores or comments? |
| Grand rounds inside and outside my home department | Note how many and where | How can I improve the CME evaluations related to these talks? Where or how many more should I seek to give? |
| Other | | |

Have you had a national reach? Would you promote yourself? If not, yet, note what four additions you would like to make to your CV. Then, write *how* you will fulfill each addition. Do this for each mission. You can use the following template to guide your self-audit (Table 9.4).

## Career Planning for Educators

Take the time to revisit your career goals to see where you are. Understand what is expected of you to get promoted. Set a timeline and reassess at least twice a year. This allows you to keep abreast of the promotion criteria. During the annual evaluation, assess progress made, and revise deliverables. Do the duties allow you to meet the requirements for promotion? This goal setting also serves as a promotion milestone in your journey to associate professor. Remember that mentorship matters, and networking is essential to being invited to serve on regional or national committees or grand rounds. Keep in mind and ask yourself if you have the skills to carry out the activity. Whether initially or after being hired, faculty development is always essential, moving you along the continuum of becoming an expert educator tailored to the area of responsibility. To assist you, consider using a faculty development plan. We present some of the key components from the Rutgers New Jersey Medical School Faculty Development Plan as a guide [13]:

Step 1: Clarify your values: what drives you, such as being an educator.
Step 2: Set Your Mission: be succinct—Think BIG—consider it fitting a T-shirt slogan.
Step 3: Assess Your Skills using SWOT analysis for selected areas; define your developmental needs (writing skills, presentations).
Step 4: Planning Your Career: How will you demonstrate expertise as a clinician educator in Scholarship, Teaching and Learner Development, Professional Skills, Leadership, Patient Care, and Service?

What are your professional goals for the upcoming year?
What are your long-term career goals (3–5 years)?
What are some motivating factors for pursuing these goals?
Are there any circumstances or barriers that may make it more challenging to achieve your goals for the upcoming year?
Which of the above goals did you meet? If you did not meet a goal, why?

By definition, any professional development opportunity should help LHS+ faculty understand their role in education and how to improve or acquire relevant knowledge and skills that better prepare them for a successful academic career.

Common pitfalls related to planning for promotion readiness include a focus on salary, while incredibly important, cannot be the sole priority; insufficient time to carry out the educational activities; and insufficient mentorship [22]. Several challenges can impede progression in an academic career if not managed thoughtfully:

1. *Neglecting Scholarship and Documentation*: Many faculty members excel in teaching and clinical duties but may overlook the need to document these contributions as scholarly work. Converting daily teaching efforts into impactful scholarship, such as peer-reviewed publications or educational materials, is essential for promotion. Document all your work and strive to publish it.
2. *Insufficient Mentorship and Networking*: Faculty who do not actively seek advisors, mentors or network broadly may miss key guidance and opportunities that can enhance their professional development. This can lead to missed promotion criteria or a lack of visibility in regional and national circles. Also, by expanding your network, you can identify potential recommendation letter writers for promotion.
3. *Overcommitting without Strategic Focus*: While it may be tempting to take on numerous roles, overextending oneself can dilute focus and prevent achieving the necessary benchmarks in each promotion area. Balancing roles and aligning them with long-term goals are critical for sustainable advancement.
4. *Underestimating Institutional Requirements*: Academic institutions often have nuanced requirements for promotion, which may vary by track or rank. Failing to thoroughly understand these can result in missing essential steps in documentation or focusing efforts on less impactful activities.

Additionally, there are many challenges for the LHS+ faculty when it comes to persistence and social integration into the academy [23]. However, in our opinion, these seven could be the most relevant for your educator journey:

1. *Misinformation and Stereotypes:* LHS+ medical educators often face harmful misconceptions and stereotypes about their ability to teach effectively, leading to a hostile work environment and a real impact on their ability to provide students with the best education. The representation of LHS+ faculty in different roles and capacities in the institution can help decrease stigmas surrounding LHS+ identities in society as a whole.
2. *Lack of Inclusivity:* While many medical schools and healthcare centers have policies that promote inclusivity, there is still a lack of support for LHS+ medical

educators in many institutions. This leads to a sense of isolation and a loss of connection with coworkers and the wider educational community, affecting opportunities for growth and collaboration. The support of allies within the education system is vital in bringing authentic change and creating opportunities for LHS+ faculty members. Allies not only support the professional and emotional well-being of LHS+ medical educators but also help to improve the educational outcomes of students.

3. *Mental Health and Well-Being:* LHS+ medical educators also face unique stressors due to systemic oppression and discrimination, which can negatively affect their mental health and well-being. Addressing this through inclusive work practices can help improve their job satisfaction and promote the success of their students.

   Developing stronger faculty networks or associations that advocate for LHS+ inclusivity is a great way to provide support for LHS+ faculty and connect them with a wider community of medical educators. This also ensures that institutional changes in support of LHS+ faculty are sustained.

   LHS+ faculty have unique assets that can transform medical education. These individuals bring diverse perspectives and experiences that enrich the learning environment. Their cultural background, language skills, and understanding of health disparities can help bridge the gap between healthcare providers and underserved communities. The following are some assets that these individuals bring to the institution:

4. *Cultural Competence*: LHS+ individuals have a deep understanding of their culture and traditions. This knowledge can help healthcare providers develop cultural competence and provide better care to patients from diverse backgrounds. By incorporating cultural competency into medical education, LHS+ individuals can help reduce health disparities and improve patient outcomes.

5. *Language Skills*: LHS+ individuals are often bilingual or multilingual, which is a valuable asset in any healthcare setting. By speaking the same language as their patients, they can improve communication and build trust. Incorporating language skills into medical education can help future healthcare providers communicate more effectively with their patients and provide better care.

6. *Health Disparities*: LHS+ individuals are more likely to experience health disparities due to systemic inequalities. Their experiences can help healthcare providers understand the root causes of these disparities and work toward eliminating them. By incorporating the perspectives of LHS+ individuals into medical education, future healthcare providers can be better equipped to address health disparities and provide equitable care to all patients.

7. *Community Engagement*: LHS+ individuals have strong ties to their communities and can serve as advocates for better health care. By engaging with their communities, they can help healthcare providers better understand the needs of underserved populations. Incorporating community engagement into medical education can help future healthcare providers develop a deeper understanding of the social determinants of health and the importance of community-based care.

LHS+ individuals have unique assets that can transform medical education and improve healthcare outcomes for all patients. By incorporating their perspectives and experiences into medical education, we can create a more inclusive and culturally competent healthcare system.

## Conclusion

Remember how you will demonstrate your excellence, and that you are in control. Know the benefits of your track and the countless opportunities available. It is your time to make a difference while at the same time being noticed for the work and impact you have on so many others. By advancing yourself, you can change the "status quo" by opening the door of opportunities for others.

The journey from Assistant to Full Professor is a multifaceted path, particularly for those on the educator track who are focused on enriching medical education. For LHS+ faculty, this journey offers an incredible opportunity to influence and reshape medical education, bridging cultural gaps and addressing health disparities. By understanding institutional expectations, setting achievable milestones, and leveraging resources like mentorship and faculty development programs, LHS+ educators can navigate this path with clarity and purpose. The diversity and unique skills they bring are invaluable in creating an inclusive, culturally competent healthcare workforce prepared to meet the needs of an increasingly diverse patient population. As you advance in your career, remember that each achievement not only propels you forward but also paves the way for future generations of educators and leaders in medicine. Your dedication to excellence in teaching, scholarship, and service will leave a lasting impact on students, institutions, and communities alike. Never lose sight of what an educator's reach can be. Scholarly engagement and promotion position you to seek leadership roles: division chief, chair, residency/fellowship directorships, associate dean positions (education, faculty affairs, faculty development, graduate medical education), and provost.

## Personal Narratives

### Alvaro Perez, MD-MS-MMEL
Assistant Dean for Curriculum Development, Accreditation, and Licensing
Universidad Central del Caribe, School of Medicine

I am a physician by training and originally from Colombia in South America. After finishing medical school, I continued my education as a researcher, aiming to become part of a clinical/translational investigative team. As such, I subsequently obtained my master's degree in Pharmacogenetics. Upon completing my master's training, I was hired at my home institution in Colombia, where I started my journey as a researcher, teacher, and clinician. After a year, the chief of the department encouraged me to apply for a position as both a teacher and researcher in a basic science department at a medical school in Puerto Rico. I was curious and applied. In an exciting turn, the medical school hired me in less than a month as my academic journey moved to the United States.

I started as an assistant professor in the Biochemistry department, in charge of biochemistry, cell biology, and genetics courses, and developing the molecular biology and pharmacogenetics lab. Everything seemed to be on track for me. However, 3 years later, and after one major hurricane, my experience took a turn. Sadly, I learned that my freezers and other equipment were not attached to the emergency power supply system. As a result, I lost all my samples, materials, and a portion of my equipment. I was now in the situation of restarting my career. In a serendipitous experience, the dean of the medical school requested assistance with administrative projects. I utilized this opportunity to explore other facades of an academic career, while I redirected my career plans. I was pleasantly surprised by the options.

At the time of my exploration and administrative service with the dean, the School of Medicine was deeply immersed in institutional accreditation, program accreditation, renovation of operations licensing, developing a new strategic plan, and starting a curricular review. I had little experience in these areas, but the challenge was so appealing. I made a goal to strengthen these areas to have a better foundation for my aspiring role as a leader in academic affairs. I, then, became a member of various committees and attended conferences and professional development after the first successful accreditation. After the accreditation experience, my academic career took off! I assumed multiple leadership positions, to the tune of being appointed as director of institutional research, leading the planning team, and cochairing the curricular review. At that moment, I was satisfied. I decided to keep the administrative responsibilities in addition to my teaching responsibilities.

After 10 years in the role, my career mentor advised me to go up for a professorial promotion to the next academic rank. My mentor also encouraged me to invest in continuing formal education for further advancement. After some research and values exploration, I applied to the Certificate in Medical Education and Leadership from the AAMC. This is a 2-year experience that led me to apply to a master's program in medical education. As part of the program, my mentor and I decided that such upskilling would improve my portfolio and increase my competitiveness for a higher position at another institution. Upon completing it, I put it to the test. I sent my CV to other medical schools, and in less than 1 month, I received an invitation for an interview for the position of Assistant Dean of Curriculum Development at another medical school in Puerto Rico. This career move added a new chapter to my career wherein I became part of the institution's presidential cabinet while maintaining an educator's footprint in teaching and course planning.

I continued with this formula and invested more time in professional development from national programs. I subsequently finished my Healthcare Executive Diversity and Inclusion Certificate (HEDIC) at the AAMC and served as the first Chief Diversity Officer of the university under the direct supervision of the president.

**Maria Soto-Greene, MD**
Professor and Executive Vice Dean
Rutgers New Jersey Medical School

Reaching the upper rungs of the promotion ladder can be onerous. It is a path that can be laden with hurdles that may cause one to alter their direction. Yet, in sharing this story, the advancement in medicine is indescribably fulfilling. As I reflect on both the joys and setbacks in this professional journey, I recognize the impact that mentorship has had on my career when combined with my resilience, perseverance, and work ethic. Today, in my leadership role and as a full Professor with tenure, I dedicate myself to making the invisible visible and providing those who aspire to careers in or advancement in medicine with the tools they need to be successful.

In this promotion journey, it is essential to consider the milestones in your personal life that have contributed to your success. For me, the story begins with my Puerto Rican grandmother, who left an indelible footprint in my life. She was a quiet, kind, gentle woman who selflessly cared for the family through depression, poverty, and as a single parent in Puerto Rico. She, like my mother, came to the USA with a dream of a better life and worked in a factory, providing for a growing family. My parents divorced at a young age. However, the traditions rooted in the meaning of family prepared me for life's twists and turns. I was the second to finish high school, the first and 1 of 2 of 11 cousins to enter college, and subsequently the first and only MD.

Senior year of high school proved to be the most memorable challenge. My brother, only 11 months younger, became ill and bed bound. He died with only a presumptive diagnosis, awaiting an appointment with a "super specialist." Years later, as a physician, I wonder whether he would still be alive if we had insurance or the financial resources to pay for his care. This experience has served as my lifelong commitment to addressing the social determinants of health.

As I transitioned from being a chief resident to faculty, I knew I had clinical competence. I was known for addressing every administrative and service challenge put before me. In many ways, I told myself that if I could face life's hurdles, then I could handle any academic challenge. The first rung in the ladder from instructor to assistant professor was a smooth one. I was the Director of our Medical Intensive Care Units, already homing in on the importance of teamwork and collaboration within medicine, specialties, and across professions. Academically, in addition to training residents and fellows, I was actively involved in medical education for second and fourth year medical students and committees that spanned the hospital, school, and university levels. I also immersed myself in professional development with a focus on my identity as a minority and attended AAMC development conferences. As I look back, all the work I did fueled my desire to make a difference, especially in the lives of the underrepresented and underserved. This reinforced my commitment to focusing on the social determinants of health from many vantage points.

It is equally important to periodically self-assess, asking yourself when it is too much and whether these contributions will allow you to balance your passion with the expected upward mobility requisite of academia. It is indeed doable, but you need to have a plan that you revisit regularly. This leads me to the next rung of Associate Professor. It also proved to be relatively smooth, largely supported by the work that I had done as an assistant professor. At this time, I became nationally active and generally received almost every grant that I applied for, focusing on diversity and workforce development across the continuum from precollege to college and pre-matriculation to faculty.

I transitioned from intensive care to primary care with a focus on leadership as an associate dean. I continued to be tapped at the school, university, and national levels as someone who was contributing to new strategies and practices impacting those like me. I joined like-minded colleagues who, as products of the pipeline, wanted to make a difference that leveraged our historically underrepresented communities. A pivotal point was to remember the influence of family. While I knew that my dean, school, and department were behind me, it was the support from family, specifically my husband and parents, that made the career a success. It allowed the type of partnership to raise children, who, as they were growing up, were also part of the team.

Moreover, it is pivotal to recognize the teamwork and trust my staff and colleagues, both junior and senior, had in collectively meeting our shared goals. Additional leadership training through the Executive Leadership in Academic Medicine Program, dedicated to the advancement of women, allowed me to further advance my skills and contributed to my successful promotion. As Senior Associate Dean, I expanded my portfolio spanning across all components of undergraduate medical education and diversity affairs. I had always been involved in curriculum and, through my grants, was able to introduce and support the evolution of "cultural competency" education, now known as the health equity and social justice curriculum spanning all 4 years.

While one learns to navigate hurdles, my promotion to Professor did not flow as smoothly. I did not initially succeed and used the setback to learn from colleagues how to address this roadblock. While I had excelled in certain areas, including a highly successful and sustained record of attaining peer-reviewed federal grants along with other private grants, I needed to engage in more scholarship. It was taking this advice, along with having experts in diversity assess my work, that made a difference. I subsequently was promoted to Professor with tenure in keeping with the guidelines for promotion at the time. This leads me to a critical takeaway. Please revisit your promotion guidelines and use them as your guidepost for discussions with your supervisors, including your chiefs and chair.

At present, I have spent over 15 years as a senior administrator, moving from Vice Dean to Executive Vice Dean with a broad portfolio which now encompasses undergraduate medical education, faculty affairs, diversity affairs, and the academic departments. I have also served simultaneously as an interim chair on several occasions. My sense of duty to others has never wavered. With this responsibility, I am reminded of the humility and love of humanity that my grandmother instilled in me long ago.

In conclusion, the path to success doesn't have to be linear, as is typically illustrated in the promotion rungs from instructor to professor. I invite you to listen to a wonderful TED Talk, "The best career path is not always a straight one," that permits us to explore "squiggly" career paths. In my journey, I explored a range of possibilities, which also allowed me to navigate and achieve promotion. Moving from the frontline of care as director of the intensive care units in a clinically intensive setting to present day as a senior academic administrator sheds light on the many opportunities that lie before us. To take a leap in your career path, I recommend you navigate this journey with input from mentors, support from sponsors, the influence of networks, and, as needed, coaching to sharpen the skills to be successful for the tasks at hand.

As we present our stories, we leave you with the statement that your advancement as an educator will not only influence what is taught, how it's taught, what is endorsed, and what is needed to drive institutional change. You hold the key to preparing future generations of physicians equipped with the capacity to tackle the health disparities and inequities of our nation.

# References

1. Skochelak SE, Lomis KD, Andrews JS, Hammoud MM, Mejicano GC, Byerley J. Realizing the vision of the Lancet Commission on education of health professionals for the 21st century: transforming medical education through the accelerating change in medical education consortium. Med Teach. 2021;43(sup2):S1–6. https://doi.org/10.1080/0142159X.2021.1935833.
2. Association of American Medical Colleges. New AAMC report confirms growing physician shortage. 2020, June 28. Retrieved October 29, 2020, from https://www.aamc.org/news-insights/press-releases/new-aamc-report-confirms-growing-physician-shortage
3. Terregino CA, Byerley J, Henderson DD, Friedman E, Elks ML, Kirstein IJ, Leep-Hunderfund AN, Fancher TL. Cultivating the physician workforce: recruiting, training, and retaining physicians to meet the needs of the population. Med Teach. 2021;43(sup2):S39–48. https://doi.org/10.1080/0142159X.2021.1935832.
4. McOwen KS, Whelan AJ, Farmakidis AL. Medical education in the United States and Canada, 2020. Acad Med. 2020;95(9S A Snapshot of Medical Student Education in the United States):S2–4. https://doi.org/10.1097/acm.0000000000003497.
5. Council on Graduate Medical Education. Third report: improving access to health care through physician workforce reform. Rockville: Department of Health and Human Services, Health Resources and Services Administration; 1992.
6. Council on Graduate Medical Education. Eighth report: patient care physician supply and requirements: testing COGME recommendations. Rockville: Department of Health and Human Services, Health Resources and Services Administration; 1996.
7. Council on Graduate Medical Education. Fourteenth report: COGME physician workforce policies: recent developments and remaining challenges in meeting national goals. Rockville: Department of Health and Human Services, Health Resources and Services Administration; 1999.
8. GlobalData Plc. The complexities of physician supply and demand: projections from 2021 to 2036. Washington, DC: AAMC; 2024.
9. Acosta D, Ackerman-Barger K. Breaking the silence: time to talk about race and racism. Acad Med. 2017;92(3):285–8.

10. Rodriguez JE, Lopez IA, Campbell KM, Dutton M. The role of mentorship in advancing Latino representation in academic medicine. JAMA J Am Med Assoc. 2022;328(10):982–4.
11. García GE, Velez L. LHS+ individuals in graduate medical education. In: Sánchez JP, Rodriguez D, editors. Latino, Hispanic, or of Spanish Origin+ identified student leaders in medicine, Sustainable development goals series. Cham: Springer; 2024. https://doi.org/10.1007/978-3-031-35020-7_12.
12. Triemstra JD, Iyer MS, Hurtubise L, Poeppelman RS, Turner TL, Dewey C, Karani R, Fromme HB. Influences on and characteristics of the professional identity formation of clinician educators: a qualitative analysis. Acad Med. 2021;96(4):585–91. https://doi.org/10.1097/ACM.0000000000003843.
13. Rutgers New Jersey Medical School. Faculty development plan. Rutgers Biomedical and Health Sciences, Rutgers University. 2024. Retrieved April 29, 2025, from https://facultyaffairs.rbhs.rutgers.edu/faculty-development/
14. Díaz DHS, Garcia G, Clare C, Su J, Friedman E, Williams R, Vazquez J, Sánchez JP. Taking care of the Puerto Rican patient: historical perspectives, health status, and health care access. MedEdPORTAL. 2020;16:10984. https://doi.org/10.15766/mep_2374-8265.10984.
15. Ortega P, Francone NO, Santos MP, Girotti JA, Shin TM, Varjavand N, Park YS. Medical Spanish in US medical schools: a national survey to examine existing programs. J Gen Intern Med. 2021;36(9):2724–30. https://doi.org/10.1007/s11606-021-06735-3. Epub 2021 Mar 29. FMID: 33782890; PMCID: PMC8390604.
16. Sánchez JP, Guilliames C, Sánchez NF, Calderon Y, Burton WB. Video tool to promote knowledge of syphilis among black and Hispanic men recruited from clinical and non-clinical settings. J Community Health. 2010;35(3):220–8. https://doi.org/10.1007/s10900-010-9239-4. FMID: 20151183.
17. Hill KA, Desai MM, Chaudhry SI, Fancher T, Nguyen M, Wang K, Boatright D. National institutes of health diversity supplement awards by medical school. J Gen Intern Med. 2023;38(5):1175–9. https://doi.org/10.1007/s11606-022-07849-y.
18. Nunez-Smith M, Ciarleglio MM, Sandoval-Schaefer T, Elumn J, Castillo-Page L, Peduzzi P, Bradley EH. Institutional variation in the promotion of racial/ethnic minority faculty at US medical schools. Am J Public Health. 2012;102(5):852–8. https://doi.org/10.2105/AJPH.2011.300552.
19. Boyer EL, Moser D, Ream TC, Braxton JM. Scholarship reconsidered: priorities of the professoriate. Wiley; 2015.
20. Sánchez JP, Rodriguez D, editors. Latina/o/x/e, Hispanic or of Spanish Origin+ (LHS+) identified student leaders in medicine: more than 50 years of presence, activism, and leadership. Accepted for Springer Publishing September 2023; 2023. Open Access via link https://link.springer.com/book/10.1007/978-3-031-35020-7
21. De Luca SM, Escoto ER. The recruitment and support of Latino faculty for tenure and promotion. J Hisp High Educ. 2012;11(1):29–40. https://doi.org/10.1177/1538192711435552.
22. Raldow AC, Siker ML, Bonner JA, Chen Y, Liu FF, Metz JM, Movsas B, Potters L, Schultz CJ, Wilson E, Wang X, Romero T, Steinberg ML, Jagsi R. Assessment of differences in academic rank and compensation by gender and race/ethnicity among academic radiation oncologists in the United States. Adv Radiat Oncol. 2023;8(5):Article 101210. https://doi.org/10.1016/j.adro.2023.101210.
23. Kaplan SE, Raj A, Carr PL, Terrin N, Breeze JL, Freund KM. Race/ethnicity and success in academic medicine: findings from a longitudinal multi-institutional study. Acad Med. 2018;93(4):616–22.

**Open Access** This chapter is licensed under the terms of the Creative Commons Attribution 4.0 International License (http://creativecommons.org/licenses/by/4.0/), which permits use, sharing, adaptation, distribution and reproduction in any medium or format, as long as you give appropriate credit to the original author(s) and the source, provide a link to the Creative Commons license and indicate if changes were made.

The images or other third party material in this chapter are included in the chapter's Creative Commons license, unless indicated otherwise in a credit line to the material. If material is not included in the chapter's Creative Commons license and your intended use is not permitted by statutory regulation or exceeds the permitted use, you will need to obtain permission directly from the copyright holder.

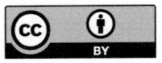

# Chapter 10
# Succeeding Along the Researcher Track from Assistant to Full Professor

Hector Rasgado-Flores, Cristina R. Fernández, Saira A. Mehmood, John Paul Sánchez, and Ramon Gilberto Gonzalez

> **Learning Objectives**
> - Clarify the criteria and expectations for promotion from assistant to full professor on the research track (tenure and nontenure).
> - Identify barriers faced by LHS+ scientists and physician-scientists in the promotion process and strategies to address the barriers.
> - Summarize institutional and external resources to support the advancement of LHS+ faculty on the research track.

H. Rasgado-Flores (✉)
Chicago Medical School at Rosalind Franklin University, Chicago, IL, USA
e-mail: hector.rasgado@rosalindfranklin.edu

C. R. Fernández
Division of Child and Adolescent Health, Department of Pediatrics, Columbia University Vagelos College of Physicians & Surgeons, New York, NY, USA

S. A. Mehmood
American Association for the Advancement of Science (AAAS), Washington, DC, USA

J. P. Sánchez
Latino Medical Student Association Inc., Chicago, IL, USA

Building the Next Generation of Academic Physicians Inc., Rye Brook, NY, USA
e-mail: exec.director@lmsa.net

R. G. Gonzalez
Massachusetts General Hospital, Harvard Medical School, Boston, MA, USA
e-mail: rggonzalez@mgh.harvard.edu

## Introduction

A successful career in academic medicine conducting basic or clinical research by LHS+ physicians and scientists requires unraveling several fundamental issues, including the following:

- Fully understanding what a research track in academic medicine entails
- Knowing why a physician/scientist would embark on this academic medicine research path
- Identifying and accomplishing all the necessary steps to attain success
- Recognizing and overcoming the obstacles that physicians in general and LHS+ physicians in particular encounter
- Identifying and taking advantage of the opportunities that a career in science offers, especially for LHS+ physicians
- Asserting and expanding the contributions that LHS+ physicians/scientists make to US society

## What Is a Research Track in Academic Medicine?

A research track in academic medicine consists of training Ph.D. students, physicians, or MD/Ph.D. students to significantly contribute to the research effort of an educational institution (hospital and university) forming healthcare providers. The investigation focus can be clinically oriented, basic science, or translational. For Ph.D. students, this track formally starts in graduate school. For physicians, this track can start during medical school via an MD/Ph.D. combined program, research electives/years built into the school curriculum, and become more focused during residency and fellowship training. Research residency programs with specific physician-scientist tracks or medical research tracks typically have a substantial (e.g., 80%) component of protected time to conduct research during at least 1 year of the residency program [1]. At this level of training, the residents are mentored by seasoned physicians/researchers in multidisciplinary research to gain experience using state-of-the-art techniques to answer important scientific questions with clinical and public health significance. For MD-only physicians who are not on specific residency research tracks, it is feasible to prepare to join an academic research track in fellowship or with the first academic position and to be successful with appropriate research training, such as a scientific Master's level degree or rigorous research training and fellowship experiences.

## Why Would a Physician Embark on the Research Path?

The most common reasons physicians have for undergoing research training include the following:

- Satisfying their curiosity about learning first-hand how scientific research is conducted

- Gaining state-of-the-art knowledge and treatment options for specific diseases
- Using this training stage as a bridge to pursue a medical specialty
- Hoping that one's research work can contribute to a better understanding and curing of diseases
- Making this step the first phase of a lifelong career dedicated to research

This chapter focuses on this latter approach to an academic medicine career.

A career in science is simultaneously extraordinarily challenging and rewarding. The challenges arise from needing time and effort to be clinically productive, teach, and engage the broader scientific and academic communities while meeting all the expectations for successful research endeavors. These expectations include the following:

1. Achieving grant funding
2. Maintaining a cohesive, motivated laboratory/research team
3. Publishing in high-impact scientific journals
4. Gaining international recognition and promotions while accomplishing well-being and life-work balance

The rewarding component originates from the exceptional privilege of having a career where an essential element consists of being creative. Few professions offer this opportunity; scientists and artists are two professions where creativity is their main driving force.

A successful researcher must have, first and foremost, a true passion for seeking knowledge through science. This goal is critical, because successful scientists work far beyond regular office hours. Scientists willingly and patiently dedicate their time and effort to their research enterprise without expecting immediate results. In addition, they are willing and ready to face the rejection of grant applications and manuscripts submitted to peer-reviewed journals. They endure and do not give up easily. Without genuine passion for research, one is unlikely to be successful along an academic medical research career track.

## Which Are the Necessary Steps to Become a Physician/Scientist?

The first step in becoming a physician/scientist is cultivating a true passion for research. If this is accomplished, the following actions consist of gaining appropriate research training and creating the building blocks for a productive career.

Being educated as a physician already provides the foundations for being a scientist. Physicians learn to apply the scientific method to plan a path for the treatment of their patients. During the first patient/physician interactions, the signs and symptoms that affect the patient are revealed. Subsequently, ideally, the physician/patient team proposes a hypothesis explaining the etiology of the disease affecting the patient. The next step consists of offering and carrying out a clinical experiment: the treatment. Data is subsequently collected, and the hypothesis is tested. If the predicted results are attained, the thesis remains plausible. If the results do not support the idea, the physician/patient team modifies the proposed hypothesis and carries out a new experiment. If the findings are novel and may benefit other patients, the results are disseminated at seminars, grand rounds, and journal publications.

The foundation of evidence-based medicine is the scientific method. All clinician physicians are scientists; they practice the scientific method during patient interactions. Furthermore, the progress in treatment and the development of more efficient therapies require a continuous deepening in our understanding of the molecular, biophysical, and physiological basis of cellular, tissue, and organ behavior under normal and pathological conditions. The driving forces for the generation of this new knowledge are basic and clinical research.

If a physician starts a research career during residency, clinical or postdoctoral fellowship, or as a new junior faculty, this required research training will be supervised by a seasoned physician/scientist mentor. The next stage requires the mentee to decide whether to embark on an independent research career path or to remain closely associated with an established principal investigator. The benefits of the latter option are that the trainee does not necessarily have to apply for their grants and would instead focus on efficiently supporting the supervisor's laboratory and research program. The degree to which the mentee contributes to generating original ideas, designing and performing experiments, analyzing results, and publishing the outcomes would vary greatly depending on the level of interaction and mentorship developed with the principal investigator. The main pitfall of this kind of partnership is the likelihood of the mentee never reaching their full research potential and remaining as a perennial subordinate to the principal investigator. If, on the other hand, the mentee decides to pursue an independent research career, numerous requirements must be met to succeed along this productive and rewarding path.

The first stage consists of asserting the independence of the new investigator. This stage takes time as the mentee will usually have to develop an initial research program with scientific questions that partly overlap with the focal research program of the research mentor. The mentee successfully transitions to research independence either by obtaining a faculty position as an independent scientist in a research institution with start-up funds and federally funded grants or, if the mentee is already a junior faculty, by obtaining large federally funded grants to support a research laboratory or team separate from the research mentor. At this stage, a delicate balance must be created between establishing self-assertion and maintaining productive collaborations with the former research mentor and new collaborators.

The early career investigator's goal is to establish a sustainable research program, create a niche in the scientific community, and leave a significant scientific legacy on society.

## Which Are the Components of a Sustainable Research Program?

To become a successful, productive scientist, several components must work efficiently and synchronously. The main features are as follows:

1. Creating original, essential ideas which can be articulated as testable scientific hypotheses
2. Planning pertinent well-designed experiments or study procedures to test the hypotheses
3. Obtaining funds to conduct experiments or research procedures to test the hypotheses
4. Generating a cohesive research team that is well-staffed, supplied, and equipped
5. Establishing strong, reliable interdisciplinary collaborations where all parties benefit significantly
6. Performing straightforward experiments or conducting validated study procedures leading to reproducible results
7. Correctly analyzing the experimental or study results
8. Timely research presentations at scientific conferences and publication of the results in high-impact, peer-reviewed journals
9. Understanding the fitting and significance of the research study and findings as advancing scientific knowledge
10. Creating new ideas again

The sustainability of the research effort depends on always maintaining the cycle functioning. This process, known as the research cycle, clearly establishes the main components that must work in synergy to create a thriving research enterprise [2]. If one of the components fails, the entire research program risks collapsing. It is essential to recognize that early-career scientists may go through periods of decreased or lapsed grant funding and ebbs and flows in team member support if relying on trainees on research electives or summer students. While these bumps in the road will not permanently derail one's success along the research track, it is essential to (a) establish strong research mentorship support to guide during these challenging periods and to (b) apply to many different types of funding mechanisms over and over again to obtain sufficient funds to stabilize, grow, and then sustain the research program. This includes the assembly of a more stable research team.

## Which Are the Traits of a Successful Research Laboratory or Research Team?

Biomedical research laboratories differ significantly depending on the type of research institution and which model of shared resources they follow. For basic science and translational investigators, sharing research technologies is the best practice for performing research. Modern laboratories are designed with a shared resources laboratory model that significantly reduces the laboratory setup time for a new investigator. For clinical and patient-oriented researchers, striking a balance between individual innovation and pursuing more complex scientific advances with a collaborative interdisciplinary team science approach is critical. Clinical research teams may be physically housed in a laboratory or office space within an academic department or a center.

Despite the substantial differences between laboratories and research teams, the following characteristics are commonly shared as best practices:

1. Promote creativity among the laboratory/team members.
2. Provide clear job assignments to each member.
3. Attain sufficient funding.
4. Hire a laboratory manager who is efficient, competent, and sincerely committed.
5. Attract enthusiastic and committed graduate and medical students, residents, and clinical and postdoctoral fellows who will engrain ownership for their projects.
6. Maintain organization and effectiveness using printed or online tools for project management and communication.
7. Nurture a friendly environment.
8. Create a culture of generosity.
9. Make all members accountable for their responsibilities.
10. Ensure that all members comply with academic center and laboratory/team expectations and regulations.
11. Publish efficiently and engender support and resilience in team members.
12. Establish strong collaborations.

## Promotion of Cohesiveness in a Laboratory

To promote creativity in a laboratory or among a clinical research team, it is necessary to create an environment where all members feel safe to express their ideas, make mistakes, and learn from each other. Best practices include the following:

1. Creating a culture where all members partake in a common cause, easily identified via a mission statement.
2. Have regular, organized progress report meetings that allow for team members to provide updates, ask questions, get feedback, and keep members on track as to how their task or project supports the overarching laboratory or team mission. Have regular brainstorming sessions. Passion for presenting novel ideas should be encouraged. These meetings are likely to be disruptive. The laboratory/research team principal investigator should not be intimidated by this! On the contrary, discussions should be encouraged and embraced.

3. Develop a culture of mutual respect despite differences in opinions and approaches.
4. Have fun activities where members relax and get to know each other better.

## Engagement or Commitment?

Like any leader, laboratory/research team principal investigators should assess whether they prefer an engaged or committed team. There are significant differences between these options. Building an engaged team entails defining expectations, having team members understand these expectations, and nourishing the group members' sense of obligation to fulfill a pledge. An engaged group is busy at work trying to meet expectations effectively.

On the other hand, a committed team's work is driven by a positive attachment to the group's goals. Rather than being focused on fulfilling expectations, the team's work is triggered by an urgency to accomplish an objective. Building this kind of team demands developing a sense of ownership, purpose, and passion for reaching a common goal.

The group's character usually starts under an engagement platform during team building. Eventually, in the hands of an efficient leader, it can evolve into an environment of commitment.

## Types of Leadership

According to emotional leadership theory [3], several types of leadership styles readily apply to a research team or laboratory setting:

1. Coaching: leading by mentoring
2. Affiliative: leading by creating harmony
3. Commanding: leading by setting procedures
4. Pacesetting: leading by example
5. Democratic: leading by encouraging participation
6. Visionary: leading by inspiring

The best practice for a laboratory or research team principal investigator is to resist sticking to only one emotional leadership style and to adopt any of the styles, depending on the team's circumstances at any given time. For example, if the team members are neophyte scientists, the coaching and pacesetting styles may be the most appropriate. In contrast, the democratic style may be the most fitting and conducive to creativity for a seasoned group. Under tension among team members, the affiliative type may be the most suitable.

## Promotions on the Research Track

Climbing the academic ladder should always result from a scientist's efficient hard work and commitment. Unfortunately, this is not always the case, especially for LHS+ researchers.

As mentioned above, achieving success along the research track demands the successful and simultaneous attainment of numerous distinctions. Promotion to a higher academic position implies that the academic institution envisions rewarding and retaining the scientist to enhance the institutional research, educational and administrative efforts. This situation is particularly true if an academic institution has a tenure structure and the physician-scientist is granted tenure.

Although institutions have different requirements for promotion, the majority expect that the candidate demonstrates collegiality and efficiency in advancing the institution's mission. In most institutions, the candidate for promotion must demonstrate the ability to balance scholarship, teaching, and clinical and academic service duties.

The scholarship component is evaluated by the research performance, which includes obtaining and *maintaining* external grant support, publishing in peer-reviewed journals, and gaining recognition by being invited to:

Present one's research at national and international scientific meetings.
Serve on study sections for grants review.
Be invited by journal editorial boards to review manuscripts submitted for publication, serve as a guest editor for a special edition, and submit invited commentaries.
Perform significant and prestigious administrative duties for scientific, clinical, and educational societies.

The teaching aspect is assessed by the quality and quantity of content development and delivery, interactions with students, and, in some cases, curriculum development. The teaching expectations should be commensurate with the institution's teaching mission. Peer and student assessments evaluate the quality of teaching.

The service category includes participation in the institution's committees and mentoring junior faculty.

Candidates under consideration for promotion (either tenured or nontenured) must show meaningful contributions in scholarship, teaching, and service areas, though not necessarily in equal weight. The relative importance of each category will vary depending on the level of promotion. For promotion along a research track (with consideration of tenure or nontenured), research/scholarship achievements are generally given the most significant weight.

Regardless of the balance between scholarship, teaching, and service, promotion requires that a candidate's scholarly activities provide compelling evidence for future creative contributions.

# What Are the Challenges That LHS+ Research Track Faculty Encounter?

In addition to the obstacles that aspiring independent academic scientists must overcome, LHS+ scientists have additional barriers to surpass to succeed. These obstacles include the following:

1. Foreign-born LHS+ scientists speaking English as a second language must learn to write and speak this language fluently to compete with US-born, native English speakers. This ability is essential for writing manuscripts and grant applications, teaching effectively, and communicating ideas to the scientific community. Not speaking English fluently or speaking with a heavy accent can severely undermine the research career of foreign-born LHS+ scientists. Overcoming this obstacle requires great effort and training. To prevail over writing limitations, it is critical to write profusely and ensure peer mentors review, which constructively corrects the LHS +'s writing pieces. Finding strong peer mentors and writing support is essential for the progress of foreign-born LHS+ scientists. Unfortunately, this may not be easy to accomplish.
2. Another significant limitation that foreign-born, and perhaps to a lesser extent, first-generation US-born LHS+ scientists may face is that many cultures, e.g., Latinx, discourage self-assertion. In these cultures, collectivism (i.e., uplifting of the group over individual achievement), profound humility, and self-devaluation can be seen as attributes rather than hindrances. The historical fact that many of these countries were subjugated by the USA further compounds this situation as it may create an image of a conqueror/conquered dichotomy, which could lead to a sense of "inferiority" in some LHS+ scientists.
3. A successful scientist must be self-assertive. There are two main paths for LHS+ scientists to develop this critical skill: (i) identifying LHS+ role models and mentors from one's institution or other institutions who look and have had similar life experiences to the LHS+ scientist and (ii) becoming the role models and mentors that previous LHS+ researchers never had.
4. Generating a critical mass of LHS+ scientists who will become role models and mentors for younger generations in a pipeline fashion will take time. At this moment, it is essential to recruit and maintain the ever-increasing participation and growth of LHS+ as successful independent scientists.
5. A third barrier that LHS+ scientists encounter, whether foreign or US-born, is imposter syndrome. Imposter syndrome can occur in any person of any background at any point along the research track. However, cultural and racial isolation in any environment is a poignant experience that may generate doubts about one's hard work, skills, and accomplishments to deserve a position of opportunity. Being LHS+ significantly increases the likelihood and severity of experiencing imposter syndrome [4], potentially severely dampening the attainment of LHS+ scientists' full potential. Overcoming imposter syndrome involves recognizing colleagues also experience self-doubt, being patient with oneself and not

constantly comparing oneself with others, reaching out to trusted peers and senior mentors to talk about one's feelings and experiences, and reframing bad news about grant applications and rejected manuscripts and failed experiments or studies as learning opportunities to improve one's science and impact.

## Need for LHS+ Physicians/Scientists in the USA

In the USA, 18.5% of the population is LHS+. However, only 5.8% of active physicians are LHS+ [5]. This underrepresentation of LHS+ physicians and scientists is further exacerbated along the research track, as only 2% of physician/scientists are UiM [5]. As discussed above, there are many reasons explaining these statistics. However, an additional and very significant explanation is that the education system in the USA, from kindergarten to higher education, is designed to efficiently support higher socioeconomic status students while hampering the development of their low socioeconomic status peers [6]. Since the ratio of proportion in poverty relative to total population is greater for LHS+ (overrepresented by a ratio of 1.5) compared to an underrepresentation for non-LHS+ Whites with a ratio of 0.7, the LHS+ population is severely overrepresented in the low socioeconomic status category. Consequently, this cohort is impacted by the potential for persistent lower quality primary and secondary education from a dearth of resources, insufficient or lack of expectations by educators, systemic racism, and racialization of schools and universities [7].

## Why Does This Matter?

There are many important reasons to bring all population sectors to parity in education and economic opportunities. Some of them are the following:

1. Social Justice. A society can only be sustainable if it offers equal opportunities and resources to all its members. Unequal distribution of resources generates anger and mistrust. Eventually, this translates into social unrest.
2. Economic growth and competitiveness. In a global economy, education and the well-being of the population in each country are critical for attaining world competitiveness. If 18.5% of the people in the USA are LHS+, failing to provide resources and means to accomplish the full potential of this group will have dire social, political, and economic consequences as it would place the USA at a disadvantage over other developed countries, which provide attainable higher education to all their population groups.
3. Missing creativity from diversity. Numerous studies demonstrate that workplace diversity significantly increases a group's effectiveness [8]. This happens, because the participation of members from different ethnic and socioeconomic

backgrounds enhances the ability to analyze situations and propose solutions that would have otherwise been out of the realm of a given group.

Science is a method and, as such, is universal. However, scientific perspective and creativity are not universal; they result from individual scientists' personal experiences, endurance, resilience, and opportunities. Based on their life experiences and cultural background, LHS+ scientists have a rich perspective to share with the world. The scientific enterprise in the USA cannot afford to lose the participation and wisdom of this societal group.

## What Are the Opportunities for Being an LHS+ Research Track Faculty Member?

The National Institutes of Health (NIH) and the National Science Foundation (NSF), as the US's premier biomedical, public health, and science agencies, recognize the dearth of racial and ethnic diversity in the biomedical workforce [9]. To begin correcting the historical remnants of racism and ethnoracism within the US biomedical science community, these powerful agencies are developing programs to increase the diversity of their grantees to enhance the development and sustainability of a diverse biomedical workforce [10, 11]. Society in general and LHS+ scientists are increasingly scrutinizing implicit bias in the grant review and awarding system, given the lower award rates of independent funding mechanisms for LHS+ scientists compared to White scientists [12, 13]. It would require a bold affirmative-action type of program to catalyze this process. Unfortunately, the current administration in the US is quickly dismantling these efforts.

LHS+ physicians/scientists should communicate, organize, and create mutual support mechanisms to enhance their opportunities for promotion and research career success. These mechanisms should also mutually create positive alliances with non-LHS+ peers to support their research tracks. The Latino Medical Student Association, National Hispanic Medical Association, the National Hispanic Science Network, National Institutes of Health Office of Intramural Research Hispanic Health Research Scientific Interest Group, and the Society of Latin American Biophysicists are excellent examples of LHS+ physicians, physicians-scientists, and scientists working together to promote each other's research success, career advancement, and well-being.

## LIDEReS in Research: Advancing the LHS+ Academic Workforce

A critical component of fostering a diverse and inclusive academic research workforce is the development of structured programs that support early-career researchers from underrepresented backgrounds. The LIDEReS (LHS+ Identity,

Development, Empowerment, and Resources Seminar) in Research initiative exemplifies how strategic partnerships between federal agencies and national organizations can create meaningful opportunities to prepare early-career LHS+ researchers through a structured seminar, focusing on health disparities, research career navigation, federal grant processes, and networking.

## *Program Design and Implementation*

LIDEReS in Research was developed through a collaboration between the Latino Medical Student Association (LMSA) Faculty/Physician Advisory Council and a federal agency. The partnership resulted in (1) applying a Community-Based Participatory Education (CBPE) model and Kern's Six-Step Approach to adapt LMSA's LIDEReS to a novel program titled LIDEReS in Research, consisting of a new LHS+ and research focused curriculum [14, 15], and (2) a federal agency's provision of a travel award to support the participation of aspiring LHS+ interns, residents, fellows, postdoctorates, and junior faculty interested in biomedical research careers. This initiative provided interactive workshops, plenary sessions with federal agency representatives, and career development planning tailored to the unique challenges faced by LHS+ researchers.

The inaugural seminar, held in Puerto Rico in April 2024, included 30 fellows from a competitive applicant pool for the LIDEReS in Research Travel Award. An additional four participants attended the seminar using their own funding sources. Participants engaged in discussions on health disparities, federal grant processes, and strategies for navigating research careers. A structured career mapping exercise allowed fellows to draft individualized professional development plans, ensuring they left the seminar with actionable goals.

## *Outcomes and Impact*

Post-seminar evaluations indicated a strong positive impact, with 100% of respondents agreeing that the program met its objectives. Attendees highlighted the program's emphasis on mentorship, networking, and culturally tailored career guidance as key strengths. Feedback suggested enhancing session interactivity and extending networking opportunities to further improve the experience.

Beyond its immediate impact, LIDEReS in Research represents a scalable model for increasing LHS+ representation in academic research leadership. The program's success underscores the importance of sustained investment in training initiatives that address health disparities through a diverse and well-equipped scientific workforce.

## *Future Directions*

Building on its initial success, LMSA can expand LIDEReS in Research with other federal agencies and professional organizations across all five LMSA regions and integrate its curriculum into institutional faculty development programs. Long-term engagement with fellows will be critical in assessing career progression and ensuring continued support for LHS+ researchers.

By providing structured training, mentorship, and networking opportunities, LIDEReS in research contributes to the broader effort of diversifying the academic research landscape. Applying a community-based participatory education model helped to create a novel seminar for advancing the LHS+ workforce, and this approach sets a precedent for additional partnerships between federal agencies and national organizations in advancing career development programs that are culturally responsive though community-informed educational innovations.

## Conclusions

A research career as a physician-scientist is simultaneously gratifying and challenging. Minoritized populations are very much underrepresented in the medical field, especially in research. Many complex reasons have led to this situation. LHS+ physicians/scientists encounter even more obstacles than their non-LHS+ peers to become successful scientists. Practical steps and opportunities are available to overcome career path barriers. Leveraging existing networking and pipeline programs spearheaded by national LHS+ organizations, LHS+ physicians/scientists can and should take full advantage of opportunities to foster career success along the research track and support initiatives to uplift the next generation of physician-scientists.

## Personal Narrative

### Hector Rasgado-Flores, PhD

My journey as a scientist started several years before I was born. My father (my hero) was a peasant from Oaxaca, Mexico. Although he was born with humble resources, he had two big dreams: becoming a musician and a physician. The only path to attaining his first goal was to join the seminary. A nun appreciated his potential and gifted him a professional violin. A few years later, he became the concertino of the Oaxaca Symphonic Orchestra. This orchestra was so remarkable that famed Maestro Leopold Stokowski conducted it. Following this accomplishment, he realized that the only way he could become a physician was to become a military doctor. My father became a plastic surgeon and developed innovative procedures for skin grafts for burned patients. He operated on the nose of a beautiful woman, my mother, and married her. They had seven sons. My father trained all of us in music. Two of us studied medicine, and one of my brothers and I followed professional music training.

When I was very young, I had severe asthma. I remember waking in the middle of the night, jumping out of bed, and gasping for air. Fortunately, albuterol inhalers arrived in Mexico, and I was one of the first kids to get one. However, my physical activities were minimal. I missed many days of school and could not play like other kids. I found consolation in playing the piano and composing music. I eventually won national composition, mathematics, and literature contests.

I wanted to understand and manage my disease better and simultaneously studied medicine, music, and a master's and a doctorate in Neuroscience. I decided to concurrently follow my passions for science and music to the best of my abilities.

Because of a life of many remarkable privileges, I was commissioned by the American Physiological Society to write a symphony about the human life cycle which several orchestras have performed. I have also been commissioned by the Colegio Nacional (Mexico) to compose a piano suite about chemical elements.

As a scientist, I have studied the transport of ions across cell membranes, cell volume regulation, cystic fibrosis, and the use of music as a therapeutic tool.

As an administrator, I founded the Society for Latin American Biophysicists and was the Chair of International Physiology of the American Physiological Society, Co-Chair of the Research Council of the American Heart Association, and Director of Diversity, Outreach, and Success at my Medical School. I am a member of the National Faculty/Physician Advisory Council of the Latino Medical Student Association.

Most importantly, the work I am the proudest of is to contribute to bringing to higher education minoritized students from the community where my medical school is located.

I have been privileged to have had amazing mentors: Drs. Hugo Gonzalez-Serratos, David Erlij, Mordecai Blaustein, Martin Frank, Robert Rakowski, Richard Hawkins, and Robert Bridges.

At least as important, I have been very fortunate to have my partner/wife, Cecilia. She is the first woman to graduate as a physicist from her University (Universidad Autonoma of San Luis Potosi, Mexico).

**Cristina R. Fernández, MD, MPH**
My family moved to the States from Panamá when I was an infant. I experienced early childhood in downtown Chicago surrounded by Spanish-speaking family, friends, and community members involved in engineering, transportation, education and teaching, and government. No doctors. In high school I fell in love with science and wanted to study biology in college. While I was a strong overall student, math had always been my most challenging (and lowest graded) subject; I was dismayed to learn that biology programs required calculus prerequisites! When I grew discouraged, my mother reminded me that people can learn in different ways and strongly advocated for me to get math tutoring and additional help in school. I

learned from my mother that society's default low expectations bias for people from racial and ethnic minoritized backgrounds is to be swatted away as we work to achieve our goals.

I attended Washington University in St. Louis for my undergraduate studies as a John B. Ervin Scholar, a program that offers tuition scholarships and stipends to students who advance the goals of academic excellence, leadership, community service, and diversity. I developed close friendships with scholars from Washington University's other signature scholarship programs—the Danforth Scholars Program and the Annika Rodriguez Scholars Program—who were also Biology majors and many of whom were on the "pre-med" track. We formed study groups and tutoring teams to pull each other through the agony of Organic Chemistry and Biology labs.

After completing a Master of Public Health degree in epidemiology of microbial diseases and considering a career in public health with the Centers for Disease Control, I ultimately turned back to pursuing medicine due to a desire to use public health perspectives to improve individual- and family-level health and well-being. During medical school, I was active with our school chapter of the then National Boricua-Latino Health Organization (NBLHO), now Latino Medical Student Association (LMSA). I took advantage of the annual House of Delegates meetings and national conferences to meet other Latino medical students, submit my early developing research as scientific abstracts for poster presentations, and learn important skills for preparing residency applications. As a pediatric resident and then academic fellow, I participated in the regional activities sponsored by the National Hispanic Medical Association (NHMA) Council of Residents and then Council of Young Physicians and learned about health disparities science, health equity and policy, and post-trainee transition fundamentals at the NHMA's national conference sessions. All of these experiences well prepared me to pursue an academic pediatrics research career with goal to mitigate early child obesity risk through examining the biologic and behavioral pathways through which prenatal and early life nutrition, adversity, and socio-structural determinants of health influence child feeding, growing, and development, especially among historically and socioeconomically marginalized communities.

As an early-career physician scientist at the Assistant Professor level, I was successfully awarded an institutional KL2 mentored career development award from our university Clinical and Translational Science Award (CTSA) hub. I also leveraged the research skills and scientific knowledge I obtained through participation in the Health Disparities Research Institute hosted by the National Institute on Minority Health and Health Disparities (NIMHD) to successfully be awarded NIH Loan Repayment Program awards (original plus two renewal awards) that were applied to repayment of my educational loans and enabled me to focus on developing an academic research career. Yet my research career trajectory has had several bumps, since I joined the faculty. I had my first child during fellowship and my second child as a first-year faculty member, and I had to adjust how I did research writing at home to ensure time for my family. Early on, I also had increased clinical responsibilities during a staffing challenge in my clinical area, impacting my time to conduct research and write manuscripts. I leaned heavily on supportive and trustworthy peer mentors during these challenging periods. These peer relationships, research mentors, and a department that believes in me and my work help me remain engaged in research even when manuscripts are rejected, and grant applications are not funded. I also developed peer mentorship and writing accountability groups with colleagues outside of my institution through participation in the Association of American Medical Colleges (AAMC) Minority Faculty Leadership Development Seminar. A successful research career requires tons of resiliency, drive, and determination. Next steps to aim for: promotion to Associate Professor and independent research funding!

**Saira A. Mehmood, PhD**
My parents immigrated to the USA from Pakistan in the early 1980s, and I was born and raised in New Orleans, Louisiana. Although they did not have college degrees, my parents always encouraged me to prioritize education. Initially, I pursued a premed track and spent the summer after my freshman year working in a microbiology and immunology lab at the LSU School of Medicine. However, two pivotal moments in 2005 shifted my career trajectory toward anthropology.

The first occurred in early 2005 when Dr. Jameela Arshad, a respected member of the New Orleans Muslim community, witnessed a bicyclist get hit by a car. As a physician, she stopped to help—but as a Black woman, she was met with suspicion by local police. Instead of recognizing her medical credentials, the police arrested her. She died while in custody. The second moment came later that year when Hurricane Katrina forced me to evacuate my home. I saw firsthand the systemic failures of local, state, and federal governments in their response to the flooding and their lack of coordination in evacuating the city's most vulnerable residents. Both events illuminated the deep racial inequities embedded within social systems.

My anthropology courses provided a framework to make sense of these injustices. I received my first research grant from Tulane University's Department of Anthropology to complete my senior honors thesis on the emergence of community-based clinics in New Orleans following the state's closure of Charity Hospital. That research solidified my interest in understanding how social systems shape individual and community outcomes, ultimately leading me to pursue a PhD in medical anthropology. However, my academic path was not always linear.

As a first-generation college student, I had to navigate academia's "hidden curriculum" without prior exposure to its unspoken rules and expectations. Fortunately, I found mentorship and support along the way. At Tulane, the Office of Multicultural Affairs played an instrumental role in helping underrepresented students thrive, and I later worked there as a program coordinator, developing initiatives to support first year and transfer students. During graduate school, I was elected to serve as the student representative on the executive board of the American Anthropological Association (AAA), the largest professional society for anthropologists. That experience deepened my understanding of the systemic challenges students face in academia and allowed me to advocate for graduate students' needs.

After earning my PhD, I taught at Spelman College for 2 years. Teaching at a historically Black women's college, particularly during the COVID-19 pandemic, reshaped my understanding of mentorship—not just as guidance but as a practice rooted in epistemology (how we know what we know) and phenomenology (how we become who we are). Spelman, the largest producer of Black women who go on to earn PhDs in STEM fields, taught me invaluable lessons about effective mentorship, partnership, and the power of community.

In 2021, I was selected as an American Association for the Advancement of Science (AAAS) Science & Technology Policy Fellow, a program that places scholars with terminal degrees in scientific fields within federal agencies to engage in policy work. After my fellowship, I remained at my agency and collaborated with colleagues and the LMSA Advisory Council to develop LIDEReS in research. Recognizing the urgent need for more LHS+ individuals in academic medicine, we created a program to support and empower the next generation of researchers.

Through my experiences—from undergraduate and graduate school to teaching and working in diverse environments—I have come to believe that centering the voices of those most marginalized benefits everyone. When we prioritize equity, everyone thrives.

**Ramon Gilberto Gonzalez, MD, PhD**
I was born and raised in the Mexican border town of Nogales, Arizona, in the heart of the Great Sonoran Desert. My parents did not go beyond middle school, but they always encouraged me to pursue higher education. My Tio Humberto, an orphan who became a surgeon, inspired me to pursue medicine. While attending the University of Arizona, my life changed after joining a chemistry research lab. The joy of working in a lab to solve a problem using the scientific method was unexpected and transformative. To further explore research, I entered grad school at the University of California at Santa Cruz, receiving a Ph.D. in biophysical chemistry followed by a postdoc in molecular biophysics at MIT. During my research, I developed expertise in nuclear magnetic resonance and MRI.

My medical training was nonlinear. I attended Harvard Medical School, did a medical internship and radiology residency at the Brigham and Women's Hospital in Boston, and completed a neuroradiology fellowship at the Mass General Hospital. My training was regularly interrupted by stints in the lab, including working on my Ph.D. and doing my postdoc. I joined the MGH Radiology research faculty, built a lab, and was the principal investigator of multiple NIH R01 grants.

I practiced neuroradiology while leading my lab and was asked to lead the Neuro Division, which I did for 25 years. My research turned to more clinical pursuits, advancing the utility of brain imaging. Currently, I am a Professor of Radiology at the Harvard Medical School and Associate Chief of Imaging Sciences at the Massachusetts General Hospital. I am focused on developing deep learning algorithms for the interpretation of neuroimages.

My lifelong great good fortune was made possible by scholarships, fellowships, grants, and mentors' generosity at critical points of my life. Cornelius Steelink at the U of A, Tom Schleich at UCSC, Leo Neuringer at MIT, Harry Mellins at BWH, and Jim Thrall at MGH all saw promise in me and encouraged me to pursue my dreams. Most significant has been my family's support; above all, my wife, Michele, an atmospheric chemist, whom I met at the MIT Magnet Lab.

## References

1. Williams CS, Iness AN, Baron RM, Ajijola OA, Hu PJ, Vyas JM, Baiocchi R, Adami AJ, Lever JM, Klein PS, Demer L, Madaio M, Geraci M, Brass LF, Blanchard M, Salata R, Zaidi M. Training the physician-scientist: views from program directors and aspiring young investigators. JCI Insight. 2018;3(23):e125651. https://doi.org/10.1172/jci.insight.125651. PMID: 30518696; PMCID: PMC6328016.
2. Jerome WL. Br Dent J. 1994;177(11–12):401. https://doi.org/10.1038/sj.bdj.4808633.
3. Goleman D, Boyatzis R, McKee A. Primal leadership: learning to lead with emotional intelligence. Moscow: Alpina Business Books; 2008.
4. Bravata DM, Watts SA, Keefer AL, Madhusudhan DK, Taylor KT, Clark DM, Nelson RS, Cokley KO, Hagg HK. Prevalence, predictors, and treatment of imposter syndrome: a systematic review. J Gen Intern Med. 2020;35(4):1252–75. https://doi.org/10.1007/s11606-019-05364-1. Epub 2019 Dec 17. PMID: 31848865; PMCID: PMC7174434.
5. AAMC diversity in medicine: facts and figures 2019. Figure 18. Percentage of all active physicians by race/ethnicity, 2018 | AAMC.
6. Carnevale AP, Fasules MG, Quinn MC, Peltier Campbell K. Born to win, schooled to lose. Georgetown Univ. Center on Education and the Workforce; 2019.
7. De Brey C, Musu L, McFarland J, Wilkinson-Flicker S, Diliberti M, Zhang A, Branstetter C, Wang X. Status and trends in the education of racial and ethnic groups 2018 (NCES 2019–038). US Department of Education. Washington, DC: National Center for Education Statistics; 2019. Retrieved [date] from https://nces.ed.gov/pubsearch/
8. 5 Advantages of Diversity in the Workplace. https://www.indeed.com/hire/c/info/benefits-of-diversity#:~:text=Five%20benefits%20of%20diversity%201%20Expanded%20creativity%20and,and%20human%20by%20a%20greater%20number%20of%20people. Accessed on 5 July 2025.
9. Mervis J. NSF grant decisions reflect systemic racism, study argues. Science. 2022;377:455–6.
10. National Center for Science and Engineering Statistics. Women, minorities, and persons with disabilities in science and engineering: 2021, Special report NSF 21-321. Alexandria: National Science Foundation; 2021. Available at https://ncses.nsf.gov/wmpd
11. Valantine HA, Lund PK, Gammie AE. From the NIH: a systems approach to increasing the diversity of the biomedical research workforce. CBE Life Sci Educ. 2016;15(3):fe4. https://doi.org/10.1187/cbe.16-03-0138. PMID: 27587850; PMCID: PMC5008902.
12. Hoppe TA, Litovitz A, Willis KA, Meseroll RA, Perkins MJ, Hutchins BI, Davis AF, Lauer MS, Valantine HA, Anderson JM, Santangelo GM. Topic choice contributes to the lower rate of NIH awards to African American/black scientists. Sci Adv. 2019;5(10):eaaw7238. https://doi.org/10.1126/sciadv.aaw7238. PMID: 31633016; PMCID: PMC6785250; indeed, 2022.
13. Ginther DK, Schaffer WT, Schnell J, Masimore B, Liu F, Haak LL, Kington R. Race, ethnicity, and NIH research awards. Science. 2011;333(6045):1015–9. https://doi.org/10.1126/science.1196783. PMID: 21852498; PMCID: PMC3412416.

14. Fritz CDL, Naylor K, Watkins Y, Britt T, Hinton L, Jones J, Curry G, Lam H, Kim K. From community-based participatory research to community-based participatory education: the implementation of community participation in cancer disparities curriculum development. [abstract]. In: Proceedings of the sixth AACR conference: the science of cancer health disparities; Dec 6–9, 2013; Atlanta/Philadelphia: AACR. Cancer Epidemiol Biomarkers Prev 2014;23(11 Suppl):Abstract nr A49. https://doi.org/10.1158/1538-7755.DISP13-A49.
15. Thomas PA, Kern DE, Hughes MT, Chen BY. Curriculum development for medical education: a six-step approach. 3rd ed. Johns Hopkins University Press; 2016.

**Open Access** This chapter is licensed under the terms of the Creative Commons Attribution 4.0 International License (http://creativecommons.org/licenses/by/4.0/), which permits use, sharing, adaptation, distribution and reproduction in any medium or format, as long as you give appropriate credit to the original author(s) and the source, provide a link to the Creative Commons license and indicate if changes were made.

The images or other third party material in this chapter are included in the chapter's Creative Commons license, unless indicated otherwise in a credit line to the material. If material is not included in the chapter's Creative Commons license and your intended use is not permitted by statutory regulation or exceeds the permitted use, you will need to obtain permission directly from the copyright holder.

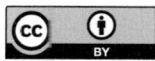

# Chapter 11
# Striving to Become a Department Chair

Monica Verduzco-Gutierrez, Julie Ann Sosa, Ruben J. Azocar, Rolando De Leon, and A. Orlando Ortiz

**Learning Objectives**
- Factors for LHS+ physicians to consider in aspiring to become a departmental chair at an academic medical center.
- Create a framework, using the chair's roles and responsibilities, that LHS+ physicians can use to assess their motivation and potential for becoming a department chair.
- Assemble strategies and tools that LHS+ physicians can apply as they prepare themselves for promotion to department chair.
- Value the important impact that this clinical leadership position can have along the healthcare continuum for LHS+ physicians, trainees, and patients.

---

M. Verduzco-Gutierrez (✉)
Department of Rehabilitation Medicine, Long School of Medicine at the University of Texas at San Antonio, San Antonio, TX, USA

J. A. Sosa
University of California San Francisco (UCSF), San Francisco, CA, USA

R. J. Azocar
Department of Anesthesiology and Perioperative Medicine, Tulane University School of Medicine, New Orlenas, LA, USA

R. De Leon
Division of Obstetrics and Gynecology, Kiram C Patel College of Allopathic Medicine, Nova Southeastern University, Ft. Lauderdale, FL, USA

A. O. Ortiz
Albert Einstein College of Medicine, Bronx, NY, USA

© The Author(s) 2026
J. P. Sánchez et al. (eds.), *Advancing Latino, Hispanic, or of Spanish Origin+ Leadership in Academic Medicine*,
https://doi.org/10.1007/978-3-032-07570-3_11

## Introduction

"What is your ten-year plan?" Is it in your plan to become a department chair? For many, it may not be a clearly paved road with a perfectly mapped-out plan that leads one to become a department chair. For some, the inspiration to seek this responsibility may occur at some point in their academic career. The role of department chair in medical schools or academic medical centers is critical to the success of a department. Department chairs must address multiple stakeholders, including trainees/learners, faculty, administrators, and patients, to name a few. Chairpersons manage and are responsible for the clinical, educational, research, and programmatic innovation that occurs in an academic medical center department at any given time. It can be a powerful position and is often not filled by a person of Latina/o/x/e, Hispanic, or Spanish Origin+ (LHS+) lived experiences. Recent data from the AAMC shows that only 5% of department chairs are held by LHS+ individuals (Table 11.1) [1]. This number is even lower than that (~10%) calculated over a 2-year period from 2018 to 2020, for all underrepresented minorities that were clinical department chairs [2]. Another study compared the percentage of Latino chairs in 2007 (3.4%) to 2019 (3.6%) [1]. These suboptimal figures are clearly asynchronous with the growing Latino population. This representation gap reflects an unfavorable supply–demand function in which there is a low percentage of potential candidates combined with a system that does not cultivate and support their academic promotion. The proportion of Hispanic faculty and chairs has remained low compared to their White cohorts over a four decade period, from 1980 to 2019, and the percentage of Hispanic chairs shows a proportional representation relative to the number of Hispanic faculty [3]. In other words, the percentage of LHS+ chairs is what one might expect given the small number of available LHS+ faculty. It is also likely that there will be a paucity of LHS+ mentors within their institution to guide them in the process. With few LHS+ academic leaders, it is also likely that selection committees will be devoid of members who can make a case for the recruitment of a prospective LHS+ chair candidate [1]. Given that there is a growing population of

**Table 11.1** Modified AAMC Faculty Roster, December 31, 2024, snapshot as of December 31, 2024, for LHS+ chairs in the basic and clinical sciences [5]

| Discipline | Hispanic/Latino or Spanish Origin+ | | Multi-race or multiethnicity Hispanic origin | | Total | | |
|---|---|---|---|---|---|---|---|
| | Women | Men | Women | Men | Women | Men | All LHS+ |
| Basic sciences | 15 | 16 | 11 | 13 | 26 | 29 | 55 (6.9%) |
| | | | Subtotal: | | 243 | 558 | 801 |
| Clinical sciences | 28 | 76 | 5 | 37 | 33 | 113 | 146 (5.7%) |
| | | | Subtotal: | | 598 | 1964 | 2562 |

Hispanic/Latino individuals in the USA, and it is known that this patient population is underserved, it is imperative that there be representation in academic leadership to help address healthcare disparities [4].

## Why Might You Want to Become a Department Chair?

There are many reasons to consider the position of department chair. You may want to lead a group of faculty, learners, and staff in enhancing patient care, advancing clinical research, or training culturally competent practitioners. You may have an interest in leadership or possess a desire to improve a department or favorably impact the institutional mission. From a personal growth perspective, you may value the recognition and status that are derived from being a department chair. For the ambitious, it may also serve as an interim step on a path to another position (i.e., medical school dean, CEO of a healthcare company, chief medical officer, etc.). Lastly, never discount the obvious favorable impact of this position on your financial compensation package. You will certainly deserve and earn every dollar!

## What Are the Roles and Responsibilities of a Department Chair?

A department chair has numerous responsibilities and is either assigned or takes on any number of roles depending on institutional priorities [6]. At a minimum, the department chair is involved with strategic planning, programmatic development, monitoring and reporting, and human resource management. With respect to strategic planning, the department chair helps to determine the immediate and future course for the department. This is influenced by the chair's vision for their department which will in turn influence the department's missions in the context of institutional objectives. To varying degrees, the chair may be involved in different types of internal and external marketing endeavors. Programmatic development and maintenance pertains to clinical, educational, research, and institutional or community-related activities. These involve the educational training programs for students, residents, fellows, and allied health fields that work with the department. Research programs span the gamut from basic clinical projects to any number or type of grant or industry-funded projects. Community outreach and institutional citizenship, serving on and assisting numerous institutional committees, also are important components of the chair's job. The provision of optimal clinical service and service-line development and collaboration are additional programmatic responsibilities. Quality management has evolved into an important aspect of the department's operations and is now one of the chair's priorities, since the chair must serve as a key patient advocate (Table 11.2).

**Table 11.2** Additional chair roles and responsibilities

| Quality management | Financial management |
|---|---|
| Policy and procedure | Accounting |
| Compliance | Budgets |
| Patient relations | Fiscal planning |
| Patient safety | Fundraising |
| Risk management | Equipment/program acquisition/maintenance |
| | Performance/efficiency scorecards |

A chair has significant fiscal responsibility for the department's finances and must monitor and report on these activities regularly. Academic chairs are involved with many types of departmental financial activities including budgeting, conducting monthly reviews of departmental financial performance, and approving expenditures. They must ensure compliance with relevant regulations and stay informed about changes in reimbursement policies for clinical services from both governmental and private payers.

Another key chair responsibility is human resource management. The chair is responsible for adequately staffing their department, focusing on recruitment and retention of staff, hiring new staff, and, when necessary, firing staff. The chair oversees the appropriate credentialing of their staff. A critical chair function is faculty and staff development; the chair is constantly counseling and mentoring. The department chair is a coach; they manage and operate a successful team. The chair is there to help others perform and grow professionally and inspires and gives guidance when needed. The chair will get out of the way of early-career faculty when they are doing a great job and will applaud these successes. The chair does not use the power of the position to dictate what others need to do, since this will not lead to the creation of multipliers/leaders but will continue to promote followers. The chair facilitates collaboration with other departments and helps to sustain the department's service lines or "turf." The chair is a perpetual ambassador for the department and institution both within and outside the academic community. Lastly, the chair is a communicator, and there will be no shortage of important meetings with leadership at the hospital and/or medical school, faculty and other staff, researchers, students, industry representatives, and so many others. As a mid-level manager, the chair provides bidirectional communication and interpretation of directives and concerns between senior-level administration and the department staff.

## Considerations and Qualifications in Preparing to Become a Department Chair?

There is not a secret formula to become a department chair, and the trajectory to chair is different for everyone who earns this position. Experience in the four pillars (clinical service, research, education, and institutional citizenship) of academic medicine is necessary, but excellence in all four is not necessary (see Table 11.3 for personal and professional prerequisites). "Leaning in" at the appropriate time on your way to becoming chair—whether that is becoming a leader in your national specialty society, having a role in your specialty's journal editorial board, or holding a position of vice chair—will give you vital familiarity with certain aspects of the role of chair. Serving as interim chair or as a prior chair at another institution is obviously beneficial. Regarding clinical care, have you been involved in clinical enterprises, whether at a department or hospital level? It can be very advantageous to have previous leadership roles that have allowed for oversight of clinical operations, compliance, and quality. Roles such as vice chair of clinical operations or vice chair of quality and compliance are possibilities that do demonstrate leadership experience. Also, hospital or community center-based roles, such as medical director, can be helpful in the chair role. Furthermore, leadership programming can be helpful in building skills and acquiring competencies needed on your road to department chair.

Train to be a chair: read and increase your fund of knowledge [7]. Formal courses are available through the Association of American Medical Colleges (AAMC) (including those directed to faculty from traditionally underrepresented groups), through several national societies, as well as numerous leadership courses and workshops at major universities (see Resources section of this chapter). Some of the courses require in-person attendance, while others consist of online modules with periodic remote workgroups, and still others utilize a hybrid attendance format. These courses can be accessed prior to attaining, or while retaining, the position of chair. Many professional schools also provide opportunities, including workshops and educational programs, to obtain additional skill sets or additional degrees such

**Table 11.3** Some personal and professional prerequisites for the chair role

| Personal characteristics | Professional prerequisites |
| --- | --- |
| Caring (for the human condition) | Leadership experience |
| Integrity | Prior chair |
| Objective | Interim chair |
| Consistent | Vice chair |
| Organized | Quality-assurance officer |
| Meticulous | Highly competent |
| Follow through and follow-up | Recognized expertise |
| Comfortable with change | Clinical |
| Ambitious/driven | Research |
| Visionary | Academic |

as an MBA, MPP or MPH. Professional coaches are readily available and can be a valuable resource for aspiring or developing chairs. The value of mentorship in this process cannot be understated. Always seek out guidance and support from those individuals, whom you value and respect, who have been or are chairs. In the end, regardless of the amount of preparation and education, expect and be open to some on-the-job training.

Research and innovation are key strategic priorities of an academic medical center. It is valuable to have experience in research funding—both federal and nonfederal grants—and in clinical trials. Being a primary investigator on multiple funded grants can look very favorable on an application for chair, especially at an institution with an established reputation for research. Also, holding a role such as vice chair of research can be helpful. While LHS+ individuals tend to be underrepresented in research, scholarship, and grant funding [8], showing scholarship, publications, and knowledge of the process, and being willing to work with collaborators at your institution will help you in your quest to become a department chair. In the education arena, there is both undergraduate and graduate medical education that must be considered. Being involved in undergraduate medical student education (UME) and/or graduate residency education (GME) is also imperative to a person striving to become a department chair. Evidence of teaching excellence, program development, or GME leadership (such as associate program director or program director), will be helpful tools when becoming a department chair. Also, a commitment to justice, advocacy, community engagement, diversity/equity/inclusion (DEI), and wellness issues are important when striving to be a department chair. Understanding institutional finance and reporting structures and revenue cycle is one of the most essential roles of the department chair. Knowing and asking about these topics will also be important during the interview process and negotiations. The current emphasis on clinical quality and value necessitates an understanding of quality metrics in your field, and how it is measured and incentivized is also crucial. Public performance reporting and patient ratings should be known for your own practice and for the institution you may be applying to. An approach to population health should be recognized especially in the context of addressing healthcare disparities.

Most importantly, it is necessary to have a clear vision of your future department and imagine the steps it will take to make that vision come to fruition. What is your dream for the department that aligns with the institutional priorities and best serves the community, faculty, and trainees? The department chair needs to have a vision that guides strategic goals. This forethought and planning—inclusive of DEI, population health, and social justice—will guide you through what can easily become rough waters and impact our community in a positive way.

## Some Personal Considerations When Deciding to Become a Department Chair

It is important to think about your goals and timing if you are thinking about becoming a chair. Do consider if you really want to be a chair or if you are pursuing this because you were told to. Follow your heart, know yourself along with your strengths and weaknesses, and pursue being a chair if that is truly your goal. If you want to be a chair, think about where you want to be a chair. Your relative strengths and weaknesses must be well suited to the community you would be serving and to the institution that you would be working for. You must also have a passion for the work, community, and people you will serve. Communication is a critical skill, and compassion is essential. Contemplate what is most important to you and your family, personally and professionally, and pursue it. It is not always, or all, about the finances.

Practice makes you better and more effective; we all make mistakes, and it is important to always learn from them. Like any other occupation, the job is associated with a learning curve [9]. Do not be afraid to ask for help. Seek the input and advice of mentors, sponsors, and colleagues throughout the process. Be patient. Change is hard for everyone including the chair, and the cadence of change is as important as its content. Be flexible. The day of a chair rarely reflects what the Outlook calendar predicted it would be the day before. Crisis management is a large part of being a chair. Emotional intelligence and financial savvy will be much more important than your amount of grant funding, publications, or RVUs. In many ways, serving as a chair is a continuation of the concept of self-sacrifice that is initiated during the process of becoming a physician. When you become a chair, make sure that you are fully prepared to drop the "I" and use the "we" pronoun in nearly everything you say and do. You need to be prepared to often step away from your own professional development priorities to prioritize others. This selflessness and generosity are critically important and require maturity… are you at that tipping point?

As a department chair, think of a long-term race, a marathon through a mountain where you run a mile every day for many days to come and where you will have to use different tactics to reach the objective—somedays you will have to run slowly, and some days you may have to run a little bit faster, but it is about understanding what the terrain will be in the mile and whether or not there are cliffs and/or other areas that may require you to slow down. As a leader, work toward developing long-term coping strategies instead of short-term solutions or reactively putting out fires. This will give those around you a sense of vision, mission, and inspiration that will allow them to lead, and therefore you create multipliers as you do this. Many times, we want to make decisions right away, and we do not give opportunities to our team members to make those decisions and sometimes learn from their own mistakes. When presented with this situation, give advice instead of orders, share experiences, and let your team members make their own decisions. In the long run, you will enjoy more success, and those around you will continue to grow. Inspire and guide, but do not micromanage your team. Always strive to clearly communicate your expectations [10]. It may be uncomfortable at times but in the long run, your colleagues will be appreciative and will know what is expected of them. They will then work much more expeditiously toward goals. Sometimes if you first ask them what their goals are, you will notice that their goals will often align with yours. So, if you just say "Go for it," then they will feel validated and empowered to act. Accountability can be challenging, as it is much easier sometimes to be the nice person and not hold those around you accountable. If you do this, then you are not fulfilling your role as a leader and you are not allowing your team members to develop to their full potential. Hold your team accountable for performance, and hold yourself accountable for performance and leadership. Get regular evaluations that are blinded, so you know your own gaps and opportunities for improvement. Give effective feedback regarding performance, and if you see strengths and opportunities in a team member, do not hesitate to let them know how much you value their work and admire what they are doing, and do not be reluctant to tell them that maybe there are other things they would consider doing to continue to improve.

In addition to helping your colleagues, it is essential to consider your own well-being while embarking on this journey. Taking care of your health, maintaining a balance between personal and professional life, and committing to continuous growth are key elements of success at all levels. It can sometimes be lonely at the top and as a chair, you will encounter hard choices and hard times. To overcome professional isolation, mental fatigue, and/or emotional stress, it will be important to establish and build relationships with other leaders, not only at your institution but at other institutions. These individuals will become an integral part of your professional support network and can help you maintain focus and balance during challenging situations in your tenure as chair. Your leadership team (i.e., vice chair(s), residency program director(s), and senior department administrator(s)) will be another group of individuals that will be there to assist before, during, or after crises or impending events (such as a major department inspection, reaccreditation, etc.). Suppose you have gone about setting up your table of organization correctly. In that case, there should be at least one or two individuals on your team who can cover for you when you need to be out of the department, for whatever reason (meeting, vacation, illness, personal family situation).

## Next Steps: Job Application and Interviews

Congratulations! If you have gotten to this point in this chapter, it is reasonable to assume you are interested in becoming a department chair. The application process for a potential job occurs via a solicitation process. This may be a job posting, an email notification, a contact from a recruiter, or word-of-mouth through your professional network [6]. A healthy reminder: think before you apply. Again, ask yourself if the timing is right and if the position is right. If the opportunity passes this screening test, then you will submit a cover letter and a copy of your curriculum vitae. While anonymity can be requested at the outset, keep in mind that as this process moves forward, your application is subject to becoming common knowledge. The cover letter should express your interest in the position and the qualifications that suit you as an excellent and appropriate candidate for the opportunity. Once you apply for the position, start doing your homework on the department, the institution, its leadership and staff, and its culture. Review their websites and their professional social media. Talk to your confidential contacts. Learn about changes, both positive and negative, that are taking place and why they are seeking a new chair. Do your due diligence regarding a prospective job opportunity. Was the last chair successful? Why or why not? Talk to that person if possible. Talk to people in the department and outside of the department at the institution. When possible, talk to people there and to people who have left. Beware of any red flags that suggest problems that may not have a solution, but that will quickly become your problems if you accept the position. The benefit of this initial investigation is to get you organized and prepared. This will provide insight into the degree of presence of that specific department within your field—in other words, its reputation. This will also start to give you a sense of the department and institutional cultures and is the forerunner to your subsequent SWOT (strengths, weaknesses, opportunities, threats) analysis of that department.

Within a few weeks of applying for the position, you may hear back from the institution, usually the chair of the search committee. This communication may take place via email, telephone conversation, or web-based conference. You should treat this initial encounter as if it is your first interview for the position. The search committee is contacting you, because they are interested in your application and want to arrange for a visit. In general, you will have two formal interview sessions. The first visit will consist of meetings with key members of the department and the search committee. You will also have an opportunity to tour the department to get an overview of the department and the institution. During this visit, ask questions that will provide meaningful information on issues or changes that impact the department's daily or future operations [11]. It is also important to identify all key stakeholders that will either evaluate you and directly or indirectly benefit from your success as chair. During this process, it is important to assess the department's current situation. Are you being asked to create a new department? Is it a relatively stable department that only needs some realignment to sustain success? Are you being asked to accelerate growth as part of the institution's strategic plan? Or is it a turnaround situation that requires deep and significant changes [12]? If there is mutual interest, a second visit will be arranged at which time you will have the opportunity to share your vision of the department with the selection committee. Your observations, both what you see and hear and, equally important, what you do not see and hear, along with the information you obtain before and during the visit should help you craft your presentation to the selection committee. Do understand whether there is a true commitment to ensuring safe, quality care for all communities, including the LHS+ diaspora. Is it meaningful, and is the job resourced to allow you to succeed and advance your vision and mission? During the interview process, are you asked questions about supporting accessibility and success for all communities? In the end, all of us should try to pay it forward. Will this chair position allow—and support—you to do such?

## Negotiating a Job Offer

You are offered the job. This is great news, but what should you do next? This is a continuation of your preparation and homework. You now must reinvent your department in the context of your vision and strategic plan. Several key resources must be addressed in the negotiation. The negotiation may take place with the chief executive officer, the dean, or other key leaders who determine or control the financial operations of the department and institution. You will negotiate for people (staff), equipment, space, and programs. This is what will determine the success of your department. You should also consider the department's table of organization and if any specific additions or changes are necessary. A department chair must be knowledgeable in the components of academia—clinical, education, and research—and the various functions of an academic medical center. You do not have to be an expert in each but need to have experience and skills around these core missions. You can always complement your leadership team with others who are strong in areas where you are not. For example, you notice that there is no quality assurance officer and know that this is not your strength, so you negotiate for that position with the appropriate salary line so that you can either promote someone from within or hire someone else. The next negotiation deals with currency: your time commitment and your compensation. This is the moment when you can optimize the package on behalf of the department and yourself. Do not be shy but do be realistic in the context of your department and institutional assessment. This is the opportunity to clarify how you will be evaluated and just exactly who will be evaluating your performance [9].

## What Strengths Do LHS+ Chair Candidates Have to Offer?

The role of department chair is not for the weary. An LHS+ academic physician might be well suited for this role, since they have often thrived despite multiple adversities in life and work.

As an LHS+ potential chair candidate, remember that you bring a lot to the table in terms of not only ability, but a wide breadth of cultural skill sets and an inherent grit that will make you an asset to your institution and an angel to your community! LHS+ physicians can better understand racial, ethnic, and cultural differences in the communities from which they originated [2]. This applies to Latino communities where English may not be the primary language for communication. It is reasonable to expect that an LHS+ physician is in an optimal position to not only better relate

**Table 11.4** Reflection exercise on your academic and professional journey to becoming a department chair

| Category | Prompt |
|---|---|
| Personal connection | Have you ever thought about becoming a department chair? Why or why not? |
| Representation and impact | How do you perceive the current representation of LHS+ physicians in academic leadership? What impact do you think an LHS+ department chair could have on patient care and trainee development? |
| Motivation and readiness | Based on your experiences and values, what aspects of the department chair role resonate with you the most? What qualities or skills do you already possess that would support you in this role? |
| Barriers and strategies | What challenges might deter you from considering this path? What strategies could you use to overcome them? |
| Long-term vision | If you were to actively consider this leadership role, what steps could you take in the next 5–10 years to prepare? |

to Latino patients but also to more effectively communicate with them. The implications for improved diagnostic accuracy, treatment choice, and compliance in this scenario are significant [2]. As an educator, an LHS+ department chair can advocate for these patients and include identity-based training as an integral part of healthcare education, so that compassionate care can be provided at the highest level to these historically marginalized patients [13]. The LHS+ chair will also be able to help tailor clinical service lines that support preventive care strategies in Latino-based communities and develop research initiatives that contribute to a better understanding of healthcare trends and management strategies.

## Reflection Exercise

Considering the Department Chair Pathway—Take a moment to reflect on your academic and professional journey. Consider the following questions, and jot down your thoughts (Table 11.4).

## Skills Exercise

Building a Readiness Framework for a role as Department Chair—Using the department chair's roles and responsibilities as a guide, assess your readiness and identify areas for growth (Table 11.5).

**Table 11.5** Skills exercise on readiness framework for a role as department chair

| Category | Prompt |
|---|---|
| Self-assessment | Review the quadripartite missions of academic medical centers (clinical care, education, research, service) <br> Rate your confidence in each area on a scale from 1 (limited experience) to 5 (highly experienced) <br> Identify one strength and one area for improvement in each category |
| Leadership attributes checklist | Review the quadripartite missions of academic medical centers (clinical care, education, research, service) <br> Rate your confidence in each area on a scale from 1 (limited experience) to 5 (highly experienced) <br> Identify one strength and one area for improvement in each category |
| Action plan | Identify 2–3 concrete actions you can take in the next year to strengthen your preparation for a future chair role. Examples may include seeking mentorship from a current chair, leading a departmental initiative, or engaging in leadership training programs |

## Summary

There has not been a more difficult time to be a leader in academic medicine than now. The COVID-19 pandemic contributed to significant financial strain and sky-high levels of burnout among our faculty, staff, and learners [14]. While many of us expect our leaders to be immune to human struggles, this is not the case, and leaders can be the most vulnerable given their accountability and responsibility. Moreover, the business of medicine has created a healthcare industry in which corporate models are at play and in which nonmedical personnel may be the key stakeholders in enterprise-wide decisions that will likely impact your department. There is a significant risk to being chair; you will almost certainly not be popular all the time or to all people if you commit to principle and doing the right thing. Do you have the integrity, strength, and courage to expose yourself to those risks? How willing are you to confront, compromise, or negotiate? Preparation, patience, and persistence will guide you [15]. In the end, you will enjoy the satisfaction of watching your faculty, trainees, and staff flourish, your programs grow, and your patients benefit from the fruition of your vision [16]!

## Resources

National Professional Development Opportunities Supporting the Development of Prospective and Current Department Chairs:

- Becoming a Successful Department Chair resources page. AAMC. https://www.aamc.org/career-development/leadership-development/toolkits
- Organizational Leadership in Academic Medicine for New Associate Deans and Department Chairs. AAMC. https://www.aamc.org/career-development/leadership-development/organization-leadership-program

- The *Hedwig van Ameringen* Executive Leadership in Academic Medicine. ELAM. https://drexel.edu/medicine/academics/womens-health-and-leadership/elam/
- Harvard Macy Institute—Leading Innovations in Health Care & Education https://harvardmacy.org/courses/leaders
- American Association for Physician Leadership (AAPL) https://www.physician-leaders.org/

## Personal Narratives

### Monica Verduzco-Gutierrez, MD

Early on in my career, I was asked where I would be in 10 years. I never imagined it would be getting prepared for a chair role. I am a small-town girl who had big-town dreams. I am the only person in my family who is a physician and was the first in my family to be in medicine. I am thankful my parents allowed me to focus on my education and be successful in school. As long as I remember, I always wanted to be a doctor. You may have heard, "You can't be what you can't see," and I was able to see just a few Latino physicians in my community (that was 95% Hispanic). But those two inspired me to be a physician. I thought I was going to be a pediatrician and now I am a Physical Medicine and Rehabilitation (PM&R) physician. I had no idea what that field was before going into medicine, nor did I know what academic medicine was, and what these different roles were. Why was someone just an assistant professor? What did it mean to be a tenured professor? These words were foreign to me with my background. But I always looked up to those around me, and even if the lessons were harder, my tenacity helped me get to the top. One of the biggest eye-opening moments in my career was when I did not go for promotion to Associate Professor. I was told by the vice dean of faculty that I only had a 50% chance to be promoted. I did not like those odds. My colleague—a man—went to the same vice dean and was also told he had a 50% chance. That academic year, he went through the promotion process, and I decided to wait. He got promoted and of course, I remained as an Assistant professor for another year. This was definitely a lesson in "you miss 100% of the shots you don't take." Years later, when the role of chair opened at the University of Texas Health Science Center at San Antonio, I read the criteria: "We are looking for tenured professors of Physical Medicine and Rehabilitation." I was not tenured nor a professor at that time and almost did not apply. I talked to a close mentor who told me, "What is there to lose? You have an interest in being a Chair. You can at least learn from the process." And I did have a dream. I had a lifelong vision to return to my roots in South Texas to further improve access to health care for those who are underserved in our community, as my own grandfather did not get stroke rehabilitation and stayed in a nursing home for the rest of his life. This position aligned with a personal leadership vision and with the priorities of the institute. I went for the position and became that tenured professor and distinguished chair. I became only the third Latina in the USA to become a professor of PM&R. I then started my role as Chair on April Fool's Day 2020. Literally when everything shut down at the start of the COVID-19 pandemic (Was the joke on me?). It was a challenging time, and my leadership vision had to take a short detour, and my priorities had to shift to a holding type of leadership. Keep the team together, preserve everyone's health and sanity, stay within an extremely tight budget, maintain relevance to the hospital system during a difficult pandemic, and care for patients who are suffering. The pandemic is a school of hard knocks for new chairs. But despite the challenges, I remained committed to creating a physiatric community that is creating leaders, supporting faculty and trainees, eliminating health disparities, and promoting equity at all levels.

**Julie Ann Sosa, MD**
I have several different identities that together make me who I am as a leader in academic surgery. While many of us focus on financial disclosures and conflicts of interests in medicine, I believe it is much more important to understand people's identities, as they almost certainly impact their thinking and approach to life.

So let me introduce myself; my pronouns are she/her/hers/ella. I'm a woman. I'm also a surgeon; as an endocrine surgeon, I specialize in caring for patients with benign and malignant conditions of the thyroid, parathyroid, and adrenal glands.

I'm a scientist; I spend a good part of my time conducting health services research, clinical trials and translational research, especially focused around optimizing the management of thyroid cancer.

I'm Latina; my father and his family are from Guatemala.

I'm an immigrant; I was born in Montreal, Canada, and my mother is Canadian.

I'm LGBTQ and have been with my partner for more than 20 years.

Taken together, this makes me a very intersectional person, and I believe that this intersectionality is a superpower, as it allows me to share personal truths with colleagues and friends and better understand more people for their similar life experiences. Intersectionality also enhances my courage but certainly does not eliminate fear when advocating for change in academic surgery.

My path to becoming Chair of Surgery at the University of California San Francisco (UCSF) was a very long and serpentine one. It was perhaps longer than it needed to be, because I did not have any (repeat, any!) role models who looked like me. I was blessed to have mentors or sponsors, but because they did not share my life experience, it was hard to ask them to walk in my shoes. Perhaps as a result, I was late deciding to go into medicine and was actively pursuing a career as a labor economist until after college. I was also late deciding to go into surgery, anticipating a career in internal medicine because my father was a cardiologist. Finally, I was late deciding to become an endocrine surgeon, because almost everyone in my residency training program became a pancreatic surgeon, in large part because that was what the Chair and the senior faculty members had for their specialty. I certainly don't regret any of the switchbacks that I've taken in my professional life, but I do wish that I'd had better guidance to follow my own heart and passion rather than that of my parents, or my department chair, or my coresidents. It might have made my professional development a little more efficient!

I started my career as a faculty member at Yale University, where I spent 11 years until moving to Duke University for a leadership opportunity. I was there for 6 years before coming to UCSF Surgery in 2018 as Chair. Change is hard, and moving is challenging for you and for your family; I have only moved for significant leadership opportunities. Coming to UCSF as Chair was literally my "dream" job; when I was a learner, I had interviewed at the mystical and magical place called UCSF, where there was a woman Chair of Surgery, Dr. Nancy Ascher. At that time, UCSF was unique for having a woman leader, and this was empowering. While there are still too few women chairs of surgery in the USA, there is only one department that has had two consecutive women Chairs of Surgery—UCSF. This speaks to the importance of institutional and departmental culture, and the critical ingredient of "belonging." UCSF is in the minority-majority state of California, and more than half of the incoming students to the School of Medicine are underrepresented in medicine (UIM). As a department, we are aligned with the school in striving to be the most diverse, equitable, and inclusive surgical community…and thereby the most spectacular! More than half of our residents are women, and half or more of our last two incoming classes of general surgery interns have been UIM, the majority of whom are Latino/Latina.

Milestones like these are possible in academic surgery with strategic goals and planning, resources, a community with shared values committed to prioritizing inclusivity and PRIDE (Professionalism, Respect, Integrity, Diversity, and Excellence) values and social justice, and unwavering leadership. I believe department chairs are important agents for change when they deploy their power to empower the disempowered. While I am proud of the changes in our department, I also know there is so much more work to do. I am so happy to have made my way West to UCSF; it is the first time in my personal and professional lives that I feel like I am "home." I am committed to creating a surgical community where Latino/Latina colleagues want to come and also want to stay.

### A. Orlando Ortiz, MD, MBA, FASSR

As I reflect on my career pathway and choices, when I was attending medical school, I would never have imagined myself, a Puerto Rican, as the chair of an academic department. But sometimes goals can be the seeds of dreams that occur during our professional development. It was not until I became chief resident during my radiology residency that I became sensitized to one of my qualities—whenever I saw a problem or challenge, I wanted to do more than just complain about it, and I wanted to bring about change and make the situation better. Previously, as a medical student, my intent was guided by the same principle, as my active involvement in the then Boricua Health Organization exposed me to so many committed physicians and political leaders who were interested in improving the health of Latino communities. This involvement also engaged me with the academic leadership at Harvard Medical School which, in turn, served as a sound learning experience in interacting with deans, directors, and senior administrators.

After completing my residency in radiology and a 2-year fellowship in diagnostic and interventional neuroradiology at the Neurological Institute at Columbia

University, I realized that I enjoyed teaching and research and decided to become an academic radiologist. My first job was certainly the result of divine intervention, as straight out of fellowship I became a director of a division, in diagnostic and interventional neuroradiology, within the Radiology Department at West Virginia University School of Medicine. I immersed myself in the program, building the section; starting a fellowship exposed me to graduate medical education and the ACGME, and starting a medical student elective in my section got me involved in medical school teaching experiences. My clinical, academic, and research activities, catalyzed by mentorship and collaboration, quickly gained momentum and within 3 years I was promoted from assistant to associate professor. Then one day, in keeping with my credo to get involved, I was elected to the hospital's medical board by my clinical colleagues. Attending those meetings was an eye-opener for me, because I witnessed the operation of the entire healthcare enterprise from a new perspective. Since I wanted to contribute to this group, I decided to obtain an MBA at WVU as I really wanted to understand the business of medicine and its implications for healthcare delivery. The combination of my leadership experiences at this juncture, in the medical school, at the hospital, and in the classroom fomented my decision to become a department chair.

My objective was to become a department chair in 5 years. Sometimes, when traversing life's mountain range, you must get off one mountain and climb another, to enjoy the view. I developed a strategic plan which required relocation from my institution to another. I believe that I could utilize my newly acquired business skills to assist me in this endeavor. I chose to step up from division director to a vice chair position, specifically, vice chair of Finance in the Department of Radiology at the University of Maryland Medical School. I sensed that this move would bring me one step closer to my goal and would provide an invaluable experience as I had the opportunity to work with so many talented colleagues. I am reminded that my first attempt to obtain a vice chair position resulted in rejection. While I did not like this result, I cherished the lessons learned in the endeavor, stuck to my plan, and was patiently persistent while actively exploring new opportunities.

At this point in my career, I had created a national reputation for myself and had begun to cultivate a healthy network of colleagues through my active participation in regional and national specialty societies [17]. An opportunity to become an academic chair at a university hospital was brought to my attention, and I was asked to apply for the position. Even though I had only been a vice chair for 1 year, I decided to apply. This required preparation for which my MBA skill set was well-suited. I took a consultant's perspective on this opportunity, so that I could craft my vision and strategic plan for the radiology department in the context of the institution's mission. My approach was successful, and I was offered the position and promoted to Professor.

In addition to rapidly rising through the ranks to become a department chair, I also had the opportunity to serve as a chair in a different institution. This time around, for me, it was payback time, as I decided to return to the community where I was raised to make a positive difference. I had developed a favorable reputation as being a "builder" and saw an opportunity to rebuild a struggling academic radiology department at Jacobi Medical Center in the Bronx, NY. Jacobi Medical Center is part of the 11-hospital public health system that serves New York City. Jacobi serves a large Hispanic population in the Bronx, approximately 55% of the Bronx's inhabitants. My first task was to hire a full complement of fellowship-trained subspecialty radiologists to provide the appropriate level of clinical service to our colleagues and patients and to replenish the faculty-to-trainee ratios necessary to provide adequate trainee supervision and education. Simultaneously, I upgraded all of the radiology modalities to state-of-the-art equipment, so that radiology examinations could be performed efficiently and precisely. In other words, the patients, half of whom were LHS+, were getting quality imaging studies that were being interpreted by experts in the field. This meant that our department was on equal footing, fulfilling if not exceeding standard of care, with the other major radiology departments at the private hospitals in New York City. I then recruited a vice chair of research and education, and a chief quality management officer, to drive our educational, research, and quality missions. Within 3 years, our department was on the national academic map, as evidenced by our publication, presentation track record, resident board pass rate, and our 100% fellowship match rate. Furthermore, our educational programs included all members of the department to provide the best care possible to each patient. For our LHS+ patients, this also included a large complement of staff who were medically Spanish proficient to facilitate timely and accurate communication and ease patient stress.

My Jacobi chairmanship was an incredible experience, as I learned to work with so many committed colleagues, to resurrect the Department and all its programs. After I saw that I had accomplished my goal, I decided to stop being a chairman. Being a chair is not always easy: There are good days and not-so-good days. I have enjoyed my successes and lamented some of my decisions, but above all, I have taken pride in leaving each department in a better position than when I started. I have always believed that no hospital can be excellent unless its radiology department is excellent, a concept that is readily transferable to other clinical departments. This is how as a physician I chose to serve and improve the human condition. This is how as a leader I chose to get involved with my LHS+ patients and make it better for them.

**Rubén Azócar, MD**
Growing up, I always had a desire to help others, which has profoundly shaped my life and career. This passion centered around two key areas: education and medicine. My primary educational role model was my grandmother, who dedicated herself to helping hundreds learn to read, write, and develop math skills. In medicine, I was inspired by a pediatrician in Lima—where my mother is from—who made home visits, demonstrating exceptional kindness and professionalism.

This desire to serve led me to pursue medical school in my native Venezuela. During my clinical rotations, I enjoyed all specialties. I then spent a few months fulfilling my mandatory social service in the rainforest among the Yanomami tribe, where I applied everything, I learned in medical school across various circumstances.

At the end of that journey, I decided to become a surgeon. However, during the early 1990s, it became nearly impossible for a foreign medical graduate to pursue that path. After 2 years of General Surgery at the University of Miami and a Surgical Critical Care fellowship at Cook County Hospital, the route remained closed to me. Along the way, I encountered individuals who attempted to derail my goals, some of whom identified as LHS+. Fortunately, I found guidance and support from many mentors—LHS+ and otherwise—who illuminated my path and encouraged me to shift my focus to anesthesiology. This decision marked a significant turning point in my career.

A pivotal factor in this transition was Dr. Marcelle Willock, a leader in anesthesiology and medical administration, who hired me as I began my residency at Boston University (BU). Dr. Willock was the first female, Latina, and person of color to serve as chair at BU, and she remained my mentor until her untimely passing.

After completing my fellowship in Critical Care Medicine at the Beth Israel Deaconess Medical Center (BIDMC), I launched my faculty career at BU, progressing from Associate Program Director to Program Director and eventually becoming vice chair for Education and Simulation. I also advanced to the rank of Associate Professor. Clinically, I took on the role of Director of one of four Surgical ICUs.

Ten years into these roles, I conducted a self-assessment of my career and decided I wanted to become a chair. I recognized that I needed to make important changes: taking better care of myself, improving my English, and pursuing additional executive education in management. This led me to Tufts University, where I became the Executive Vice Chair. About 18 months later, I was named interim chair and then permanently appointed to the position.

My executive education not only enhanced my leadership skills but also deepened my understanding of financial principles and managerial proficiencies. This knowledge allowed me to take a different route in health care as a physician executive in the role of vice president of Perioperative Services at the Beth Israel Deaconess Medical Center in Boston.

A common question I receive is how, as a hospital-based specialist, I can address issues affecting the LHS+ community, especially since we do not directly bring patients to the hospital. The answer lies in being present and proactive. One key approach is understanding that in the Boston metropolitan area, 20–25% of the population is Hispanic, and in certain neighborhoods—like East Boston—that figure exceeds 50%. During the COVID-19 pandemic, one of our sister hospitals, located in a predominantly Latino area north of Boston, was overwhelmed by an influx of patients. The Anesthesiology Department became aware of this, and we proposed and implemented the opening of an additional ICU at our institution to care for these patients and ensure the best possible care. Another example of our proactive approach is in the care of parturients. We recognized the need for early epidural placement for pain management, and in cases of cesarean sections, we worked to ensure that the proper information and processes were in place to facilitate timely epidural administration. This included providing printed information and streamlining procedures to enhance patient care. Additionally, as chair of the department, I raised the lack of Diversity, Equity, and Inclusion (DEI) initiatives during a meeting with the hospital CEO. As a result, I was appointed the first chair of the DEI Committee within our physician organization. Among other achievements, we paved the way for the creation of a system-wide DEI vice president position. Finally, we focused on making our department more representative, significantly increasing the proportion of Hispanic faculty and trainees. This not only helped us to better reflect and understand the community we serve but also enhanced our ability to provide culturally competent care.

Looking back, I often marvel at how a kid from Caracas, Venezuela, has traveled so far. The reasons are clear: my parent's guidance and support, mentors who inspired and encouraged me; my wife Maray, who covered my blind spots; and my children J and Andrea, who were patient with me through my obligations. At times, being in the right place at the right time was also crucial. While challenges and detractors have been present, the positive influences prevailed. I remain committed to our patients and passionate about educating, developing, and growing the next generation of healthcare providers.

### Rolando J. DeLeon, MD, FACOG

Academic and clinical careers rarely follow a straight line with a constant slope. More often, they are, to borrow from the Beatles, "a long and winding road," whose destination may not be completely clear to us until we arrive. Interestingly, my road has been a combination of both, certainly not the typical path to an Academic Department Chair.

As the only child of Cuban immigrants who left Cuba soon after the Castro regime took power, I was raised in Puerto Rico by my grandparents until my parents had the means to provide for me. At 8 years old, I arrived at a strange new place called Virginia which would ultimately become my home. My academic path to medicine was certainly not one of top named institutions but rather economically and logistically driven. It turned out to be the perfect path for me. I attended Virginia Tech, because it was the least expensive university in the state and miraculously was accepted to Eastern Virginia Medical School.

I attended medical school to become an Obstetrician and Gynecologist and never wavered in my choice. I matched at my top-rank site at the University of Miami/Jackson Memorial Hospital. At the time, it was not at all difficult as Miami in the early 1980s was possibly the most dangerous city in the country and not a very desirable destination. UM/JMH, at the time, had one of the top three busiest L&D units in the country. It was here my path to medical education and leadership began to take form. I realized that as a resident, I truly enjoyed teaching and mentoring the medical students assigned to my service. For 3 out of my 4 years at UM/JMH, I was awarded the Outstanding Resident Teaching Award simply for spending time, respecting my students, and sharing what little knowledge I had acquired. Upon finishing my time as a resident, I remained on staff, paying back a national Health Service Corps Scholarship for medical school. Now, I was teaching residents! Here was when I truly fell in love with clinical teaching. Seeing the residents stretch their surgical skills in difficult cases where I was their attending and mentor was the most satisfying feeling I had experienced in medicine. If you love what you do, people will notice and gravitate toward that energy. I found this to be completely accurate as there was, almost always, a small army of students following me to the clinic, L&D, and the OR to share in the adventures.

One thing I often marvel over is the "Nature vs Nurture" aspect of leadership. In my clinical interactions with students and residents, I notice some shy away from difficult scenarios and others rush toward them. I always seemed to find myself in the thick of some clinical mayhem.

After leaving UM/JMH I settled at Mercy Hospital, a large community hospital in Miami where fate called upon me to start my own private practice, which was the last thing I ever envisioned as my business acumen was practically nil. With the help of loyal friends and family, the practice grew to where there are now nine other Board Certified OBGYNs working in the group, one of the largest OBGYN practices in the city. Each one of my partners is of LHS+ background. I was blessed to have my first two partners become the managing partners of the practice, so I could focus on my loves: patient care, teaching, and hospital leadership. My career evolved in a state with one of the highest LHS+ populations in the country. More than one-third of the state's population (33%) is of a Hispanic background, yet only 17% of the total number of physicians share this background with the general population. In Miami, my last 40 years have been spent caring for a patient population that was close to 80% LHS+. My cultural connection to my patients throughout that time made all the difference in my being able to provide the best care I could deliver for them. In Florida, Latinos make up 11% of medical school graduates. Unfortunately, a reverse trend exists nationally, in 1980, there were 135 Hispanic physicians per 100,000 Hispanic patients in the USA. However, the number of LHS+ physicians has not kept pace with the growth of the Hispanic population in the USA. In 2010, the rate of Hispanic physicians per 100,000 LHS+ population dropped to 105 [18].

I continued teaching but in a less formal role as the rigors of my own practice took me in a different direction. I became involved in my hospital's physician leadership team out of necessity. I discovered the truth to the adage, the more you do, the more you are asked to do. I moved from OBGYN Quality Assurance Chair to 16 years as OBGYN Department Chair, to Chief of Staff, and, ultimately, Chairman of the Board of Trustees of Mercy Hospital. Without looking for it, I had become the first LHS+ Board Chair in the Hospital's history. The higher I rose in the ranks, the more I held on to the concept of servant leadership. I realized my greatest strength was having respect as well as the ability to work well with the hospital's greatest asset, its medical staff, and employees.

The same formula which had worked so well years before as a resident was the strategy for success. Sharing time with my colleagues, empathy for their concerns, respect, and thoughtful interchange of ideas paved the road for my new position. During my tenure as Chief of Staff, Mercy Hospital was acquired by the largest hospital corporation in the country. In the hospital, fear was everywhere, rumors of departmental and service line closures were everyday conversations. It was my place to shepherd the flock and assure all that we would come out of this acquisition much stronger. This was no easy feat, almost 800 physicians formed the medical staff, most of whose livelihood depended on a smooth and successful transition. The physicians needed complete transparency, guidance, and reassurance. The hospital corporation was also anxious, as an exodus of physicians would abort the acquisition and force the closure of the hospital. I was trusted to be the liaison between both parties in this enormous venture. Countless meetings ensued. Taking over a year, this transition became the culmination of my role as a leader in my medical community.... or so I thought.

It was during this time that a physician friend invited me to become an OBGYN preceptor at the Florida International University College of Medicine. I accepted the position. After many years, my love for teaching was reawakened. Beyond clinical teaching, I became involved in numerous clinical and curricular committees, student advising, and preclinical teaching, in short, immersing myself in as many aspects of medical education as I could. I loved this new turn my career had taken and dreamt of a full-time, postclinical opportunity in academia.

Completely unbeknownst to me, a new medical school, in its fetal stages a few miles north in Davie Florida was taking shape. The Dr. Kiran C. Patel College of Allopathic Medicine at Nova Southeastern University had just received preliminary accreditation and was welcoming their first class. The corporation which had acquired Mercy Hospital was partnered with the new medical school to provide the clinical settings for the third and fourth years of the curriculum. Now comes the part you may find hard to swallow. Almost 5 years ago, I was invited to lunch at the Hospital's corporate headquarters which as Board Chair happened from time to time. There I met the President of the University, the Dean of the medical school, and the President of the Hospital Corporate division. I was asked to consider being the Founding Chair of the Department of Obstetrics and Gynecology of the medical school. I laughed and humbly declined stating that I truly did not believe I had the experience or background for such a position. The Dean stated that as a new school the most important criteria were significant clinical experience, a profound love and commitment for teaching, and strong ties to the South Florida medical community. The Corporate President assured me that anyone with the leadership skills I had shown him at the time of the acquisition could easily help give birth to a clinical department of a new medical school.

That was it! After multiple handshakes, the position was mine. Of course, all the credentialing paperwork had to be in order and ratified by the school. I realized quickly why I was given the job. With less than 6 months to the inaugural class's beginning clinical rotations, there was nothing in place. I mean nothing. No clinical curriculum, no faculty, no preceptors, just the hospitals which up to this point had no undergraduate medical education experience. Utilizing the experience I had gained at FIU, a blank dry-erase board, and input from several academic friends, I worked out a curriculum. I recruited the help of every OBGYN I knew in clinical practice in South Florida and in less than 5 months, we got the program off the ground. In fact, more than that, it is soaring. In the first 3 years, we had a 100% OBGYN match rate and continue to grow and improve in quality.

This is my story, no grants, minimal publications, minimal fiscal, and budgetary knowledge. All I brought was the clinical experience of thousands upon thousands of mothers and babies that I have been blessed to care for, a deep love for medicine and for sharing my passion with my students, hundreds of wonderful colleagues to help bring my vision to reality, and most importantly a very supportive family. More than 50 years ago, a mentor shared a saying with me that has carried me through my professional life: Estudiar Para Saber, Saber Para Valer, Valer Para Servir!

My path has been a very different one from almost anyone I know. In no way is my story meant to diminish the role of scholarship, research, and academic leadership, rather it is to show that the unintended path can lead us to where we always hoped to end up. Let me finish with this; every day I am grateful and strive to pay forward this incredible gift that I have been given. This has been my long and winding road to academic and clinical leadership, and I would not change a single step.

My mission in the time I have left in medicine is to help others grow in their clinical knowledge and rise to their desired leadership roles in medicine.

**Acknowledgments** The authors acknowledge the following colleagues for their early insights into the topic: Alfredo Quinones-Hinojosa, MD, of Mayo Clinic and Minerva Romero Arenas, MD of NYP Brooklyn Methodist Hospital and Weill Cornell Medical College.

# References

1. Meadows AM, Skinner MM, Hazime AA, Day RG, Fore JA, Day CS. Racial, ethnic, and sex diversity in academic medical leadership. JAMA Netw Open. 2023;6(9):1–13.
2. Xierali IM, Nivet MA, Rayburn WF. Diversity of department chairs in family medicine at US medical schools. J Am Board Fam Med. 2022;35(1):152–7.
3. Odei BC, Jagsi R, Diaz DA, Addison D, Arnett A, Odei JB, Mitchell D. Evaluation of equitable racial and ethnic representation among departmental chairs in academic medicine, 1980-2019. JAMA Netw Open. 2021;4(5):1–4.
4. Pew Research Center. Hispanic Americans' trust and engagement with science. 2022, June. https://www.pewresearch.org/science/2022/06/14/hispanic-americans-experiences-with-health-care/. Accessed on 20 June 2025.
5. Association of American Medical Colleges. Faculty Roster, December 31, 2024, snapshot as of December 31, 2024, for LHS+ individuals in the basic and clinical sciences. 2024. https://www.aamc.org/data/facultyroster/. Accessed 20 June 2024.
6. Slakey DP, Korndorffer JR, Long KN. The modern surgery department chairman. JAMA Surg. 2013;148(6):511–5.
7. Biebuyck JF, Mallon WT. The successful medical school department chair: a guide to good institutional practice. Washington, DC: Association of American Medical Colleges; 2002.
8. Masters-Waage T, Spitzmueller C, Edema-Sillo E, et al. Underrepresented minority faculty in the USA face a double standard in promotion and tenure decisions. Nat Hum Behav. 2024;8:2107–18. https://doi.org/10.1038/s41562-024-01977-7.
9. Fisher M. Being chair: a 12-step program for medical school chairs. Int J Med Educ. 2011;2:147–51.
10. Association of American Medical Colleges. GSA professional development initiative: feedback and recognition guide. 2016. https://www.aamc.org/media/23256/download. Accessed 16 Oct 2024.
11. Gunderman RB, Buckwalter KA, Farber JM. Seeking an academic department chairperson. Am J Roentgenol. 2003;181:951–4.

12. Watkins MD. Picking the right transition strategy. Harvard Business Review. 2009. Picking the Right Transition Strategy. Accessed 23 Oct 2024.
13. Evans A, Chun E. Department chairs as transformational diversity leaders. Depart Chair. 2015;25(3):1–3.
14. Lluch C, Galiana L, Doménech P, Sansó N. The impact of the COVID-19 pandemic on burnout, compassion fatigue, and compassion satisfaction in healthcare personnel: a systematic review of the literature published during the first year of the pandemic. Healthcare (Basel). 2022;10(2):364. https://doi.org/10.3390/healthcare10020364. PMID: 35206978; PMCID: PMC8872521.
15. Association of American Medical Colleges toolkit. Becoming a successful department chair. https://www.aamc.org/career-development/leadership-development/toolkits. Accessed 20 Sept 2024.
16. Sheldon GF. Embrace the challenge: advice for current and prospective department chairs. Acad Med. 2013;88:914–5.
17. Quencer RM. Orlando Ortiz: eight presidents of the American Society of Spine Radiology. Am J Neuroradiol. 2002;23(9):1611.
18. Sanchez G, Nevarez T, Schink W, Hayes-Bautista DE. Latino physicians in the United States, 1980-2010 a thirty-year overview from the censuses. Acad Med. 2015;90(7):906–12.

**Open Access**  This chapter is licensed under the terms of the Creative Commons Attribution 4.0 International License (http://creativecommons.org/licenses/by/4.0/), which permits use, sharing, adaptation, distribution and reproduction in any medium or format, as long as you give appropriate credit to the original author(s) and the source, provide a link to the Creative Commons license and indicate if changes were made.

The images or other third party material in this chapter are included in the chapter's Creative Commons license, unless indicated otherwise in a credit line to the material. If material is not included in the chapter's Creative Commons license and your intended use is not permitted by statutory regulation or exceeds the permitted use, you will need to obtain permission directly from the copyright holder.

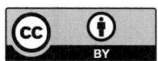

# Chapter 12
# Being a Medical School Dean: Perspectives from Past and Current LHS+ Deans

Jose Manuel de la Rosa, Pedro "Joe" Greer Jr., and Olga Rodríguez de Arzola

**Learning Objectives**
- Describe the trajectory to dean
- Describe skills that are important to develop for leadership positions, including dean
- Examples of how these skills can be developed
- Detail the why of being a Latina/o/x/e Dean

**Key Terms and Definitions**

AAMC: Association of American Medical Colleges
ACGME: Accreditation Council for Graduate Medical Education
COD: Council of Deans of the Association of American Medical Colleges—it is the organization convening deans of AAMC member medical schools in the United States and Canada to address issues affecting academic medicine and develop strategies to achieve excellence in medical education, research, and patient care. *Council of Deans (COD) | AAMC*

---

J. M. de la Rosa (✉)
Department of Pediatrics, Paul L. Foster School of Medicine, Texas Tech University Health Sciences Center, El Paso, TX, USA

P. J. Greer Jr.
Roseman University College of Medicine, Las Vegas, NV, USA

O. R de Arzola
Ponce Health Sciences University School of Medicine, Ponce, Puerto Rico
e-mail: orodriguez@psm.edu

| | |
|---|---|
| ELAM: | Executive leadership in academic medicine—it is a year-long, part-time fellowship for women faculty in schools of medicine, dentistry, public health, and pharmacy. The program is dedicated to developing the professional and personal skills required to lead and manage in today's complex health care environment, with special attention to the unique challenges facing women in leadership positions. *Executive Leadership in Academic Medicine—Drexel University College of Medicine* |
| CME: | Continuing medical education |
| GME: | Graduate medical education |
| HHS: | Human health services |
| LCME: | Liaison Committee on Medical Education |
| MBA: | Master of business administration |
| MHOM: | Master of health occupation management |
| MMM: | Master of medical management |
| MPA: | Master of public administration |
| MPH: | Master of public health |
| MSCHE: | Middle States Commission on Higher Education |
| PHSU: | Ponce Health Sciences University |
| PSM: | Ponce School of Medicine |
| PUH: | Ponce University Hospital |
| UPR: | University of Puerto Rico |
| SOM: | School of Medicine |
| THCHAN: | Harvard T.H. Chan School of Public Health |

## The Long Road to the Deanship

The dean is often defined as the chief executive officer for the college of medicine. She or he often reports directly to the president of the university or the Vice President for Health Affairs. As a chief executive or administrative officer, the dean sets the tone for the college and will provide leadership for all programs and missions. The majority of schools of medicine in the United States have tripartite missions of clinical education, clinical service, and research. However, the way each school defines these missions also defines the emphasis that school's dean will place on her/his administration. Thus, to facilitate a dean's success, the mission of the school must be strongly intertwined with the personal preferences and styles of the person selected by the university leadership to serve as the dean.

Each one of us has personal preferences. Some of us prefer the mission of acquiring new knowledge or research. Others prefer the mission of serving patients and expanding healthcare to underserved populations. Some are highly motivated by the mission of educating and teaching the next generation of students in undergraduate, graduate, or community settings in innovative ways. Additional motivators include advancing diversity, equity, and inclusion principles or the school achieving a strong financial footing.

If you are reading this chapter of this book, you obviously have a desire for a leadership position in the school of medicine. As noted above, it is imperative that you seek a school whose mission coordinates with your professional values and motivations for practicing medicine. Thus, your first priority as you seek the deanship is to know yourself and recognize your motivation for being the dean.

## *Exercise #1: Know Yourself*

If you had a magic wand and could imagine yourself as the ex-dean tomorrow, what would be the legacy that you would want to leave on the school? In three words or less fill in this epitaph.

Dean .... *your name here*... **was** a GREAT Dean.
She/He/They really set the school up to become a national leader in ... *max three words here.*

As the leader of the school of medicine within the university, there are some skills that a physician may find helpful. The first step for young faculty on the road to the deanship is to acquire those skills (Table 12.1).

Certainly, the skills associated with leadership are of paramount importance. Developing leadership skills takes practice and often requires acquiring new knowledge through education in communication, behavior change, emotional intelligence, motivation, negotiation, and other facets of human behavior.

Many physicians recognize that the leadership skills of decision-making, directing, delegating, influencing, motivating employees, and actively managing change

| Table 12.1 Skill requirements for the aspiring dean | |
|---|---|
| | Leadership |
| | Conflict resolution |
| | Financial acumen |
| | Practice management |
| | Understanding research |
| | Management and administration |
| | Mentorship |
| | Curriculum design |
| | Role model |
| | Faculty recruitment, retention, promotion, and mentorship |
| | Fundraising |
| | Marketing |
| | Government relations, especially for public institutions |

can be learned. A successful leader always leads by example and becomes an inspiration for his employees when they role model the values of the medical profession and the organization, which include integrity, respect, accountability, and teamwork.

Other skills are critical for the day-to-day survival of the dean. One of the most useful is the art of conflict resolution. Frequently, the dean must be the arbiter between competing visions, missions, viewpoints, and personalities. The tenor of faculty relationships can enhance or degrade the working environment. The art of negotiation is a part of conflict resolution and can be learned and acquired by the dean.

A dean also requires financial acumen and must be responsible for recognizing, framing, and asking the appropriate questions of their chief financial officer in order to support the financial well-being of the institution.

Balancing the tripartite mission requires recognition and understanding of each of the areas. Physicians believe that they inherently recognize how to run a practice. Unfortunately, the majority are not trained in practice management. The aspiring dean must pursue opportunities to gain additional skills. In a similar manner, the life of the academic researcher in the discovery, translation, and implementation of new knowledge must be a familiar topic for the aspiring dean. Certainly, the concepts behind faculty development, including principles behind curriculum design, healthcare education, and the multiple types of adult learning theory, should be familiar topics for the accomplished dean. The successful dean must not only role model for certain behaviors but must actively take on the role of mentorship. Building a network of trusted mentors and mentees is part of the road to the deanship. The arts of networking, mentorship, and sponsorship is a talent the dean should cultivate actively. The dean is not only expected to be inwardly facing toward his own school but must also look out into the community. Whether it be with a goal of fundraising, recruiting faculty, or engagement with community partners, shaping the face and presentation of the school to the public requires specific talents of communication and marketing for all deans.

Leadership training is often a part of clinical specialty or clinical subspecialty programs. Many public universities offer senior executives in their universities training in leadership (e.g., governor's executive leadership programs). These are often targeted to general interdisciplinary skills designed for educational programs in a general academic university but are quite useful for all deans.

However, there are specific executive programs that focus on specific leadership skills for medical programs (Table 12.2). These programs are major steps on the road to the deanship. The Association of American Medical Colleges (AAMC) offers these leadership courses focusing on the different stages of individual faculty careers and qualifications. The AAMC midcareer and early-career leadership programs are examples of such programs. AAMC leadership programs for department chairs are also available. There are two programs specifically designed for senior faculty considering the deanship. The Executive Leadership in Academic Medicine (ELAM) program is a well-structured 1-year program specifically designed for female faculty already in senior positions who are discerning whether they should pursue a deanship. The program is dedicated to developing the professional and personal skills required to lead

**Table 12.2** Formal training opportunities and degree programs

| |
|---|
| I. Executive leadership programs for academic leadership |
| A. State higher education/university based |
| B. Corporations and foundations |
| II. Formal masters' degrees |
| A. Master of business administration (MBA) |
| B. Master of public administration (MPA) |
| C. Master of health occupations management (MHOM) |
| D. Master of medical education |
| E. Master of public health |
| III. AAMC leadership programs |
| A. Early career faculty development programs |
| B. Midcareer faculty development programs |
| C. Department chair |
| IV. AAMC Dean's training programs |
| A. Executive leadership in academic medicine (ELAM) |
| B. AAMC Council of Deans Fellowships |

and manage in today's complex health care environment, with special attention to the unique challenges facing women in leadership positions. Topics such as the strategic approaches to financial and resource management, personal and professional leadership effectiveness, organizational dynamics, and communities of practice that support academic organizational leadership are addressed. Admission is competitive, and about 60 new fellows are admitted every year.

A distinct program offered by the Council of Deans of the Association is the AAMC Council of Deans (COD) Fellowship Program, which has the unique capacity to afford an aspiring dean the ability to learn from senior deans across the country. This mentorship opportunity, along with the series of preparatory exercises, not only gives the aspiring dean the coursework necessary for strengthening leadership skills, but it also affords the networking opportunity that allows a potential dean candidate name recognition among leading medical schools across the country. This type of exposure or name recognition, together with the networking opportunity, is often the advantage a candidate needs to land the position as a dean. For this reason, the limited positions in the AAMC COD Fellowship are highly prized and quite competitive (only six fellows each year).

Additionally, there are designated degree programs that can strengthen a potential dean candidate's financial and managerial acumen.

The most traditionally recognized method is obtaining a master's degree for each of the different types of skills. The prototypical degree for this is the master's degree in business administration (MBA). There are specific executive MBA programs that focus on health occupations management (MBA/HOM). The MBA gives those desiring to update or upgrade their financial acumen a series of courses in finance, management, and administration.

Those who feel they need to strengthen their skills in the areas of administration could seek a master's degree in public administration (MPA). This degree is ideal for those seeking to lead public- or state-funded schools of medicine.

A master's degree in medical management (MMM) focuses on the skills needed to guide a medical practice. This would be ideal for those universities and medical schools that have large group practices or their own hospital systems.

Another possibility for those who seek to lead in deanship positions that emphasize community involvement is to strengthen one's skills in public health. The traditional master of public health (MPH) offers courses not only in leadership and public health but also in qualitative research methodologies. This is particularly true of public health degrees focused on clinical epidemiology (e.g., the MSc in clinical epidemiology offered by the THCHAN School of Public Health).

There are both universities and private foundations offering programs designed for those wishing to improve their skills in medical education. One of the best-known is the Harvard Macy Medical Education Program, which emphasizes modern pedagogy and leadership skills in curriculum reform and assessment. The skill of mentorship and coaching can be enhanced by participation in academic certification programs. The degree programs leading to a master's or certification in medical education are moderately new developments but are specifically designed to fortify the skills needed by the modern dean. An excellent example is a Master of Science in Health Professions Education degree program offered by the Massachusetts General Hospital (MGH) Institute of Health Professions.

Of course, prior to gaining access to these formalized programs, junior faculty/potential deans require senior faculty to be cognizant of a potential candidate's desire to be a dean, and therefore, one must be visible to senior leadership in one's institution. The road to this recognition and visibility is traditionally through service on medical school committees. As an aspiring dean, it is always best to utilize this service on committees to demonstrate exposure to the multiple facets of a school. *This section is the most* approachable in regard to developing skills outside of your discipline and cultivating an institutional (as opposed to division or departmental) focus. We believe these local opportunities should come before the outside training options. First local committee service activities—e.g. Promotion and Tenure, Academic Affairs, etc. then National Committee Service and combine these with formal training opportunities. Also remember, many local human resources (HR) departments offer leadership and management training, which is often at no cost to the candidate and will not involve travel, so more accessible to candidates. Aspiring deans should think of committee service as "on-the-job" training for the deanship (Table 12.3). A diversity of experience outside of one's clinical or academic area is most noted. Focus specifically on the student programming and education committees. Young faculty should volunteer to serve on the admissions committee, the student grading and promotions committee, the student affairs committees, the curriculum committee, the scholarship/financial aid committee, and the clerkship committee. These dean's committees not only allow notice from the dean but also afford on-the-job training in student programming and education.

As one obtains expertise in committee work, one should seek leadership in school-wide committees, such as the clinical practice committee, the government affairs committee, the institutional advancement (fundraising) committees, and/or the faculty research committee. Never be afraid to say "yes" to committee

**Table 12.3** On-the-job dean training through committee service, or how to get noticed as you climb the academic ladder

| |
|---|
| I. Informal on-the-job training (fill in your knowledge gaps with experience) |
| A. Committee work (fill in your knowledge gaps), promotion retention, and tenure committee |
| Admissions committee |
| Grading and promotions (ethics) committee |
| Scholarship/financial aid committee |
| Human resources committee |
| Curriculum/clerkship directors committee |
| Curriculum/preclerkship committee |
| Continuing medical education committee (CME) |
| Graduate medical education committee (GME) |
| Clinical practice development committee |
| Faculty research/faculty research organization committee |
| Institutional advancement (fundraising) committee |
| Government relations committee |
| B. Professional societies (demonstrate your leadership capacities) |
| 1. Chair affinity groups |
| Diversity and inclusion committee |
| Bylaws committee |
| Professional/ethics committee |
| 2. Service as group officer |
| a. Chair, vice chair |
| b. Finance |
| C. Staff as important informal resources for clerical and administrative "informal dean training" |
| II. Mentorship |
| AAMC mentorship programs |
| Provide mentorship |

assignments, and "punch your ticket" in all the areas of the school's affairs. As you serve on committees, do not be afraid to take on ever-increasing administrative roles. The road to the dean's title is littered with secondary signposts. Accept departmental duties as a vice chair for different department missions (education, clinical service, and research) as an enhancement to your quest for the deanship. Do not become stagnant in one area. Try to only serve two or three terms in one area, but send your message that you wish to serve and acquire knowledge as you climb the academic ladder.

Move forward *outside* your school by similar strategies within your specialty society. Develop your hard-working reputation not only within your department and school but also within your region. As you climb the academic ladder, remember that you are establishing your reputation. Your institutional leadership will take note, and your name will be at the forefront when they are asked for recommendations for deanships. Most traditional entry points for deanship are from the departmental chair position, but other venues exist. Arm yourself with expertise acquired through service.

## *Exercise #2: "Punch Your Ticket"*

Consider the outline in Table 12.3: As a series of experiences to be undertaken over the next several years,

Which have you already done? Draw a thick black line through these.
Which ones do you lack? Circle in red.
For those circled in red, PLAN: Which ones will you undertake next year (maximum two)?
Which ones will you undertake in 2 years?
Which ones will you undertake in 5 years?
Which ones will you ask your dean to appoint you next year (one max)?
Which ones will you ask your dean to appoint you in 3 years?
Which ones will you ask your dean to appoint you in 5 years?
When will you ask your dean to nominate you for the Council of Deans Fellowship or ELAM?

## Why Be a Latina/o/x/e Dean

It has been argued that the current postpandemic crisis in medical education has physicians leaving their positions within medicine in record numbers. Recent estimates range from 50% to 60% of physicians would not choose a medical field for practice if they had the chance to choose again. Some argue that leadership, and in particular the models utilized by corporate America, have no place in a health-related institution.

For these reasons, perhaps it is time to consider the leadership differences between mainstream groups and Latinos in medical education.

Several authors, chief among them Dr. Juana Bordas, argue that Latinos as a group have different styles of leadership. Table 12.4 presents 10 characteristics of Latino leadership styles that could be timely for the medical school in today's environment.

The Latina/o/x/e Deans bring a unique perspective to the leadership of a school of medicine. No matter where your Latina/o/x/e roots are, our culture nurtures collegiality, professionalism, personal awareness, trust, respect, inclusiveness, and vision. And these are characteristics, among others, that contribute to the success of deans.

Dr. Juana Bordas has listed 10 qualities that make Latina/o/x/e deans different from your traditional dean. These qualities are virtues and individually not

**Table 12.4** Ten principles of Latino leadership

| Principle | Overview | Leadership application |
|---|---|---|
| 1. *Personalismo*—the character of the leader | Every person has inherent worth and essential value. The leader's character earns trust and respect. Personalismo secures the relational aspects of leadership. | Treat each person with respect regardless of status of position. Never forget where you came from. Connect to people on a personal level first. Always keep your word. |
| *Consciencia*—knowing oneself and personal awareness | In-depth reflection. Self-examination. Integration. The psychology of oppression and "white privilege" are barriers to inclusion. | Examine personal intention: "Why do I do what I do?" Listen to your institution and "inner voice." Resolve discrimination or exclusion issues. Develop a secure cultural identity and know cultural assets. |
| *Destino*—personal and collective personal | Every person has a distinct life path, purpose, and a unique life pattern. Destino is not fatalism. Tapping into one's destino brings clarity, alignment, and a clearer sense of direction. Power leaders are in sync with their destino. | Know your family history and traditions. Explore your heart's desire. Identify your special skills and talents. Open the door when opportunity knocks. Reflect on your legacy and personal vision. |
| *La Cultura*—culturally based leadership | Latinos are a culture and ethnic group, not a race. Seven key values are the fastening points for the culture. A humanistic orientation (people come first) and diversity/inclusion are cultural mainstays. | La familia—"We" orientation drives collective shared leadership. Leaders are expected to be simpatico congenial and likable. Respect, honesty, and generosity are required leadership traits. Leaders establish personal ties and are part of the familia. |
| De Colores—inclusiveness and diversity | Latinos are connected to 26 different countries. Hispanics were added to the US Census in 1980. Hispanics are the only group that "self-identifies" on the census. Latinos embrace all ages—an intergenerational spirit. | Leaders practice Bienvenido. Because culture is learned, people can become Latino by corazon or affinity. Forging a collective identify from diversity is a leader's ongoing work. Intergenerational leadership: create allies, circular relationships, participation, social action. |
| *Juntos*—collective community stewardship | Juntos means union, being close, joining, being together. Latinos are servant leaders and community stewards. Leadership is conferred by the community of leaders and community capacity. | The leaders follow the rules. Four practices anchor the collaboration process: shared vision, integrating history and cultural traditions, shared responsibility, and paso a paso. |

(continued)

**Table 12.4** (continued)

| Principle | Overview | Leadership application |
|---|---|---|
| *Adelante!*—global vision and immigrant spirit | The United States is a nation of immigrants who bring initiative, hard work, tolerance, optimism, and faith. Latino growth has been fueled by immigration. Latinos are acculturating, not assimilating. A cultural revitalization is occurring. With ties to 26 countries, Latinos are a prototype for global leadership. | Leaders integrate the newly immigrated. Immigrants have revitalized the cultural core and are strengthening Latino identity. Immigration is a civil rights and advocacy issue leaders are addressing. |
| *Si se Puede*—social activist and coalition leadership | Economic discrepancies and social inequalities drive a social activist agenda. Si se Puede is a community organizing, coalition-building, and advocacy forms of leadership. The Latino model is leadership by the many. The inclusive Latino agenda speaks | Leaders build people's faith so that they take action. Leaders practice consistencia-perseverance and commitment. Building networks, being inclusive, and forging coalitions are leadership trademarks. Externally, leaders are cultural brokers building partnerships with other groups. |
| *Gozar la vida*—leadership that celebrates life! | Latinos re a celebratory, expressive, optimistic, and festive culture. Celebration strengthens bonds, collective identity, and reinforces people's resolve. Latinos are stirring the salsa and gusto into leadership. Communication is key for getting things done through people. | Leadership is congenial, includes good times, and time to socialize. Leaders communicate with charisma (charisma), carino (affection), and corazon (heart). Leaders speak the "people's language" and "translate" with mainstream culture. The hard and fast rule of Latino organizing is always serve food. Leaders need a "cultural balance," such as strategic thinking and problem-solving. |
| *Fe y esparanza*—sustained by faith and hope | Optimism is esperanza or hope—an essential Latino quality. Gracias (being grateful) allows people to be generous and give back. Latino spirituality centers on relationships and responsibility. Spirituality is a moral obligation to ensure others' well-being and the collective good. | Leaders must be bold and make unpopular decisions—requiring faith and courage. Humility, modesty, and courtesy are the foundation for leaders to be equal. Leaders must be clear on their purpose, put an issue or a cause first, and serve something greater. This lessens self-importance. Leaders tap into optimism, gratitude, and faith and are the "translators" to inspire and motivate people. |

exclusive to Latina/o/x/e deans but are badly needed (collectively) to begin to change the toxic environment of American medical education.

Our medical school leadership must have optimistic faith in the future and hope for the direction of the school. In the end, it is what prevents burnout, the scourge of so many medical school faculty working in a toxic environment. Bordas states her 10 principles as the uniqueness of Latino leadership. That is why we see the Latino dean has a solution to the toxic environment we see in so many schools.

This is where we see the interweaving of all Bordas' Latino leadership principles (values/virtues). Can you imagine your medical school dean coming naturally to the leadership position with the experience, knowledge, and these 10 principles to define her or his character as the method and style for leading the medical school community forward! If we accept the differences of Latino leadership, we can say more Latino deans might be the answer. This provides a solution for addressing what medical schools have become. It provides a cure for the diseases of educational and health inequity and physician burnout. It provides a solution for the future medical school. ¡Ésa si es una revolución! (That truly is the revolution!).

In true Latino-style optimism, we close with a glimmer of hope for the medical school culture and the future of medical schools in America. For we see during the last decade the number of Latino deans has grown to almost a dozen! Some in new medical schools, some in large medical schools, some in Allopathic programs, and still others in osteopathic programs.

With faith and hope we approach these new developments and exhort you, our young upcoming Latino faculty, to train and walk the long road toward the dean's office.

Todo esta en las manos de Dios…
Pray like it is all in God's hands…
Work like it is all in your hands.

## Personal Narratives

### A Journey—By Pedro José Greer Jr., M.D., Founding Dean for the Roseman University Health Sciences College of Medicine

I was asked to write about how I got be a medical school dean. So here is the story of my journey. There is no single pathway to becoming a medical school dean (much has been written about it), and I believe we should have new pathways and noble reasons for our journey.

I started out in academics and was quickly disillusioned by the toxic environment that existed in academic medicine. My first title was Associate Dean for Homeless Education. I was an internist and gastroenterologist, with a deep interest in resolving the gross disparities that existed in our American society. I resigned from the university and went into practice with my father (I still maintained my title, although now a voluntary, unpaid title). As my practice grew, so did the number of clinics we had started for the homeless, undocumented, and migrant populations in South Florida.

In my private practice, I was able to grow the practice and was making a better living than I could ever imagine, but the disparities also grew larger, as did the divide of our nation. I was becoming more and more disillusioned by what was happening in my community and country and with my profession.

Perhaps my lens was clouded; I was in Miami, and we had twice the rate of Medicare fraud as the rest of the country combined. The environment in South Florida medicine can discourage anyone. This, with the economic divide, should alarm us all.

I maintained my academic interest and expanded on it. I was and am a trustee at the RAND Corporation (America's oldest and largest think tank) and had chaired the Pardee RAND Graduate School for Policy Analysis and their Health Board. This helped me pull my lens back and see a wider view. I had also worked in two prior presidential administrations, a republican and a democratic one, advising the Secretary of Health at Health and Human Services.

It was around 2006 that I sat down with my wife (we've been married 41 years at the time of this writing) and expressed my angst with medicine, and although I was making more money than I thought I could, I couldn't be any more unhappy with my professional career. I found more satisfaction in starting and running clinics for the homeless, undocumented, and migrants. How could I change the profession to get back on track to improve the health of our nation and simply return to the virtues we so profess (humility, empathy, to name a couple)? We talked about joining the industry and trying to change from within (that idea quickly fell to the wayside, as the business world would probably eat me for lunch). Well, when I looked at ourselves, I asked what I and our profession have done wrong.

That question led me to medical education, as that is where we educate our future physicians, and what was missing in it. I thought much about how we could produce the future workforce and educate them to be the generation of change agents to improve our nation's health. At the same time, it was obvious that the industry was moving rapidly, but the education of our future workforce was not.

As luck would have it, our local public university was starting a medical school: Florida International University School of Medicine (FIU). They also chose a spectacular dean, John Rock. In 2006, I was invited to dinner with him and the provost. The next day, he offered me a job, and I accepted. I was a strand leader, and Assistant Dean for Academic Affairs.

I formed a new department of Humanities, Health and Society with various divisions: Division of Family Medicine and Community Medicine; Division of Internal Medicine; Division of Policy, Research and Community Development and Research; Division of Ethics, Humanities, Arts and Design; and Division of Library. We were fully entrenched in the communities of South Florida.

That was an incredibly rewarding 13 years, being the first Medical School in North America to teach the Social Determinants of Health and have a longitudinal plan to integrate it into the student's household visits for all their 4 years. We were invited to present at the Institute of Medicine and were featured in the Committee on

Educating Health Professionals to Address the Social Determinants of Health; Board on Global Health; Institute of Medicine; National Academies of Sciences, Engineering, and Medicine. A Framework for Educating Health Professionals to Address the Social Determinants of Health. Washington (DC): National Academies Press (US); 2016. FIU became the second most diverse medical school in the country.

When Dean Rock was ready to leave FIU, the university wanted to go on a very traditional tract and emphasize the basic sciences, even though all our graduating classes had the highest pass rate and scores on Steps 1 and 2 and the highest match rate. They hired a Harvard MD/PhD, a brilliant scientist, and we felt it was time to leave.

I decided to stay in academic medicine and began responding to headhunters. I entertained different places and went through the process, but wanted a place where we could really try to expand a curriculum, where we could educate the physicians of the future workforce, reflecting the diversity we have (from the top down), prepare the physicians to practice health, not just intervention in disease, and produce great clinicians. To instill the virtues Sir William Osler professed, we should (beginning with humility) and have our physicians become socially accountable through the experience in their 4 years of medical school. This hopefully reduces the disparities in health outcomes and prepares them for population health and the importance of analytics for the future physician.

We live in a country where we spend more than any other nation on health outcomes, yet ranked horribly. As we are the ones that produce most of the workforce and leadership of our health system, we must prepare them to improve the health of our communities and our nation.

So, in June 2020 we came out to Las Vegas to start a new medical school at Roseman University (a private not-for-profit university) of Health Sciences to do something different, expanding what we started in Miami.

Follow us and make sure we do it right, from preparing the future workforce, one that is as diverse as our communities, and one where we can get to the point where we actually treat individuals without prejudice.

Let's make America the healthiest nation in the world.

## My Pathway—By Olga Rodríguez de Arzola, MD, FAAP, Dean of the School of Medicine, Ponce Health Sciences University

My pathway to the deanship of Ponce Health Sciences University, School of Medicine has been one of passion, trust, readiness, and resilience. Being there at the right time, in the right place, and ready to accept the challenges has been key to my success.

I was born in Mayaguez, a town in the west of Puerto Rico, and raised in Ponce, Puerto Rico, the largest city in the southern area of the Island. My father had a small business, and my mother was a stay-at-home parent. They both completed high school (which was a great achievement at their time) but did not pursue further education. Their goal as parents was to provide my sisters and I with the best possible education, so we all studied in private, Catholic schools. My undergraduate education was at the University of Puerto Rico (UPR), Mayaguez Campus. Medical education was at the Medical Sciences Campus of the UPR and pediatrics at the program of the UPR. All my life on the precious island of Puerto Rico.

When I completed my specialty training, I had four personal goals: to be an excellent mother and wife, to excel as a professional in primary care, to serve the people of the southwest of Puerto Rico (my region), and to be actively involved in the education of medical students and residents.

I married right before entering medical school. I was 20 years old then. My husband completed his engineering studies while I was beginning my premed. Our first son was born the day I enrolled in my third year of medical school. This was the result of careful planning so that my time in medical school was minimally affected. Yes, it worked. And with the support of my husband, my mother-in-law, and my family, I could successfully complete my medical career and fulfill my responsibilities as a mother. I graduated from the pediatric residency program when I was pregnant with my second son. At that time, my husband and I moved to Ponce, where he obtained a new job. Ponce was great for us because I lived there during my childhood, and we both had family members living there. At the same time, I decided to take a 6-month pause to study for the pediatric specialty board, and to take care of my kids. I was cautious when I made the decision, with the fear that this would delay my professional development, but on the contrary, it helped me a lot. Not only I had a tremendous quality time with my family, but also I passed the boards. Furthermore, I planned the establishment of a private pediatric practice in Guayanilla, a 21,000-population town located 11 miles west of Ponce. This was my first experience as an administrator. I enjoyed doing primary care, while at the same time balancing work and family life. After 18 months of independent medical practice, I became pregnant with my third son.

Eventually, I had additional professional opportunities, including working in a practice with a group of family physicians, and working with the Department of Health of Puerto Rico at the Ponce Pediatric Center, providing multidisciplinary services to children with disabilities. I also had the opportunity to be part of the teaching staff for family medicine residents in a local hospital, but the interaction with the residents was limited to doing rounds with them when I had hospitalized patients, and those were no more than 1–2 per week. I visited the Ponce School of Medicine (PSM) several times to bring my curriculum vitae and let the chair of pediatrics know of my availability to contribute to the education of the medical students and pediatric residents affiliated to the school. However, the only response I got was, "Thanks, there is no need at this moment." After 7 years in medical practice, it looked like I would never be able to achieve my academic goal.

One morning I was managing my clinic at the Ponce Pediatrics Center, and I received a call from the newly designated Program Director for the Pediatric Residency Program at the Ponce University Hospital (PUH). She was looking for board-certified pediatricians to fill a vacant position in the core teaching staff, and to help the program comply with the requirement of board-certified faculty, and asked me if I was interested. Of course, I was. This was my "dream job." I was interviewed the same week of the call and was offered the job right away. Accepting was easy and the offer was good. After 2 weeks, I began as a faculty member for the residency program. A wonderful opportunity with lots of challenges and responsibilities. And a sensation of "this is a miracle, and a dream come true."

And thereafter, it was a path full of opportunities within short periods of time.

After 6 months as faculty of the residency program, the role of program coordinator, which at that time was the equivalent to the assistant program director, became vacant. The program director asked me to do the job. I was honored for the offer but surprised at the same time. I remembered asking her, "Why me and not one of the more seasoned faculty members?" and she bluntly replied, "Because I want you to do the job." Although I now recognize it was a foolish question, her answer helped me gain trust in myself and recognize the capabilities that I had at a moment when I was learning about a new professional milestone in my life—graduate medical education. I immediately accepted. This was my first administrative role in academic medicine.

During the same period, the hospital was negotiating with the Ponce School of Medicine (PSM) to be the main teaching site for PSM's students. Formerly, it served as a teaching site for two other medical schools in Puerto Rico. One of them announced it was closing its campus in the hospital. One year after beginning as core teaching faculty for the pediatric residency program and 5 months after being designated program coordinator, the chief executive officer of the hospital and the dean of the School of Medicine offered me the position of Graduate Medical Education (GME), Designated Institutional Official (DIO), and Transitional Year Program Director for the hospital. Yes, GME and program director. It would be a combined appointment where part of the salary would be paid by the school and part by the hospital. And I would be the supervisor of all program directors of the hospital. I was in shock! And the question came back to my mind: Why me? And what would happen with my responsibilities as program coordinator and the pediatric residency program? This time, after thoroughly reviewing the responsibilities as GME director and conversations with the pediatric program director, I accepted the job in which I would dedicate 50% of the time to the residency program and 50% to the GME office. And in less than 1 year after my designation as GME Director and DIO, the institution underwent an institutional review by the Accreditation Council for Graduate Medical Education (ACGME) and received full accreditation. This was my first experience with accreditation. Not bad.

During this period of time, I must acknowledge the support of the program director of the Pediatric Residency Program, Dr. Ivonne Villafañe, and that of the Associate Dean for Academic Affairs of the Ponce School of Medicine, Dr. Ana Padró. They both mentored me during my paths in graduate medical education and provided me with the tools for my personal and professional growth. Mentors are key for your success, as it was in my case.

And how did I become dean? That is a longer story. But it was not planned nor anticipated. It was not a priority in my professional life. But it happened, probably, because I knew the institution well, I was faithful to the organization, and I was at the right place at the right time.

In 1993, the government of Puerto Rico implemented the Health Reform. One of the goals of this health reform was to privatize all healthcare services formerly provided by the government and delegate those services to the private sector. The government of Puerto Rico decided to sell all its hospitals to the private sector so that most of the healthcare in Puerto Rico be delivered by private organizations. As a result, in the year 2000, the Ponce University Hospital (PUH), a government-owned institution, was purchased by the Hospital Episcopal San Lucas, a nonprofit, church-owned private institution. At the same time, the Ponce School of Medicine had a new dean, who was actively involved in the change of ownership, and with whom I worked closely to ensure that GME in the hospital was supported and programs were maintained within the new owner. With the change of ownership, the Episcopal Church committed to continue with the residency programs, designated new program directors, but asked me to stay as Graduate Medical Education Director. I was the only GME administrator from the former PUH that stayed. Within the changes in the Department of Pediatrics, a new program director was designated, who was the chair of the Department of Pediatrics in the hospital and former program director of the pediatric residency program. He chose other faculty members as members of the core teaching staff.

Although I missed my role as program coordinator and faculty for the pediatric residents and medical students, this change provided new and exciting opportunities.

I began by coordinating and teaching the Introduction to Clinical Skills course to second-year medical students. This was my formal entrance to undergraduate medical education. In a short period, the chair of the Department of Pediatrics of the School of Medicine, and a trusted colleague, was designated Associate Dean for Academic Affairs, and the position became vacant. I applied for the position, and I was ranked number two by the search committee. This is the first and only time in my professional life that I have participated in a job search. Finally, the candidate ranked number one could not reach an agreement with the dean, and I was offered the job. I was very pleased and honored and accepted the position of Chair of the Department of Pediatrics of PSM, while at the same time continuing my role as GME director of San Lucas Hospital. During my role as Chair, I participated as part of the taskforce to request the initial accreditation of the PSM by the Middle States Commission of Higher Education (MSCHE). Until that time, free-standing medical schools did not need regional accreditation. As rules changed, the school had to request it as part of the Liaison Committee on Medical Education (LCME requirements). I was designated chair of the committee that evaluated the standard related to faculty. This task required a lot of research, search for data, and analysis. But the most important to me is that through my participation in the MSCHE taskforce I was able to learn in depth about the medical school, including its administration, governance, the academic program, the student body, research endeavors, and many others.

After 2 years as Chair of Pediatrics, the Associate Dean for Academic Affairs resigned, and the dean asked me to take the job. I had been participating in his weekly leadership meetings as GME director of the school's main teaching hospital, and in monthly meetings with department chairs. He knew me well and trusted I could do the job. After getting additional information about what the work entailed, I accepted the job. And I did this for 12 consecutive years. As Associate Dean for Academic Affairs, I led the development of the strategic plan of the school and its

5-year revision. I also led Liaison Committee for Medical Education (LCME), Puerto Rico Council on Higher Education, and Middle States Commission for Higher Education self-studies and visits, and initiated the annual Scientific Meeting, a peer-reviewed activity where students and residents of the school's affiliated hospitals would present their research projects through a peer-reviewed process. And many other achievements. The dean of the school supported my application to the Executive Leadership for Academic Medicine Fellowship (ELAM) offered by Drexel School of Medicine. I was accepted and began the ELAM training during the fall of 2011.

While I was associate dean, I worked with, and was mentored by, four different deans of the school. Until 2014, the dean also held the title of president of the institution. Each one had a different personality, leadership style, and areas of professional strength, but they were all great leaders and mentors, and I learned a lot from each one of them: Dr. Manuel Martínez Maldonado, Dr. Luisa Alvarado, Dr. Raúl Armstrong, and Dr. Joxel García.

During the afternoon of March 30, 2012, while I was working at my office, I received a call from the past president of the board of trustees of the school of medicine to know if I was available to meet with the president of the board and himself at that moment. I was surprised but said yes. I had no idea about what it was related to. I had asked them to meet as part of one of my ELAM assignments and thought it may be related to that. When I arrived at the meeting site, I was surprised to find the whole board of trustees. They told me that the president and dean of the school had resigned and asked me to step up as interim president and dean of the school. They would designate a search committee to identify a new president and dean but needed me to do the job until they could identify a substitute. They estimated that it would take about 6 months.

For this role, I did not feel I was prepared. However, I recognized that I was the person that best knew the school and that I could help during the transition. So, I accepted the challenge. And believe me, it was a huge challenge, but one in which I had a lot of gratifying experiences and personal and professional growth.

However, it was not 6 months; it was two and a half years (30 months). During that period, I had to work with the financial challenges of the institution while at the same time prioritize on our academic, research, and service missions. Close communication with my leadership team, our finance team, and the board leadership was key to my success. Lessons learned during ELAM were also extremely helpful. My big project was to work with the board on a change of ownership, which was finally executed in September 2014. The school changed its name from Ponce School of Medicine and Health Sciences to Ponce Health Sciences University (PHSU), and the new president asked me to stay as Dean of the School of Medicine. Thereafter, I have continued as dean of the school, with the satisfaction that the financial challenges have been resolved, and that the institution has been reinvigorated and is on a path of growth and prosperity. This has resulted in enhancement of the academic resources for faculty and students, growth of the research and clinical services enterprise, and my dream for a new building for the medical school completed during the summer of 2023.

During my tenure as dean, the size of our incoming class has increased from 72 in 2012 to 180 in 2022. The school established two clinical campuses in Puerto Rico (Metro Campus and Mayaguez Campus) and a 4-year campus in St. Louis, Missouri with 30 students per year. We also expanded our network of affiliated hospitals and clinics in Puerto Rico and the United States to more than 60.

In summary, my path to becoming a medical school dean was a combination of passion for medical education, acceptance of new opportunities, and being there at the right place and at the right time. I have been honored to be appointed dean of Ponce Health Sciences University School of Medicine. I recognize that this role requires that you have and maintain excellent communication with your faculty, students, chairs, assistant and associate deans, staff, and administrators of the institution. That includes the president, vice presidents, the chief financial officer, and other university deans. That you be available for any one of them when needed. That you have and maintain excellent communication with your affiliated sites and are faithful to them. That you support your community at all times. That you select a good team of competent chairs and associate and assistant deans. That you advocate for the well-being of medical students, physicians, and other health care professionals. That you fully comply with your responsibilities for the optimal functioning of the school. That you ensure that the necessary resources to comply with the mission and strategic plan of the school are properly allocated and are managed in a fiscally sound manner. That you advocate for optimal health in your communities. And that you be creative, think out of the box, and prioritize those things that enhance the learning opportunities for your students. That you be humble and accept when you make mistakes. And when you see how your alumni shine anywhere they are, you understand the importance of being a really good medical school dean.

I must end by thanking my husband, Juan Francisco Arzola, and my kids, Juan Gabriel, Francisco Javier, and Ricardo Andrés, for their lifelong support. They have been the stars that guide my life and my soul. Love you very much.

## My Story—By Jose Manuel de la Rosa, MD, MSc, Vice President for Outreach and Community Engagement, Texas Tech University Health Sciences Center El Paso, Founding Dean, Paul L. Foster School of Medicine, Professor with Tenure and Interim Chair, Pediatrics

My Road to the Medical School Dean's Office—"I Am as Inbred as They Come!"

Born in El Paso, Texas and raised in Ciudad Juárez until the age of six, I spent most of my grammar school and high school days living within 3 miles of what is now El Paso's Academic Health Center. My mother's family is located primarily in Ciudad Juárez, México and my father's family in El Paso, Texas. These two cities form one geographic Borderplex on the US– Mexico border. I came to know these two cities as one entity, and that has affected my perception of many issues that are still pertinent to this day.

My parents' education was hard won as my father received his bachelor's degree as a result of the Government Issue (GI) benefits awarded to him after his role as a dental technician during World War II. Due to a shortage of teachers willing to go into certain schools, he was able to receive an emergency teaching certificate and served as a grammar schoolteacher in El Paso Public schools for over 30 years. My mother went through secondary school in Mexico, with on-the-job training as a bookkeeper and, eventually, a certificate in accounting. They saw their education lift them out of poverty and inculcated in their children a love of learning and an appreciation for the social and financial benefits of both formal and informal education.

My parents attempted to give my sister and me the best education that they could afford. They scrimped and saved to send us through private Catholic grammar and high schools in El Paso. My first school experience was actually in Mexico as I attended "El Jardin de Ninos" en Ciudad Juárez. My parents' desire for their children's education was expensive and included private music lessons, which afforded me the opportunity to play with a summer symphony at the age of 15 and to tour the great European cathedrals with the El Paso Choir of the Southwest at the age of 16. Through these experiences, I was able to see both sides of the financial divide in my community, recognizing how an exclusive class of people had the privilege of seemingly endless resources and seeing how others lived on the margins of society. My education continued, thanks to both my formal schooling and informal social network, afforded by the contacts made through the music classes, I was able to attend the University of Notre Dame. It was there that I saw that even the most exclusive education in my corner of the world was insufficient when compared to the experiences of others across the country. I met and married my college sweetheart, and she has been my formidable partner, friend, and supporter for over 45 years. We married while still in school and have lived our lives together ever since. Through her I have also seen the differences in world views and learned that no matter how different people are ethnically, how similar our needs become.

When I was admitted to two vastly different medical schools in the State of Texas, I chose to return home to El Paso, where I thought I might rely upon and help my extended family and social network. Because the presence of Texas Tech in El Paso at the time was only a clinical third- and fourth-year campus, we moved and lived in Lubbock, Texas during the basic science years of medical school. Once again, I was able to see the differences and similarities in the philosophies and approaches to life and yet recognize the similarities in needs and desires by different ethnicities.

As our family grew with the addition of our six children, we struggled like many young couples for financial resources. Because of that need, I signed up for the National Health Service Corps Scholarship Program, which afforded me the opportunity to not only receive financial support in the form of tuition books, supplies, and a living stipend during medical school but also afforded me the opportunity to give back in the form of a commitment to serve in a designated health professional shortage area with the National Health Service Corps. This experience would also become formative. When I completed the basic science training in Lubbock, Texas, we moved our young family to El Paso. My introduction to medical practice in El Paso was the NHSC Preceptorship Program, which placed me for the summer between my second and third medical school years in a federally qualified health center (FQHC) known as "Centro de Salud Familiar 'La Fe'." I completed my 2 years of clinical training and graduated from the Texas Tech

School of Medicine. Like every other fourth-year student, I despaired over the choice of where I would pursue my specialty training. Despite several opportunities to train in large academic health centers, I chose to stay once again in El Paso, choosing to not participate in the National Residency Matching Program, and took a position with potential to qualify as both a board-certified pediatrician and general internist. This was not to be as I was not able to tolerate the rigors of a dual internship but was able to choose to remain within the pediatric residency program in El Paso.

Once I completed the pediatric residency, and as a part of my obligation to the National Health Service Corp, I was able to interview across the country at multiple federally qualified health centers. Once again, I saw similarities with my experiences. Thanks to my social network and the Paso del Norte Area Health Education center (PDN-AHEC), Divine Providence, I was placed in a small double-wide trailer in the City of Fabens, Texas, approximately 40 miles from my birthplace. I thought this assignment would give stability to our young rapidly growing family as I would be ready to handle a daily commute of approximately 30 miles. In discussing my choice of rural health assignment with my department chair, I was encouraged to stay in El Paso and was offered a faculty appointment as an instructor of clinical pediatrics. I was to accept medical students in rotation and expose them to the joys and hardships of rural medicine. This assignment would be able to meet the needs of the medical school, complete my service obligation, and serve the medical needs of the children in Fabens, Texas. The coalition of the state-run medical school in partnership with two federal programs (NHSC and HRSA), and local community clinics took a lot of discussion but, in the end, became a win-win-win for all involved.

During the last year of my National Health Service Corps obligations and medical school faculty contract, a grant for training nursing students in rural areas was written by the Dean of the School of Nursing at the University of Texas El Paso (UTEP). My little double-wide trailer was a natural rotation site for the nursing students. I was glad to accept a position that included subcontracts and a small stipend. Little did I know that this was to be my introduction into the world of grant management and academic collaborations. However, my propensity for saying yes to unusual assignments and my ability to build coalitions served me well.

I had learned the power of coalitions and the necessary negotiation of agreement that made them successful. I was able to negotiate participation in clinical rounds once a month for teams of nursing, medical, and social work students from two different university systems in Texas. Students studied in their didactic classes and then participated around a big table to staff real life cases that more frequently involved problems in the social determinants of health than physical or psychological problems. Our patients were willing participants in this training of medical students, nursing students, and social work students through the logistics of accessing health care. We even arranged to start a new program that certified community health workers. It was here in the Kellogg Community Partnerships that I not only learned the impact a collaborative could yield but experienced how creative solutions could be found by newcomers to the field.

In addition to participating in the new educational collaborative, I volunteered to serve on standing committees of the medical school. Beginning with the admissions committee, I served on successive rounds of undergraduate medical school committees. These were committees that frequently had difficulties attracting junior faculty, such as the grading and promotion committees (responsible for adjudication of student grades), the finance committee (responsible for establishing budgets), and the transitional residency committee, which oversaw the curriculum, administration, finances, and logistics of our fledgling 10 person PGY1 or "transitional year" graduate medical education program "(residency)."

Getting all of these committees under my belt during my 3 years of national health service obligation gave me skills with curriculum management, exposed me to the school finances, some of the challenges and heartbreak of dealing with failing students, and the concepts of interprofessional education and social determinants of health. I was lucky to be sponsored and exposed to a community of learners through the Kellogg Community Partnerships, which aggressively believed in interprofessional education. I also attempted to meet my departmental obligations.

Once again, I was to be affected and profit from being in the right place at the right time. During the spring and summer of 1990, many of the medical school faculty on the El Paso campus were deployed to the Middle East as part of "Operation Desert Shield and Operation Desert Storm." This left a skeletal crew of faculty in the department of pediatrics. That is how I came to be appointed acting residency program director for the program from which I had graduated only 3 years previously. This appointment gave me a tremendous amount of exposure to the needs of a multitude of GME issues. From dealing with truant residents, to negotiating for resident salaries and benefits, and even feeling the joys of graduating two classes of "my" residents. It taught me tremendous lessons on being a middle manager and allowed me to experiment with curricular issues, eventually allowing me to become the designated institutional officer for the entire campus. It also taught me that not all experimentation was welcome or acceptable. When the deployed faculty returned, many of the innovations were frowned upon and were discontinued. While serving as the residency program director, I also volunteered to take the place of short-staffed residents. I was elated when the deployed faculty and residents returned not only for their safe return but also because I would no longer be taking resident calls as I considered myself a full-fledged faculty member. When I was asked to continue to cover for residents who were ill, I indulged in an adolescent temper tantrum. I told my department chair that I would take call the day after his senior faculty members would take call as a resident. I believed I would never be treated as a full-fledged faculty member and left the department to work for a community health center that had given me the luxury of completing my national health service corps in the rural town. I maintained an affiliation with the Health Sciences Center and took on the title of "Clinical" Assistant Professor of Pediatrics, a community faculty mentor.

During this time away from the health sciences center, I capitalized on my knowledge of the community by establishing an HRSA-funded program of school-based health centers, which consisted of me driving from one rural school district's school nurses' office to another on a rotating basis. The nine communities that hosted these "school-based health centers" were incredibly generous, allowing their school nurses time to assist with organizing, coordinating, and officiating over a selection of students to be seen in these half-day clinical endeavors. Through these efforts and my employment with the community health center, I was able to introduce myself into and learn from the Texas Association of Community Health Centers and even participate in the National Association of Community Health Centers. This introduced me to a completely different world and yet another network. I was able to learn the intricacies of funding and administration of a community health center and came to appreciate their priorities, their process for identifying patients, and abilities for tracking funding.

Thus, when I was asked to write a new grant through the Kellogg Community Partnership Program dealing with graduate medical education and master's level nursing, it became very natural for me to deal with and write about interprofessional education with transitional year residents and master's degree advanced practice nursing students, as well as master's level social work students and their faculty. Naturally, I placed these educational efforts within the auspices of the community health centers and school districts with which I had been working. When we received this grant, I was asked by the medical school administration to take on the role of program director for the transitional year residency and was reassured that my service had given me the skills necessary for these leadership roles. The leadership of the El Paso campus addressed my fears by committing to serve as my sponsor and mentor.

During subsequent years, I was able to move into a position as the designated institutional officer (DIO) for all graduate medical education programming on the campus. As such, I received my first "deanly" appointment as the interim assistant dean for graduate medical education. This title opened the door to be part of the dean's leadership group and learn the intricacies, challenges, and joys of the dean's office. While in this office as the only native of El Paso on the dean's team, I was asked to take on various outreach activities, including liaisons with nine school districts and several boards for faith-based and public nongovernmental entities. It was these written and unwritten, untitled, and unrecognized duties that allowed me to experience the missing links between the health science center and our communities. Simultaneously, I participated in a nationwide cohort of about a dozen young medical school faculty across the United States who led the graduate medical and nursing education components of the new Kellogg Community Partnership initiative. After approximately 3 years of establishing this initiative, the cohort of leaders seemed to be resigning one by one from the leadership positions to pursue academic roles within their home departments. After studying this phenomenon, the Kellogg Community partnership leadership at the national level came to the conclusion that these young faculty members (mostly assistant professors in the clinical medical disciplines) who were leading this multimillion-dollar interprofessional initiative had missed the opportunity to participate in the natural evolution of young faculty. None had published or contributed to the literature. Several interviews established that these young faculty had not been mentored by senior faculty within their departments and had been left out of the process of academic nurturing. Many faculty gave their input as to their perception of taking on the local leadership of the Kellogg Community Partnership becoming a potential for academic suicide and a threat to their academic careers. In their wisdom, the leadership of the Kellogg Community Partnership decided to underwrite the pursuit of a formal program of academic leadership training for each of their young community partnership leaders. It was this decision that funded me to pursue a master's degree in epidemiology through the Harvard School of Public Health (HT Chan) clinical scholars' program. My mentor in the regional dean's office facilitated my departure from my clinical duties.

The Harvard School of Public Health Clinical Scholars Program consisted of two summers in residence, attending in-person classes (usually with Harvard Medical School's subspecialty fellows), along with two semesters of off-site study design, data collection, and correspondence-style coursework toward a master's-level thesis or prepublication article. It was the coursework toward publication/thesis that pushed me to capitalize on the insights I had gained by serving on committees, both internal to the university and outreach obligations imposed by my role on the Dean's leadership team. I was able to identify a school-based data gathering questionnaire that assessed families' perception of health status, usually utilizing the SF 32 self-perception of health questionnaire. I was able to stratify on the basis of the number of generations within the United States and observed a declination of perception of health status with each subsequent generation. This formed an interesting dilemma. Simply, the longer one is in the United States, the more one expects the health status to be improved, and when that does not turn out to be the case, perceptions of one's health decline. I was able to observe the first generation's desire to work hard for their children's care and document the despair when the grandchildren can not get out of the ghettoized neighborhoods to which immigrants usually reside.

I was also able to observe the New England social networks and their value to not only the School of Public Health but also to Harvard Medical School and their academic publications. I will forever remember my interaction with the editor of the *New England Journal of Medicine* and our conversation as to how she determined which articles to publish. She reiterated that these decisions were frequently casually made in conjunction with social functions within the county medical society. She noted this occurs at all County Medical Society events across the country. Connections and social networks influence perceptions and productivity.

It was during this coursework that I found myself again in the right place at the right time. As a designated institutional officer, I became head of the graduate medical education committee and, as such, was placed in the leadership role and was tapped to lead the entirety of the continuum for medical education when the associate dean for undergraduate and continuing medical education became ill. I requested the dean combine UME, GME, and CME into one office, which I would manage.

At this stage of my career, I believed I had achieved what I had aspired to become, which was the "dean for education" for our regional campus. I thought I did not aspire to any higher role.

By capitalizing on multiple circumstances and a bit of luck, I had completed my informal education on the road to the dean's office. I had "punched my tickets," had learned valuable lessons on the inner workings of a medical school through service on multiple faculty and administrative committees, educated myself with a formal degree in a public health discipline (epidemiology), and as an inner part of the regional dean's team, I thought I had been able to observe and learn from the interactions between the community through both my formal and informal networks of contacts and observed the politics on the "main or home campus" in Lubbock. I was, therefore, quite confused when the Lubbock-based Dean of the School of Medicine, together with the Chancellor of the University, paid a surprise visit to the El Paso campus. They met individually with each of the members of the regional dean's leadership group. They asked us three questions. The first was to be an exercise on responsiveness to the legislature. Asked what I would do if the state legislature cut 30% of our budget, I responded that I would cut cost by reducing waste, combine several resident and student rotations, and launch a fundraising campaign. The next question was what advice I had for them for the future of the El Paso campus. I responded that was not my role, but noted that I had become aware of the consistent complaint of the faculty that when students came to our campus for their third- and fourth-year clinical rotations, they were woefully inadequately prepared for becoming clinical clerks and interacting with the El Paso community. I added that perhaps allowing for some educational experimentation would benefit not only the El Paso campus but also the school of medicine and its multiple campuses. Finally, they asked where my family was from, and I responded that I had grown up in both Ciudad Juarez and El Paso. They nodded and thanked me for the interview. Two weeks later, I was summoned to Lubbock and met with the dean of the school of medicine, who playfully asked me if I would be willing to take on the role of interim dean for the regional campus. Apparently, the serving regional dean had resigned over a discussion on resources, and a national launch was to be undertaken for the El Paso campus. This was in 1996. I accepted thinking it was to be a temporary (6–8 month) assignment. I would serve in the position of regional dean for over 10 years. The next step into the dean's office was what to be a combination of previous experiences and being in the right place at the right time.

In early 1998, the State of Texas received a monetary settlement from the tobacco companies. The money was to be distributed to several academic health science centers and health departments along the border and was to be used for various health interventions. The President of Texas Tech University Health Sciences Center, based in Lubbock, announced that the money allocated to the health sciences center for the border was to form the basis for a university-wide Border Health Research Institute. People in El Paso were astounded. There had already been long-standing tensions between the two physician communities since the establishment of Texas Tech's School of Medicine and the legislative decision to place it in Lubbock. At the time of the legislative act establishing the "west Texas school," it was perceived that El Paso had more of the facilities to house the medical program, but Lubbock had the political muscle to land the school. Thus, the President's announcement ignited a long-simmering fuse and launched a 2-year-long discussion between the communities of El Paso and Lubbock regarding the future governance of the two campuses and the distribution of monies allocated to the border/El Paso. The discussion was contentious. It expanded to include the long-standing tensions between the two communities over healthcare resources, including the health educational programs. (Some called it "Cussing and Discussing"). Newspaper articles and political cartoons fed the ire and resentment. It grew to include the largest higher education system in Texas (the University of Texas system), which has a thriving general academic campus in El Paso. Neither community wanted to cede control of the medical school. Tensions ran high. In a brilliant stroke of political Ju-Jitsu, the chancellor of the system said in desperation, "Let them have their own medical school. It will take them 20 years to get it approved." He then delineated all of the steps it would take to clear the multiple hurdles for accreditation, including the fact that the LCME had not approved a new school in over 30 years. In late 1999, he presented the idea to the Texas Tech Board of Regents, and the El Paso regent made the motion to pursue a "separately accredited, full four-year medical school in affiliation with Texas Tech's campus in El Paso, Texas." Everyone was appeased, and handshakes were shared figuratively and physically between the two communities. We launched into the planning phase for the new school of medicine.

As a regional dean, I participated actively in planning for the 4-year medical school. We formed an educational program planning committee, medical school faculty recruitment committees, and medical student admissions committee, all under the umbrella organization of the interinstitutional 4-year medical school planning committee. It was within these planning committees I learned the inconsistency and intricacies of an accreditation process that involved regional, local, and national accrediting bodies. We worked with the Liaison Committee on Medical Education (LCME) to develop a document entitled "New and Developing Medical Schools" to formulate a process for seeking accreditation as none had been accredited in over 30 years. We joined a group of organizations that sought to establish new medical schools and gladly participated in the Harvard Macy Foundation group for new and developing schools. We worked with SACSCOC to clarify that we did not need additional accreditation as we were only establishing another school within the existing health sciences university. We were able to obtain public funding from the state legislature to build buildings, hire faculty, and recruit students. As a member of these committees, I learn to navigate the expectations of the faculty and administration in Lubbock, who are anxious to comply with all accreditation standards and build detailed, diligent, and intricate processes while balancing the expectations of the El Paso community, who cannot understand why their dream took so long to approve. The next step was to recruit and formalize the appointment of the dean of the new school of medicine.

After 4 years of joint planning, we were ready to move on to the final stages of recruiting the founding dean. We were only the second school to name a founding dean in the last 35 years, so there was a tremendous amount of nationwide interest in our success (or failure). Our Health Sciences Center's president in Lubbock was already actively being congratulated and courted by other Health Science centers in anticipation of his success in launching a second medical school, solidifying the Texas Tech system, and expanding its influence in the Texas legislature. I felt as if the entire nation's eyes were on our fledgling 4-year medical school as we launched the nationwide search for the founding dean. The president traveled to our campus, spoke to community leaders, and issued the directive to hire a nationally known recruiting firm to assist our campus as we formed a search committee. The committee was to be populated with El Pasoans but contain key personnel from the Lubbock campus. It was to reflect the values of both communities and prioritize the traditional skills and experiences of an academic medical center. The founding dean was to demonstrate seniority and experience in directing, establishing, and managing programs that exemplify the three traditional medical school missions of education, clinical service, and research. Of course, the two communities differed in their timeline. El Paso wanted an expedited search; Lubbock anticipated a diligent, deliberate, and detailed examination of all applicants. The president directed that the three finalists be brought to him within a year.

Of course, I threw my hat into the ring. After 10 years of loyal service as the regional dean, I had the hubris to believe I was qualified to be the natural successor to lead the founding dean's office. The recruiter from the national search firm encouraged my application. Later in the year, I received a call from the president's office to discuss my candidacy. I believed that was the first step onto the road to the dean's office and reported dutifully to the "interview." The president opened by informing me that he would soon be moving on to become the president of a much larger, well-established health sciences university in the central part of United States. He noted it should not be him that should make the decision on the leadership of the El Paso School of Medicine as he would not be in a position to work with this person chosen to lead the new school. He noted that the board of regents had been notified that there would be three finalists and had assigned the task of selecting the finalists to the interim president as they move forward to select the future of El Paso. He asked me to set up an appointment with the designated interim president, who was a longstanding senior faculty member at the health sciences center.

Several months later, I was called in for another visit to Lubbock to discuss the finalists with the interim president. He informed me that three finalists had suddenly been forwarded to him and described each of them. He began the meeting by noting that the committee had appreciated and discussed my application, reviewed it thoroughly, but decided that I did not have sufficient publications to demonstrate my academic prowess. He commented that, therefore, they had decided to bring three other finalists to the campus. He then proceeded to highlight the merits of each of the candidates, ranging from the fluency of one in Spanish, the seniority and longtime departmental leadership of the other, as well as the demonstrated experience as a dean of the third.

I asked him what my role was to be in this new structure, and he reassured me that I would maintain leadership. He asked me to "hold the fort down," while the school of medicine was built as I would continue in my role as regional dean, while the new medical students were brought on under the founding dean. In other words,

I would be responsible for phasing out the clinical rotations from the Lubbock students of the next 3 years as we recruited students to the El Paso school under the direction of the new dean. I was devastated.

The interim President recognized my disappointment and gave me condolences and described his experiences with military command. He expressed his and the Regents' appreciation for the work I had done over the last 10 years and explained he would be awarding me the presidential medallion to be presented during a ceremony on the El Paso campus. I had time to think about my dilemma during the return flight to El Paso. After some examination, I recognized that, indeed, I had not published and recalled the words of the president as he left for his next position that the "founding dean was to demonstrate seniority, experience interacting in establishing and managing programs that exemplified the three medical school traditions of education, clinical service, and research". I consoled myself that in reality, I did not meet the research requirements. I relegated this episode to lessons learned and resolved myself to learn from the new dean and capitalize on his extensive seniority and reputation for mentorship.

When I arrived in El Paso, I told my team that I was not chosen to lead and gave them insight into the process. I asked their help in orienting and assisting their new boss. They are committed to working with him to continue the dream of an El Paso medical school.

We welcomed the new team as an opportunity to learn and keep the momentum for a new school going and bring the full 4-year medical school to El Paso. The new dean was enthusiastic and uniquely charming. He had a wealth of experience and brought new ideas to bear. Chief among these was a new type of curriculum, which he learned during his interactions at the University of Calgary. He was an aggressive recruiter and brought nationally known faculty to the campus. In an unprecedented move, he hired Dr. Henry Mandin as an on-site consultant and visiting professor to educate the entire campus on case-based curriculum. Our dean's team worked intently to modify our curriculum to inculcate the new principles. He had a small plaque on his desk that read, "Caution I Am Subject to Fits of Enthusiasm," justifying his leadership style, enthusiastically embracing new ideas, and rapidly incorporating them into his vision for the new school.

However, the new dean was used to working in much larger facilities. He had a way of "never taking no for an answer" and frequently would not recognize advice or even direct orders from senior leadership in Lubbock. Despite several warnings, he was determined and persistent on defining the new medical school according to HIS vision rather than collaborating with Lubbock. After 6 months, I found I could no longer work for him and applied for a sabbatical, which was granted. I was to study and bring back recommendations for how general academic campuses could work with health sciences centers. I was to relocate for a full year to the University of Wisconsin–Milwaukee to study how their collaboration with the Medical College of Wisconsin could be duplicated to benefit the El Paso medical school and the University of Texas at El Paso.

My family and I relocated to Milwaukee, Wisconsin 8 months after the new dean had started his tenure.

One month later, I began to receive communications from El Paso colleagues that the regents had finally selected the president for the Health Sciences Center, and he was to begin his tenure with a visit to the El Paso campus. Soon thereafter, I received a phone call from the Dean of the School and Medicine in Lubbock, with whom I had worked closely to navigate the separation of the El Paso school. A close and cherished friend informed me that the new president would soon be calling to offer me the position of Dean of the School of Medicine in El Paso. True to form, the very next day, I received a call from the new president's office. He informed me that he was going to relieve the El Paso dean of his position and wanted me to accept the position as the Dean for the School of Medicine. After intense negotiations on the conditions for my and my family's return to El Paso, I accepted the postponement of my sabbatical and returned to El Paso with the understanding that I was to be named the founding dean. The very next week, I was flown to El Paso and invited to participate in an "all hands-on deck" faculty and staff meeting. The new president met with me and relieved the dean of the medical school and marched directly into the largest auditorium on campus, where a standing-room-only audience had been assembled. He announced that "it is no longer in the best interest of the health sciences center that the current dean continues his tenure" and then paused before announcing my appointment as the founding dean. It was several minutes before the shocked audience ceased their murmurings, and I began to receive congratulations from faculty, staff, and learners.

That is the story of how I entered into the dean's office. There are subsequent chapters of the 7 years during which we worked intensely and not only established what was to become the Foster School of Medicine but also the School of Nursing and the Graduate School of Biomedical Sciences. The entire community was enthusiastically supportive and spectacularly successful to the point that they not only supported our fundraising campaign to the tune of $85 million (including the largest endowed gift ever given to Texas Tech by Mr. Paul L. Foster to name the medical school after his father) but also leveraged their support to gain the political capital and establish the will to convert our campus from a 2-year clinical campus to a full independently accredited Health Sciences Center. I shall forever remember the governor of the State of Texas coming to El Paso on May 18, 2013, to sign the bill establishing the Texas Tech University Health Sciences Center El Paso. Coincidentally, this occurred on my birthday.

I was to continue my career as a provost for this new university. But that is another story!

**Open Access** This chapter is licensed under the terms of the Creative Commons Attribution 4.0 International License (http://creativecommons.org/licenses/by/4.0/), which permits use, sharing, adaptation, distribution and reproduction in any medium or format, as long as you give appropriate credit to the original author(s) and the source, provide a link to the Creative Commons license and indicate if changes were made.

The images or other third party material in this chapter are included in the chapter's Creative Commons license, unless indicated otherwise in a credit line to the material. If material is not included in the chapter's Creative Commons license and your intended use is not permitted by statutory regulation or exceeds the permitted use, you will need to obtain permission directly from the copyright holder.

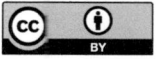

# Chapter 13
# Striving to Become a Dean of Diversity, Equity, and Inclusion

Ana Nunez and Francisco Lucio

> **Learning Objectives**
> - Describe EDI dean roles
> - Provide examples and resources to support success along an EDI leadership track
> - Reflect on one's EDI leadership trajectory and plan

## Introduction

Medicine is no stranger to talented Latina/o/x/e, Hispanic or of Spanish Origin+ (LHS+) physicians. From Carlos Juan Finlay, MD (1833–1915), who defied conventional wisdom and noticed the role of mosquito as a vector in yellow fever and enabled through his work the completion of the Panama Canal, to Helen Rodriguez-Trías, MD (1929–2001), championing the end of forced sterilization on minoritized women, we have had and continue to have numerous leaders, visionaries and champions. Their impact flies in the face of small numbers breaking barriers to training—a challenge that continues till today. LHS+ physicians are a near static number of 5.8% of all physicians in contrast to 18.1% of LHS+ people living in the United States in 2018 [1, 2]. The development of offices and support to promote LHS+ students into and through medical school is beyond the scope of this chapter.

A. Nunez
University of Minnesota School of Medicine, Minneapolis, MN, USA

F. Lucio (✉)
Health Care Advancement, University of Arizona, Phoenix, AZ, USA

© The Author(s) 2026
J. P. Sánchez et al. (eds.), *Advancing Latino, Hispanic, or of Spanish Origin+ Leadership in Academic Medicine*,
https://doi.org/10.1007/978-3-032-07570-3_13

Historically, efforts included the founding of the Office of Minority Health in 1986, funding for centers of excellence in the 1990s and 2000s, and high-visibility programs such as AAMC's Project 3000 by 2000 in 1991 [3]. Excluding LCME-accredited schools in Puerto Rico, whose majority are LHS+, mainland US medical schools established diversity, equity, and inclusion (DEI) student support offices to ensure equitable inclusion of LHS+ students. Usually, they were subunits of student affairs and populated by dedicated staff of color. Nationally, in 2008, the Group on Diversity and Inclusion of the AAMC was formulated, expanding beyond students to all aspects of academic medicine. In the mid-2000s, positions developed to promote health equity, population health, and diversity and inclusion. George Floyd's murder stood as an inflection point for society and a painful reminder that, similarly, medicine's intention of best care for all really didn't reach all. A rapid expansion of diversity, equity, and inclusion positions occurred in departments, units, institutes, and senior leadership in medical schools and health systems.

Many factors, including greater polarization in society and misrepresentation that addressing health for all would come at the expense of the majority, led to a backlash on DEI efforts with governmental encroachment and prohibitive legislation. All physicians—all—need to work with and through an equity lens for *all* of their patients. There is no partisanship there. We pledge to do no harm and care for all of our communities. Our mission in medicine, healthcare delivery, innovation, and education of the next generation remains unchanged. Our goal of best health for all likewise remains unchanged. How we address talent across the workforce and support for all groups underrepresented in medicine (URM) is yet to be optimally addressed. The future and the solutions need the best and the brightest to help disrupt health inequities, contribute and excel in missions of medicine, and lead for the future.

## Sí Se Puede: Medicine and Medical Education Can Be Better—An Unlikely and Nontraditional Leadership Story—Ana Nunez, MD

When you think about diverse communities, central Pennsylvania may not be a location that comes to mind. My family was the only Hispanic/Latinx/Puerto Rican family in the area. Living in a predominantly non-Hispanic white community was a familiar experience. Altoona had a diverse population expansion from the 1920's migration and its role in establishing the railroads in the USA There were different places of worship and different foods that represented cultures s Italian, Polish, German, Jewish, and others. But speaking Spanish at home and eating mofongo and paella were considered foreign and different. The pressure to acculturate was incredibly strong.

When asked to share my journey to become Vice Dean of an R1 land-grant, public, academic medical health center, the question was, "How did you get to a Vice

Dean position?" In fact, my path was not to a title—it was to a scope and impact. And that path was about a leadership trajectory. I chose to stay in residency in internal medicine and distinguished myself by being invited to be Chief Resident and winning teaching awards. Coming on board as a junior faculty member, I realized my general internal medicine/primary care training didn't give me all the skills I needed for a robust academic career. I had a lifelong connection with education—from, as a child, helping my mother pronounce "sheets" appropriately, to creating a chest x-ray interpretation pocket guide, to teaching as a chief medical resident in clinic. I heard about and solicited an opportunity for a medical education fellowship as a junior faculty member. After that I realized I needed more grant-writing skills and competitively sought a fellowship in health services research, where I gained qualitative and mixed methodology skills and more experience in NIH grant applications. It was here where I transformed my work in medical education to health professional and health education across the continuum by innovating interventions, applied for support to explore issues for Brown and Black Women in health, and crafted, with funding, an impactful community network alliance to promote health. During this time, I was invited to serve as an assistant dean in primary care and oversee our Robert Wood Johnson's medical school–wide primary care initiative. Later, I was invited to lead our nationally designated Women's Health Center of Excellence (WH COE) Education division. I then became WH COE Director and PI. Next, I wanted to know "where the money came from" and applied and got a DHHS Secretary of Health, Health Policy Fellowship. I expanded my leadership training with the Executive Leadership in Academic Medicine (ELAM) Program. My leadership experience grew when I became the Principal Investigator (PI) of our national center of excellence in women's health and then PI on a health promotion initiative I created, Philadelphia Ujima™, an engaged consortium across southeastern Pennsylvania that helped improve the lives of over 6000 people. After establishing the Urban Health Education and Educational Research (UHEER) office as an outgrowth of the success of our Philadelphia Ujima Collective, I was asked to serve as the inaugural associate dean of diversity, equity, and inclusion at Drexel University College of Medicine. I also assumed leadership of our premedical postbaccalaureate Drexel Pathway to Medical Schools and implemented significant educational and programmatic changes that resulted in improved success (over 90% completion and med school matriculation) for amazing, talented future physicians.

Nationally, I was very active. I engaged with colleagues to support cultural competence and women's health becoming required elements in the licensing of medical schools (LCME) and collaborated on developing core concepts (Tools for Assessing Cultural Competences—TACCT) and assessment measures of TACCT. I contributed to advances in what would later become Holistic Recruitment Practices (in both the Expanded and Simulated Minority Admissions Exercise Program, as well as Situational Judgment Testing) and provided input on the state of evaluation of cultural competence (AAMC assessing change: evaluating cultural competence education and training). I was president of the Northeast Consortium on Cross-Cultural Care and Medical Practice, a regional leadership group of educators and clinicians focused on improving health outcomes. I obtained an NHLBI K grant to develop a training program across the continuum—from community patients to learners to physicians, which included educational innovation and tool development. Also funded with our NHLBI K award and as a member of our National Multiculturalism Consortium, I served as an associate editor of a case-based approach for health professionals.

My work was singled out by being selected for the Herbert J. Nickens Award, which was a huge honor. This national award goes to an individual who has made outstanding contributions to promoting justice in medical education and healthcare equity in the United States. Dr. Nickens was a distinguished and brilliant clinician, leader, and mentor—the health services research training program was one of his many brainchildren. I had the opportunity to be an inaugural journal editor of *Health Equity* and continue to serve in a reviewer capacity to multiple journals. I was also awarded the Fierce Healthcare Most Influential Minority Executive in Healthcare for 2022. Additionally, awards include national recognition for Leadership from the National Hispanic Medical Association and the Al Dia Health Leader award in Philadelphia, PA.

A few years ago, I was recruited to join the University of Minnesota as their inaugural vice dean of diversity, equity, and inclusion. The opportunity to create an inaugural office in a much larger, public institution and lead capacity building and resilience that promotes structural transformation was compelling. The university is an amazing R1 public university, and Minnesota is graced with 11 tribal communities and unique population diversity significantly stemming from outreach to immigrants. I have the privilege to lead successful efforts in diversifying the faculty, contributing to student/trainee diversity, advocating for inclusion of everyone underrepresented in medicine and science, and collaboratively working to oversee meaningful structural transformation in the medical school. It is and continues to be important, rewarding work. The collaboration and support, as well as determination, to improve the school, university, faculty, staff, students, trainees, patients, and communities we serve feeds my passion to be communicator and collaborator in chief. Together we take on structural barriers to equity and work to improve the health and lives of all Minnesotans.

My leadership journey started with awareness and curiosity. It evolved in realizing that despite all that I knew, I had blind spots, and working with others resulted in the best outcomes. I enjoyed the challenges of learning different perspectives than mine. I came to appreciate that I have my perspective and you have yours. Yet, if we come together, we can "birth" a beautiful third that can really make a difference. Training to become a leader is hard work. It takes effort, skills, humility, and intentionality to improve. It is fueled by the inner passion to optimize the gifts you and others have been given to make a difference.

## Leadership Levels in Academic Medicine

What is the difference in leadership levels in academic medicine? Historically, there have been two academic leadership tracks—clinical, resulting in a position as chair or department head. It can also have hospital or faculty practice plan leadership positions as chief medical officer (CMO), head of faculty practice plan, and chief operations officer (COO) of health systems. The second track is the academic track. The rungs of the ladder break into several mission areas—research, education, educational service, DEI, and administration. In the research space, achieving independence as a Principal Investigator and being well-funded means that you have a successful lab and team. Leadership beyond that can include roles like departmental vice chair of research or within a dean's cabinet are positions as associate or vice dean of research.

Educational leadership can be group dependent: For students, this begins with course director or program director positions, which can lead to curricular deans. Areas beyond curricular include student affairs, admissions, and evaluation. For residents, beyond the residency director are positions such as dean of graduate medical education (GME) or institutional designated officers (DIOs). In graduate education, there are associate deans, as well. For faculty development, most departments have associate or vice chairs in faculty affairs or faculty development. There are medical school-wide positions in these areas as well. Overseeing all educational endeavors in a medical school is most often the purview of a senior associate, vice, or executive dean of education. Other leadership areas are in the finance space—from departmental to dean's cabinet.

Last, a newcomer to the leadership table is a role in DEI. These leadership roles that promote workforce diversification, more equitable processes and systems, and a more inclusive environment across our three missions—innovation and research, education and training, clinical care and community outreach—are essential if we are to improve the health of the population and serve our diverse communities. Many departments and units are looking for leadership in DEI. Those who hire are often unclear about performance expectations of DEI leaders. So, it is essential for people to "do their homework in advance" and create a menu of opportunities as they "manage up" and clarify expected outcomes sought. Moving into that space, it is important to be very clear about role, authority, expectations, and expected impact. This includes a delineation and sufficiency of resources to achieve desired outcomes. Outside of departments, in the dean's cabinets you may find associate, senior associate, or vice deans in DEI. The more senior, as in vice deans, work by mobilizing system-wide change, engaging leaders and grass roots members—"top down to bottom up." Areas of work include school- or college-wide reenvisioned recruitment, retention, support of members, and policy review and revisions, especially with an eye toward equity, structural transformation, risk management, crisis communication, advocacy, and initiatives for climate change. Success in this role takes a high level of socioemotional skills; people skills to promote buy-in and inclusion; knowledge about healthcare organization and organization change best practices; political savvy; negotiation skills; creativity, especially in problem-solving, and, most importantly, having a courageous leader as your boss.

## Lessons Learned

Reflecting, here are 12 tips that were and are guiding principles of my path:

Learn about yourself—work hard on this and figure out how to get out of your own way. Keep an open mind that is curious about learning and improving. Become a devotee of leadership principles and practices. Learn by critically observing, listening, reading, and speaking to others who've gone down the path.

As smart as you are, you don't know what you don't know. Smart people reach out for help and support.

Develop a massive, diverse network of support, colleagues, and peers locally and nationally—be connected, get support and coaching, and ask questions about everything. Cultivate your best team that roots for you throughout the journey.

Feedback isn't praise—it is about modifiable behavior—so seek it out and listen even if it isn't what you want to hear.

Pay attention—how do things work (especially for others) and what opportunities do you need to "put yourself out" for, even if that is uncomfortable?

You being "OK" matters—so self-care is essential. Don't take yourself too seriously.

Mission matters—how can you be the best (researcher, educator, clinician, clinician–scientist) in whatever area you choose? Prioritize this in your career trajectory. How can you refine your critical thinking and scholarship skills to contribute to academic medicine?

Hard work in a bubble—meaning work that no one knows about is not useful for leadership progression. In addition to doing wonderful, mission-focused work—you need to manage up and share what you are doing with others. That means spending time, building relationships, communicating your questions and getting advice and guidance, sharing your successes at regular intervals, being generous with helping others, and demonstrating your contribution to the larger mission.

Problems are easy to find. Solutions that are feasible to resolve are harder. Get into a practice of solution sharing with supervisors—not just problem identification.

The system, status quo, is bigger than any one person and their will. If not aligned, your choice is to learn to better navigate, be successful, and make changes from the inside or find another place better suited to your talents and skills.

Succeeding in your field and establishing your niche is hard work. It doesn't happen in your "covered" 9–5 time. It takes weekends and evenings and sacrifices to get there. That is true for everyone. Find ways to revisit the "fire in your belly" to reignite your passion and determination.

Deploy kindness, compassion, and grace—while clothed in thick skin. Medicine needs changes, but to do it within means navigating old and unhelpful systems. Most people are trying to do the best they can despite the dysfunction. Vent your frustration in exercise or kitten Tik Tok—but not to or at others. The more you send out kindness and compassion, the more you will get back. The boomerang effect of doing good is a powerful, replenishing energy resource.

## La Gente Unida Jamás Será Vencida: Harnessing Your Resiliency and Leading in Medicine —Francisco Lucio, JD

"La gente unida jamás será vencida" and "Si se puede" are chants that echo in my memory. I was born and raised in the farming community and lettuce capital of the world, Salinas, California. Some of my earliest memories are participating with my farm worker parents in United Farm Workers marches striving for safer working conditions and fairer wages. These experiences planted the seed that would send me on my path to serve as a dean of equity, diversity, and inclusion.

A first-generation college graduate, I had a similar experience of many others paving their path forward in education without the benefit of family members to reach out to for advice and direction. Although I started out as a biology major at San Diego State University, with a keen interest in medicine, I felt drawn to tackle the social issues posed in my political science courses. With a political science major and English minor in hand, I considered my prospects—limited by my inexperience—and decided to seek what I knew political science majors to do—attend law school. I figured if I was to continue to fight for those marginalized in society as I had with my farm worker parents, the way to do it was by learning the law. Lacking mentors or programs for career exploration, I felt the burden of making my best guesses about this career choice. Still, the voice of my parents, "Échale ganas!" pushed me forward.

I attended law school on the other side of the country and went from the sunny shores of San Diego to the gritty streets of New York City at St. John's University School of Law. I was one of two Mexican students in my class. I didn't see myself reflected in my professors, deans, or classmates. The distance from home and lack of cultural connection with peers or faculty was isolating. I learned quickly that the law in theory was fascinating, but the practice of the criminal justice system unfairly targeted and imprisoned people who looked like me and came from similar backgrounds. After graduating, eager to apply an ounce of prevention, I sought to work with underrepresented in medicine youth on programs to steer them toward careers in healthcare.

Armed with a legal background and passion for helping those who may simply need guidance and support not afforded to them by circumstance and system, I worked as program director at the Manhattan-Staten Island Area Health Education Center. Here, I continued to be inspired by the stories and resilience of the students

I guided in the pathway programs toward health careers. The work took me to Albany, New York, and Washington, D.C., where I had opportunities to advocate for ongoing support from state and federal representatives to diversify our healthcare workforce. I found a community of mentors who were from similar backgrounds and helped bridge my path to academia. The last 10 years have been spent learning about healthcare in various capacities in academia from director of career development and minority enrichment at the State University of New York (SUNY) College of Optometry, where I counseled students on career exploration and career skill building, to director of diversity at New York University (NYU) School of Medicine, where I honed my program development efforts related to diversity topics in medicine. After about 2 years at NYU, family considerations—I had a young child and hopes to continue growing my family—and a desire to lead from a position of more influence, motivated me to seek an opportunity as the inaugural associate dean, equity, diversity, and inclusion (EDI) at the University of Arizona College of Medicine-Phoenix.

The years in my role as associate dean, EDI have been a learning, challenging, and fruitful experience. Having led through the double pandemic of COVID-19 and systemic racism accelerated both the urgency and solutions needed to create more equity in medicine. Continual growth and networking have been critical to my success in the position, and participation in the AAMC Health Executive Diversity and Inclusion Certificate Program was an important national connector. Some achievements most salient during my tenure have been helping to improve our underrepresented in medicine student matriculation. This was made possible through a strategic and holistic "inside/outside" approach to EDI that relied on building the attractors inside the institution (e.g., equity-focused medical curriculum, scholarship support, and partnership with affinity groups like LMSA) and efforts outside the institution (e.g., active recruitment of URM students, pathway programs to medical school, and K-16+ student engagement). In addition, I helped establish a robust medical Spanish program that has learning opportunities for beginners looking to have simple communication with Spanish-speaking patients and an 18-month course that takes intermediate Spanish-speaking students and upskills them to an advanced Spanish-speaking level to become bilingual certified.

In 2023, I was promoted from associate dean, EDI to senior associate dean, EDI. This promotion came after a 5-year 360-degree administrative review that consisted of a self-study and survey of my performance in six areas: (1) unit culture and productivity; (2) building trust; (3) fostering collaborations; (4) maximizing resources; (5) achieving results; and (6) instilling inclusive excellence. I also participated in a committee interview to elucidate my achievements during my first 5 years as associate dean, EDI. Currently, I submitted my dossier and am under consideration for promotion from assistant professor of practice to associate professor of practice in the Department of Obstetrics and gynecology. My dossier highlighted my teaching, scholarship, and service contributions. My teaching contributions included innovations as the co-director of our health equity longitudinal curricular theme for all medical students, a fourth-year elective entitled "Structural Inequities and Health Care," and creation of an anti-racism curriculum.

My scholarship included publications that focused on EDI. My service was a combination of various institutional committees, such as the admissions committee and search committees, as well as regional and national committees, including founding a state-wide consortium of all the osteopathic and allopathic medical schools in Arizona.

The road from Associate Dean, EDI to Senior Associate Dean EDI has been facilitated by many great mentors, skill building, and resilience. Still, the most important driver to my career success was the seed planted in my youth as I witnessed the power of farmers organizing and marching toward justice—this is my fuel to address the inequities in medicine and society.

## Lessons Learned

### *Five Keys to Success as a Senior/Associate Dean of Equity, Diversity, and Inclusion*

You cannot go at it alone—collaboration is important both from within your institution and external to your institution. Whether you are creating a recruitment program for minoritized students or implementing anti-racist curricula, working with others will be necessary for success.

Develop an eye for talent and retain those individuals—if you have an opportunity to build a team, consider your strengths and opportunities and fill positions with individuals who help move your department mission and goals forward. Once you have the talent, invest in their retention by nominating them for awards, sending them to development conferences, and advocating for equitable compensation.

Use a strategic plan as your shield and your sword—clear goals that are tied to your institutional mission will serve you as you forge forward to change your institution against potential resistors or obstructers but will also help block or limit the damage related to budgetary cuts or reprioritizations that may occur.

Ask for more than you want—when negotiating for your needs, whether it is funding, personnel, or time, anchor the negotiation and ask for more than you want. Institutions have finite resources, and it may be rare to get everything you want. If you ask for more than you want, you may have a better shot of getting what you need.

Promote your successes—in the midst of all that goes on in an academic medical center, it is important to make clear what successes you have accomplished. Create your own newsletter or ensure the broader medical school newsletters are highlighting EDI achievements, publish an annual EDI report, or make regular announcements or presentations at key meetings (e.g., faculty meetings, department chair meetings, and trustee meetings). Control the stories or someone else will; or worse yet, no one will tell your stories.

## Skill Building Exercise

Strategic planning is necessary for solidifying an EDI vision, garnering broad support, and succeeding in one's professional journey. The overall process will be complex and may involve mission and vision articulation, data gathering, SWOT (strengths, weaknesses, opportunities, and threats) analysis, goal setting and metric identification, and execution. If you are tasked with creating an EDI strategic plan, the important first steps will be to identify your core group of strategic plan committee members or stakeholders. These individuals could come from existing groups (e.g., diversity committee and equity champions) or elsewhere.

Utilize the chart below to help you identify and assess stakeholders. A diverse cross-section of individuals who represent faculty, students, staff, residents, fellows, postdocs, leadership, community, etc. will be important (Table 13.1).

Although especially helpful for strategic planning purposes, the chart can also be utilized for any stakeholder group formation (curricular transformation group, inclusive excellence champions, wellness committee, etc.).

## *Reflection Exercise*

Directions: Reflect upon what impact you want to have in 10, 20, 30 years and in what EDI areas. Write your response down to both codify it and save it somewhere safe to review later.

In 10 (20, 30) years, I want have a lasting impact on (what area) and how?

Consider sending a delayed email to yourself coinciding with when you attend your national conference. The arrival of the email can then prompt you to evaluate your progress and promote further reflection.

Table 13.1 Identifying strategic plan committee members or stakeholders

| Stakeholder | Interest in Project | Engagement Readiness | Impact / Influence | Needed Contribution | Stakeholder Engagement Strategy | Person Responsible for Recruitment |
|---|---|---|---|---|---|---|
| | | | | | | |
| | | | | | | |
| | | | | | | |

Adapted from AAMC Diversity and Inclusion Strategic Planning Toolkit: Stakeholder Identification, 2016 [4]

## The Future of DEI

As mentioned earlier, a confluence of factors has intersected to fuel a recent backlash against DEI, and the future of DEI remains uncertain. As of August 30, 2024, 86 anti-DEI legislative bills have been introduced in 26 different states, and 14 of those bills have become law. The restrictions to DEI range from the prohibition of the use of "diversity statements" in employment applications to disallowing the use of any state funds to maintain an office of DEI or DEI roles. At the federal level, an anti-DEI bill, surreptitiously named the EDUCATE Act (Embracing Anti-Discrimination, Unbiased Curriculum, and Advancing Truth in Education), was introduced to the House of Representatives that specifically targets DEI efforts in medical schools [5]. The EDUCATE Act seeks to withhold federal funding, including student federal financial aid for medical schools (both public and private) that engage in certain DEI policies and requirements. The US Supreme Court also ruled in June of 2023 that the use of race in admissions decisions in higher education was unconstitutional. Most recently, a change in the political landscape from the executive and legislative branches of government and the composition of the US Supreme Court further threaten the efforts of DEI.

Although the path forward for DEI may seem unclear and perhaps perilous, it is these paths that call for a new generation of trailblazers, pavers, and individuals with the courage to stand for change. The LHS+ and other racial/ethnic representation deficits among medical school students and faculty remain; the health disparities for LHS+ and other populations remain; the dearth of LHS+ and other minoritized groups in clinical research trials remain; and the inequities in care remain. Today, more than ever, LHS+ leaders in DEI are paramount to quell the erosion of progress promised by anti-DEI efforts, to set a brighter and healthier future for tomorrow.

## Appendix (Table 13.2)

**Table 13.2** Examples of leadership topics [6–8]

| | |
|---|---|
| Balance (resilience) | Management |
| Emotional intelligence | Equity and change management |
| Openness and humility | Ethics |
| Service leadership skills | Mission, vision |
| Communication | Healthcare quality |
| Negotiation | Strategic thinking |
| Conflict management | Iterative quality improvement process and systems approach |
| Crisis communication | Leadership development opportunities |
| Building communities of practice | Work–life integration |
| Team building | Career development and succession planning |
| Budgeting | Culture by design principles |

# Example of Leadership Positions in an Academic Health System

President of Health Sciences and Medical Affairs and Dean

    Senior Director for Executive Communications
    Executive Vice Dean for Research Chief Scientific Officer,

        Senior Associate Dean for Research

            Associate Dean for Clinical and Translational Research
            Associate Dean Research Information Technology
            Assistant Dean Clinical Research
            Assistant Dean Research

    Executive Vice Dean for Academic Affairs, Chief Academic Officer

        Executive Director for Administration, Chief Operating Officer
        Senior Associate Dean Education and Global Initiatives

            Associate Dean Graduate and Postdoctoral Studies
            Associate Dean Graduate Medical Education
            Assistant Dean Graduate Medical Education
            Assistant Dean Continuing Medical Education and Lifelong Learning
            Associate Dean Medical Student Education

                Assistant Dean Curriculum
                Assistant Dean Admissions
                Assistant Dean Student Services
                Assistant Dean Assessment, Evaluation, and Quality Improvement

        Senior Associate Dean Faculty and Faculty Development

            Assistant Dean Instructional Faculty
            Assistant Dean Research Faculty
            Assistant Dean Clinical Faculty
            Senior Director of Faculty Affairs

        Associate Vice President and Associate Dean Health Equity and Inclusion
        Associate Dean Regulatory Affairs

    Executive Vice Dean for Clinical Affairs, President, U-M Health System

        Senior Associate Dean, Clinical Affairs, Executive Director, Medical Group

            Associate Dean, Clinical Affairs

    Department Heads—Clinical and Basic Science
    Institutes and Center Leads

## References

1. The Hispanic population in the United States: 2018. Bureau, U. S. C. In: U.S. Department of Congress. https://www.census.gov/data/tables/2018/demo/hispanic-origin/2018-cps.html. Accessed on 5 July 2025.
2. Association of American Medical Colleges. Diversity in medicine: facts and figures 2018. 2018. https://www.aamc.org/data-reports/workforce/data/figure-18-percentage-all-active-physicians-race/ethnicity-2018. Accessed on 5 July 2025.
3. Nickens HW, Ready TP, Petersdorf RG. Project 3000 by 2000. Racial and ethnic diversity in U.S. medical schools. N Engl J Med. 1994;331(7):472–6. https://doi.org/10.1056/nejm199408183310712.
4. Association of American Medical Colleges. Diversity and inclusion strategic planning tool kit. Stakeholder identification. 2016. https://www.aamc.org/services/member-capacity-building/diversity-and-inclusion-strategic-planning-toolkit#task1. Accessed on 5 July 2025.
5. Embracing anti-discrimination, unbiased curriculum, and advancing truth in education. H.R. 7725. 118th Cong. (2023–3034).
6. Detert JR. What courageous leaders do differently. Harvard Business Review Digital Articles; 2022. p. 1–6.
7. Nunez AE. Negotiation skills for new leaders. Atlanta: AAMC Organizational Leadership in Academic Medicine for New Associate Dean and Department Chairs; 2018.
8. Servey JT, Hartzell JD, McFate T. A faculty development model for academic leadership education across a health care organization. J Med Educat Curri Develop. 2020; https://doi.org/10.1177/2382120520948878.

**Open Access** This chapter is licensed under the terms of the Creative Commons Attribution 4.0 International License (http://creativecommons.org/licenses/by/4.0/), which permits use, sharing, adaptation, distribution and reproduction in any medium or format, as long as you give appropriate credit to the original author(s) and the source, provide a link to the Creative Commons license and indicate if changes were made.

The images or other third party material in this chapter are included in the chapter's Creative Commons license, unless indicated otherwise in a credit line to the material. If material is not included in the chapter's Creative Commons license and your intended use is not permitted by statutory regulation or exceeds the permitted use, you will need to obtain permission directly from the copyright holder.

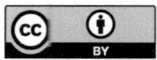

# Chapter 14
# Striving to Become a Dean of Undergraduate Medical Education/Curriculum

John A. Davis Rodríguez

> **Learning Objectives**
> 1. Describe the typical leadership structure of medical education within medical schools
> 2. Describe the typical activities of the curriculum dean (or equivalent within a medical school
> 3. Contextualize one's work, especially LHS+ work, into a framework that shows how the work might apply to the skillsets needed to be a curriculum dean
> 4. Describe a framework for navigating "facultyhood," especially along a medical educator path

## Introduction

Welcome to this chapter, and *felicidades* on making it through what many consider to be the hardest parts of the education process. I hope that your presence means you have at least some interest in becoming a dean involved with medical education and ideally centered on the curriculum that medical students (like many of us were, once upon a time) would/should complete in order to become the physicians of tomorrow. The first step is to learn more, and that's exactly what I hope this chapter will help you do, ideally also helping to clarify some aspect of your journey in leadership as part of the Latina/o/x/e, Hispanic, or of Spanish Origin+ (LHS+) community in medicine and medical education.

---

J. A Davis Rodríguez (✉)
University of California, San Francisco, San Francisco, CA, USA
e-mail: John.DavisRodriguez@ucsf.edu

## Scope of This Chapter

This chapter is organized around seven common questions that many people have when they are getting started on a path in medical education. Through answering these questions, I hope to introduce you to the role of undergraduate medical education (UME)/curriculum deans in general and give you a sense of how you might approach learning even more about the role at an individual institution, and how you might start yourself on a path to becoming one.

What this chapter will not discuss is as important as what it will. There are many articles and other works written about how to get started in medical education in general [1, 2]. Likewise, there are publications about how to get involved in leadership in medicine [3]. This entire book is more about how to become involved in leadership within the context of medical education and/or academic medicine (and has the benefit of considering how to do that as a member of the LHS+ community).

This chapter will focus on the UME/curriculum dean role specifically, and we will start by describing how a UME/curriculum dean role fits within the structure of other deans in a medical school.

One last thing before we get started. You will notice that I will often make use of first-person pronouns here, especially plural ("we/us"). While this chapter will describe something that I have personally navigated, I firmly believe that we are all on this journey together: a journey of discovery, opportunity, and, most importantly, community.

¡Vámonos!

## What Is a UME/Curriculum Dean?

We should first start by outlining the leadership structure of medical schools as academic entities. It is important to say up front that every medical school is different. That said, there are some important commonalities. Every medical school has a dean. The dean. This is the person ultimately in charge of the operations and success of the academic entity that houses the medical school (usually called a school of medicine, or sometimes a college of medicine). Usually, the school has many focus areas, often called departments, and these are usually headed by chairs. Departments can be clinical (e.g., internal medicine and surgery), basic science (e.g., pharmacology and biochemistry), and other (e.g., bioethics, epidemiology, and even medical education).

Aside from the departmental structure within a school, the dean usually needs help attending to leadership within certain key mission areas, such as research and education. For these areas, a school usually has vice deans, or sometimes senior associate deans, to help with leadership at the school level for each of those areas. Within the education mission area, there are often many important roles, and these are usually delegated to associate or assistant deans. Common examples of roles

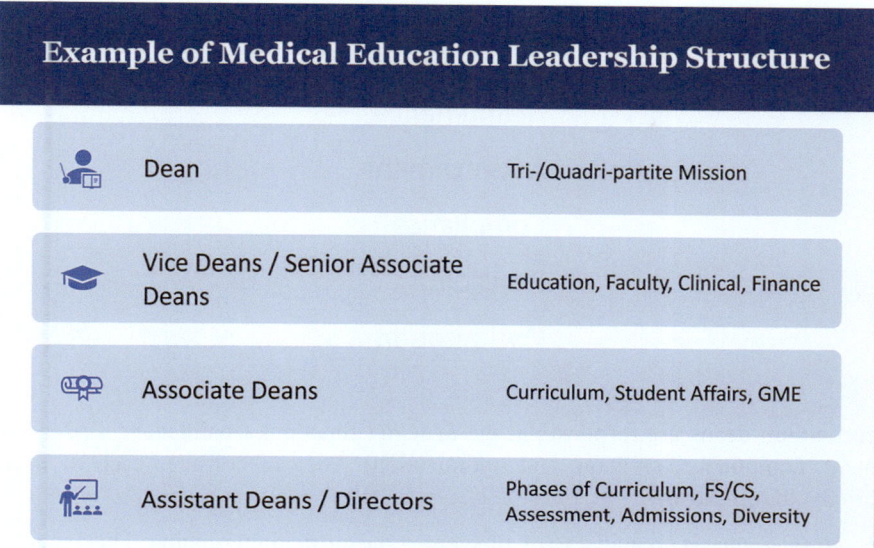

**Fig. 14.1** Example medical school decanal administrative hierarchy. Abbreviations: *GME* graduate medical education, *FS* foundational science, *CS* clinical science

within education include UME admissions, UME student affairs, UME curriculum, graduate medical education (GME, meaning residency/fellowship), and continuing medical education (CME). The number and exact purview of the different deans depend on the needs and resources of the institution. For instance, some institutions have one person as both the student affairs and admissions dean. Others may have associate deans in charge of a larger area, such as curriculum, with assistant deans in charge of subsections of the curriculum, such as an assistant dean for preclerkship curriculum and an assistant dean for clerkship/postclerkship curriculum. A brief example of a generic organizational chart is shown in Fig. 14.1.

There can be many additional and complex reporting structures within any particular academic setting, so it is worthwhile finding the organizational chart for your own institution to see how it matches up, and what nuances help distinguish it from other institutions. For now, we will turn our attention to the UME/curriculum dean role, hereafter called just "curriculum dean" for brevity, to learn more about the functions usually assigned to someone in that role.

## What Does a Curriculum Dean Do?

Broadly speaking, the curriculum dean oversees the operations and improvements to the UME curriculum. However, that charge entails lots of duties that it can be helpful to consider using some framework; one that I created as part of my work in this area is shown in Fig. 14.2. This framework enumerates five key areas for which

**Fig. 14.2** Functions of a curriculum dean: The MACRO view

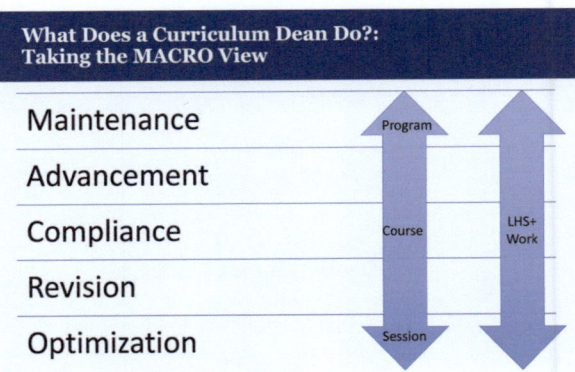

curriculum deans are responsible: the *MACRO* functions (maintenance, advancement, compliance, revision, and optimization). We can consider each of these briefly, in turn, below:

- *Maintenance* is about the work of keeping the curriculum running. This includes overseeing staffing needs, budgeting, and faculty resources, to name just a few. These managerial tasks are often also referred to as administration of the curriculum.
- *Advancement* is about trying new things—innovation and attendant scholarship. There are always opportunities to do what we do in a scholarly way, and we should, as leaders in academic medicine, always be pushing things forward, informed from that scholarly lens.
- *Compliance* is about the reporting that we often have to do to a variety of organizations. The most important compliance function for curriculum deans is that required by the Liaison Committee on Medical Education (or the LCME), the primary accrediting body of medical education programs. Curriculum deans are particularly focused on Standards 5–7 found in the LCME publication of requirements for medical school accreditation [4]. In addition, however, there are often local, state, and even national agencies that may require reporting on various aspects of the curriculum (usually what is taught and where) and how it functions.
- *Revision* is the work of changing the curriculum and its operations to meet extant circumstances. One very important example of this was the change needed to keep medical education programs running when the COVID-19 pandemic began. For many institutions, this required changes to curriculum (offering courses at different times, altering graduation requirements) as well as to operations (shifting classes and some outpatient patient visits to the remote context).
- *Optimization*, the last area, is about gathering and incorporating feedback about the curriculum. This is often referred to as program evaluation, or educational continuous quality improvement.

It is important here to note that these different categorizations can be helpful for understanding the scope of the work of the curriculum dean, but they are not at all mutually exclusive. Rather, there is significant overlap in the work done. For example, there are often compliance considerations to the work we do in each of the other categories. Likewise, any change required, whether driven by revision or optimization, is often simultaneously an opportunity for advancement of the curriculum as well.

## Who Becomes a Curriculum Dean?

In general, the types of people who are interested in this role are those who like the combination of medical education, specifically curriculum, and leadership/administration. Most often, this means people who teach because they are passionate about it, who are identified as good at teaching by their learners and by others, and who have had some exposure to medical education leadership (e.g., directing a course or clerkship or part of the curriculum) and found that both interesting and rewarding (and ideally have a passion for it as well).

In the past, those who became curriculum deans were usually clinicians who were not necessarily otherwise interested in (or beholden to) a research program. That was usually because either they weren't interested in research in general, or they had tapered down their research activity for a variety of reasons. Some curriculum deans were also found from the ranks of basic science PhDs and not just MDs. Over time, this has shifted, and more curriculum deans are MDs, and many have been on dedicated clinician–educator pathways and have thus been on a trajectory toward medical education leadership from early on in their careers.

It is important to mention here that there are significant disparities in the demographics of faculty in academic medicine, people in medical leadership, and that includes medical education leadership, when compared to the demographics of the general population, or even of medical students. In particular, people from underrepresented-in-medicine backgrounds are even less well represented in medical leadership, and again, that includes medical education leadership [5–7].

## What Are the Usual Qualifications of a Curriculum Dean?

The usual qualifications for someone in a curriculum dean role are those that speak to the areas of interest mentioned above. Some content expertise on the training path is usually required; that typically means having an MD/DO or equivalent, though some deans have a PhD in a medical science and have taught extensively in a medical/health professions curriculum as a way of obtaining that expertise. Likewise, experience in medical education is critical. Most people seeking these roles have either done a degree or specific training in education (e.g., a master's program in education) or have had significant experience in these types of roles before.

For beginners on this path, it would be very helpful to start with professional development in medical education. Often this will be a class or set of lectures/

**Table 14.1** Examples of professional development in medical education[a]

| |
|---|
| Specialty-specific organizations, for example: |
|    Infectious Diseases Society of America |
|    American College of Physicians |
| Specialty-specific educational organizations, for example: |
|    Association of Surgical Education |
|    Alliance of Academic Internal Medicine |
|    Society for Academic Emergency Medicine |
|    Society of Teachers of Family Medicine |
| Medical education organizations, for example: |
|    The Association of American Medical Colleges (AAMC) |
|    The International Association of Health Professions Education |
|    The International Association of Medical Science Educators (IAMSE) |
|    ChangeMedEd (initiative of The American Medical Association) |
|    Generalists in Medical Education |

[a]Note that many institutions have a list of organizations; see, e.g., https://www.omed.pitt.edu/medical-education-organizations

workshops offered through your own institution. Sometimes these are offered as part of a specialty/subspecialty professional organization's regular conference. You may also choose to attend a dedicated medical education conference, either regional or national, perhaps as part of your specialty organization or outside of it. Some examples of these types of conferences and professional development venues are listed in Table 14.1.

It is common for those interested in medical education leadership, after having done significant faculty development in education, to ask about the utility of progressing on to a master's degree (or even a PhD) in education. This is something that should be considered carefully, primarily because of both the time and money investments required. These can be very helpful with the acquisition of a broad and useful set of skills. However, it is important to remember that a degree does not substitute for academic productivity or leadership experience, whereas success in the latter two can often speak to the presence of the skillsets needed. In general, talk to your advisors, mentors, and sponsors to help get the best picture of what would be best for you based on your goals and current context.

## What Is the Typical Pathway to Becoming a Curriculum Dean?

It is good to state at the outset that there is no "pathway" to becoming any type of medical education curricular leader. I prefer to say that there are journeys that can lead one to consider medical education leadership, including being a UME/curriculum dean, as a career option. As above, there are qualifications that are important, skillsets that are needed, and desired attributes that speak to both the general position and its context within a particular institution. It is also true, though, that there are some people who follow a usual training and experience pathway in order to gain their skills and experiences.

Many people start as junior faculty by giving lectures (residency, medical student, etc.) and eventually with obtaining some leadership position within medical education. While this may be at any trainee level, most often this would be in the UME space, either in the preclerkship curriculum or within a clerkship that aligns with the faculty member's appointment(s). In these types of positions, if the faculty member does well, enjoys the role, and is interested in advancing, the process of "rising through the ranks" of medical education leadership usually begins. A higher leadership position opens, the faculty member decides to apply, and advances if selected.

At each level, the key question is whether one is interested in the next leadership level. If so, the process usually begins with accumulating experiences and skills that might be needed for the next level. With each subsequent level of advancement, there is usually a decrease in the amount of direct teaching in the role, and a concomitant increase in the administrative tasks allocated to the role.

## How Do I Prepare Myself for This Path?

The steps for preparing for the path to a role as a dean of UME/curriculum often depend on what experiences one has had to date. The framework I use to help consider this developmental process articulates four, usually sequential, tools/skills that can be leveraged in preparing for advancement along a medical education leadership path. Let's start from the perspective of someone who is a new faculty member (or about to be one) with relatively little experience in medical education, aside from teaching medical students and perhaps interns/residents in a clinical setting as part of team-based care.

**Saying "Yes"** In general, for the new faculty member or about-to-be new faculty member, this process starts with teaching opportunities. Usually, one must establish oneself as an excellent teacher before moving on to administrative roles. This starts with saying yes to any and all incoming opportunities to teach. Particularly in the world of medical education, relatively soon offers will come in for even some smaller leadership opportunities, such as being in charge of a set of lectures, or a set of small group activities, etc. The priority at this point is to continue to refine and demonstrate your skills as a teacher, so it is important to get evaluations of your teaching. These may come automatically, but not always. It's good to ask the person in charge of the session or course to find out. Sometimes they will be able to observe you teaching directly and then be able to write a personal evaluation of your teaching. Letters like these can be very important for advancement and promotion. The challenge with this time period is that it is relatively short-lived. Quickly, one's time can become full of teaching opportunities, which leads to the next important skill.

**Saying "No"** At some point we realize that we can be easily stretched too thin with the number of teaching opportunities that come in. Sometimes, that includes other "opportunities" such as committee work and/or other service work. It is important to refine the skill of evaluating the relative benefits and detriments of a particular offer and saying (politely) no when necessary. This is particularly important for any faculty who hold a minoritized identity, as we know that the minority tax operates within all aspects of medicine, including medical education. It is helpful to have a mentor (or mentors) to help cultivate that skill of evaluating when and how to say no.

**Saying "Yes, and…"** Sometimes, an offer will come our way even when our plates are full. Perhaps, though, it really aligns with our expertise and passions, and/or might be a really rare advancement opportunity. This is the time to deploy the next skill: how to say yes, but with conditions. Sometimes this takes the form of saying yes on the condition that another current responsibility be reassigned. For instance, taking a leadership role in a course might mean needing to give up a particular committee assignment, or another teaching activity. These decisions can be challenging, and again, mentors can be helpful in critically evaluating a teaching portfolio to determine priorities. Another time it is helpful to say "Yes, and…" is when there is an opportunity that might seem "early" for us. Perhaps a position is open or offered to us, and we feel like we haven't necessarily had the experiences needed to be successful or may feel like we're too junior for such an opportunity. Again, mentors can be helpful in two specific regards: first, to help counter any aspect of impostor syndrome that might be at play, and second, to help with articulating what resources might be needed to be successful in the role. These can be important considerations in ensuring that the work is not undervalued and is set up for success.

**Saying "*Adiós*"** This last skill is not intended to sound as dramatic as perhaps it does. It is really a reminder that we all need to be reflective and aware when it is time to let something go. Perhaps it is a particular lecture that we have been giving for a while. Or maybe it is a course we have directed. In some cases, as in the section above, our plates might have gotten too full, and we might not be devoting the time to it that we should. In other cases, perhaps we have lost some of our passion for it. And in still other cases, perhaps we are getting comfortable in our current leadership role and are looking for the "next thing" in our developmental path. Many writings on leadership discuss how leaders usually share a drive to continue growing. The concept behind "saying goodbye" is knowing when to start looking for that "next thing" and what that "next thing" might be. Perhaps it is a promotion. Perhaps it is an equal but complementary role. As with all of the other steps, mentors can be helpful in exploring this space, and good mentors will be able to discuss these topics openly and constructively.

## What About My LHS+ Identity and/or My LHS+ Work?

Many of us with marginalized or minoritized identities, including those of us with at least one LHS+ identity, do not have a choice about whether these identities are part of our work, whether inside or outside of medical education curricular leadership. They are part of our lives and expressions of ourselves. We do (should) have a choice, however, about how much of our academic work centers around our *identidad* and/or work about diversity/equity/belonging.

With respect to LHS+ identities, because of how differently these impact us and what they mean to each of us, there is no single correct answer for how these should be considered in our pursuit of curriculum leadership roles. For some, particularly in certain roles (e.g., leading a research project on the impact of a novel medical Spanish elective on quality of care in student volunteers in a local LHS+-serving clinic), LHS+ identities will directly impact work and leadership, and thus will play an important part in a leadership path. For others, and in different roles (e.g., overseeing a curricular thread on biochemistry or cellular biology), the application may be more indirect. In all instances, it is useful to consider the impact of LHS+ identities on leadership in general—an area that has been the subject of articles and other publications.

With respect to our work, being faculty at an academic institution means we have at least one area of scholarly interest and expertise we are cultivating at any given time. That interest may change and evolve over time, but there should not be any time without such an effort. Some of us may choose to make an aspect of LHS+ identity central to our scholarly work/focus. For the vast majority, that will *not* be about LHS+ topics/identities and medical education. This begs the question of how one's scholarly work, if focused on LHS+ topics, would apply to medical education, particularly if we are applying for roles in medical education. It is important to remember that every time we are giving a lecture or a talk, we are teaching, and direct teaching is one of the main components of the medical educator's portfolio. Particularly in a UME or GME setting, if we are invited to give lectures, there are learning objectives and instructional methods associated with our work. It is always helpful to find out if evaluations will be completed by learners to get feedback about our teaching and to accumulate these for both advancement/promotion/tenure purposes and for inclusion on applications for education leadership positions. In addition to this, if this is a new learning activity that has, by definition, not been done before, then this activity presents, additionally, the opportunity for scholarship and publication. The same data we would use for evaluation of the lecture can be used as outcome measures for publication purposes in venues such as MedEdPORTAL, among others.

## *Conclusion*

I hope this chapter has given you some useful descriptions, frameworks, and suggestions as you continue your journey as a faculty member involved with academic medicine. Most importantly, I hope it has served to dispel some of the mystique around being/becoming a UME/Curriculum Dean. Being involved with education, and especially education leadership, is full of opportunities to both influence the future of medicine and help serve as a role model for the next generation of physicians. Remember that you are already an important and valued member of the community of medicine, and whatever way you contribute will be meaningful to others who look up to you and will follow in your footsteps. For some of you, I hope that will include work in an education leadership capacity.

*¡Buena suerte, y un abrazo fuerte!*

## Reflection Questions

1. Take a moment to be critically reflective of your own medical education role models. Which ones have been formative to you, and what have their qualities been? What are the aspects you try to emulate?
2. Now that you've read the chapter, think of some things you have done that would be helpful on the path to becoming an associate dean for UME/curriculum, if you wanted to apply for such a position.
    (a) What do the things you have done say about where your passions lie?
    (b) What things are missing, and how might these represent growth opportunities for you?
3. Based on your answers to 2b and keeping in mind other chapters that have intrigued you, think of one thing you'd like to do next—one skillset to acquire, experience to have—that might set you up for success as a UME/curriculum dean (and ideally be useful in other positions as well).

## *Personal Narrative*

### John A. Davis Rodríguez, PhD MD

I grew up in Houston, Texas, a second-generation Mexican American and son of two police officers. While my parents were working, I spent most of my time growing up with my Mexican grandparents and larger family, and while I learned so many important and wonderful life lessons from them—things that continue to shape my character to this day—I also witnessed first-hand how the health care system treated people who looked a certain way, who had certain names, and especially who spoke primarily a different language.

Later, in college, as a first-generation student coming from a public-school background, and coming out as a gay man in the 1980s at the height of the HIV/AIDS pandemic in the United States, I witnessed how challenging higher education could be for those of us who looked different and even loved differently. I also witnessed how our healthcare system failed people, especially gender and sexual minority people, and the nation as a whole, in those early days of HIV/AIDS in the United States.

These experiences strengthened my resolve to go into medicine, especially with an eye toward service to members of my communities: LGBTQ+ and LHS+, and especially those who live at the intersection of these two. I decided then that I wanted to be a physician caring for those living with HIV.

After college, I went to graduate school and earned a PhD in chemistry as a way to prepare myself for the rigors of medical school. This was before postbaccalaureate programs were really popular, and it had the added benefit of allowing me to explore science deeply and reflect carefully on what path I would like to take in service to others. Ultimately, I realized that I wanted the direct human interaction that medicine as a profession would provide. I then went to medical school and subsequently into internal medicine residency, infectious disease fellowship, and did specialized training in HIV care and transplant infectious diseases.

Along the way, I took every opportunity I could to help others in their learning journeys. I was a teaching fellow while I was a senior in college; I taught every semester while I was in graduate school; and I participated in teaching medical students while I was a resident and fellow in training. The wonderful expressions of gratitude from the students I would interact with, punctuated with occasional teaching awards, reinforced my calling to teaching as a profession, along with medicine.

During my first faculty position, I combined my love of clinical care with teaching by giving lectures for infectious disease fellows, internal medicine residents, medical students, and even other health professions students, all on areas of infectious diseases that fit within my expertise (primarily HIV). Slowly, my teaching opportunities branched out to include tutoring students in basic/foundational sciences, and I was eventually offered a position as an assistant dean for students. After about a year in that leadership position, I applied for and was selected to serve as the associate dean for medical education.

It was a few years later when an opportunity arose at my current institution to serve as associate dean for curriculum, and while here, I have also had the opportunity to serve as associate dean for students, associate dean for assessment, and even vice dean for education over UME. Thanks to these experiences, I was recently selected in a national search to be our inaugural vice chancellor of education and student affairs.

Using my own framework here, I will note that my story is one of saying a lot of "yes" to opportunities that arose and learning as much as I could from those growth opportunities. It also included a little saying "*adiós*" as needed.

In addition, writing this narrative as part of this book offers me the opportunity to reflect on how my *Latinidad* has influenced me and my leadership as part of my journey. Juana Bordas, in her book The Power of Latino Leadership, articulates a ten-dimensional framework for thinking about some of the unique cultural aspects we bring to leadership positions as Latinos [8]. It includes characteristics such as *personalismo, conciencia,* and *destino* and some principles such as diversity, community stewardship, immigrant spirit, and coalition leadership. Many aspects of that framework resonate with me, and I see aspects of many of those pieces at work in my own style of educational leadership.

I want to conclude by expressing gratitude to those of you reading, as you are on a noble path of service, and we are all fortunate to have you as part of *nuestra comunidad*. I hope that sharing some of my story will also invite you to explore within yourself to see what types of leadership, education or otherwise, you might be called to.

*¡Seguimos adelante!*

# References

1. Gordon RJ. Launching your career in medical education [Internet]. Waltham: Massachusetts Medical Society; 2017. Mar 16. Available from: https://resident360.nejm.org/expert-consult/launching-your-career-in-medical-education-3
2. Rougas S, Zhang XC, Blanchard R, Michael SH, Mackuen C, Lee B, Nocera M, Hilliard RW, Green E. Strategies for residents to explore careers in medical education. J Grad Med Educ. 2019;11(3):263–7. https://doi.org/10.4300/JGME-D-18-00985.1.
3. Sklar DP. Leadership in academic medicine: purpose, people, and programs. Acad Med. 2018;93(2):145–8. https://doi.org/10.1097/ACM.0000000000002048.
4. AAMC. U.S. medical school deans by dean type and race/ethnicity (URiM vs. non-URiM). AAMC; 2024. https://www.aamc.org/data-reports/faculty-institutions/data/us-medical-school-deans-trends-type-and-race-ethnicity
5. Kaplan SE, Raj A, Carr PL, Terrin N, Breeze JL, Freund KM. Race/ethnicity and success in academic medicine: findings from a longitudinal multi-institutional study. Acad Med. 2018;93(4):616–22. https://doi.org/10.1097/ACM.0000000000001968.
6. Nobles A, Martin BA, Casimir J, Schmitt S, Broadbent G. Stalled progress: medical school dean demographics. J Am Board Fam Med. 2022;35(1):163–8. https://doi.org/10.3122/jabfm.2022.01.210171.
7. Bordas J. The power of Latino leadership. Oakland: Berrett-Koehler Publishers; 2013.
8. LCME. Functions and structure of a medical school, 2024. 2024. https://lcme.org/wp-content/uploads/2024/08/2025-26-Functions-and-Structure_2024-08-01.docx

**Open Access** This chapter is licensed under the terms of the Creative Commons Attribution 4.0 International License (http://creativecommons.org/licenses/by/4.0/), which permits use, sharing, adaptation, distribution and reproduction in any medium or format, as long as you give appropriate credit to the original author(s) and the source, provide a link to the Creative Commons license and indicate if changes were made.

The images or other third party material in this chapter are included in the chapter's Creative Commons license, unless indicated otherwise in a credit line to the material. If material is not included in the chapter's Creative Commons license and your intended use is not permitted by statutory regulation or exceeds the permitted use, you will need to obtain permission directly from the copyright holder.

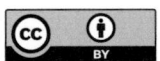

## Chapter 15
# Striving to Become a Dean/Designated Institutional Official of Graduate Medical Education (GME)

Larissa Velez, John Paul Sánchez, and Maricarmen Cruz

> **Learning Objectives**
> - Describe the landscape of LHS+-identified individuals in graduate medical education (GME)
> - List graduate medical education leadership opportunities that exist within clinical departments at US medical schools
> - Detail opportunities for career development that allow LHS+ community members to be prepared for leadership in GME
> - Review how leadership development better prepares individuals to serve a multicultural world

**Key Terms and Definitions**

- *Graduate medical education (GME)*: The period of training in either a core specialty (residency) or subspecialty (fellowship) after finishing medical school.
- *Accreditation Council for Graduate Medical Education (ACGME)*: The national organization that sets and monitors professional accreditation standards that

---

L. Velez (✉)
Department of Emergency Medicine, University of Texas Southwestern Medical Center, Dallas, TX, USA

J. P. Sánchez
Latino Medical Student Association Inc., Chicago, IL, USA

Building the Next Generation of Academic Physicians Inc., Rye Brook, New York, USA
e-mail: exec.director@lmsa.net

M. Cruz
Veteran Affairs Caribbean Healthcare System, Guaynabo, Puerto Rico

© The Author(s) 2026
J. P. Sánchez et al. (eds.), *Advancing Latino, Hispanic, or of Spanish Origin+ Leadership in Academic Medicine*,
https://doi.org/10.1007/978-3-032-07570-3_15

guide institutions and programs in preparing physicians to deliver safe and high-quality care.
- *Sponsoring institution (SI)*: The entity that holds the authority to oversee, support, and administer residency and fellowship programs and ensures that these programs are in substantial compliance with the ACGME accreditation standards and lead to a high-quality clinical learning environment.
- *Designated institutional official (DIO)*: The individual appointed by the SI who has the authority and is responsible for the oversight and administration of the ACGME accreditation standards, including institutional and common program requirements.
- *American Association of Medical Colleges (AAMC)*: A nonprofit organization that represents medical schools, teaching hospitals, faculty, residents, and students from organizations in the United States and Canada.

## What Is Graduate Medical Education?

Graduate medical education (GME) is the period of training in either a core specialty (residency) or subspecialty (fellowship) after finishing medical school, where a physician receives specialized education in a particular clinical specialty [1]. This education is mostly overseen within a medical school and/or hospital by program leadership that includes a program director and their team and the GME Office of the Sponsoring Institution (SI). The SI oversees and supports all ACGME-accredited training programs through the role of the designated institutional official (DIO).

The DIO is the recognized individual who is in charge of the GME office of the Sponsoring Institution and who is granted the authority to oversee that ACGME accreditation standards are fulfilled at the program and institutional level and that the clinical learning environment (CLE) promotes the conditions for trainees' development of core competencies [2]. Depending on who is the sponsoring institution for these GME programs (a university, a hospital, or a private organization), the DIO's role will be assumed by the dean of the medical school, an associate to the dean, the GME dean, or a designated education officer (DEO). The name may vary, but the role and responsibility for the DIO do not change and will always be overseeing the CLE.

The CLE is the atmosphere where residents and fellows enrolled in postgraduate medical education programs get trained as physicians to care for patients through a safe and high-quality approach [3]. The ACGME describes that this is attained by engaging trainees in educational activities that promote [3]:

1. A culture of patient safety
2. Healthcare quality
3. Teaming
4. Diversity, equity, and inclusion
5. Promotion of well-being
6. Professionalism

**Table 15.1** ACGME data resource book: Academic year 2023–2024

| ACGME data resource book: Academic year 2023–2024 | |
|---|---|
| Accredited residency and fellowship programs | 13,393 |
| Accredited specialties and subspecialties | 146 |
| Sponsoring institutions housing accredited programs | 905 |
| Active full- and part-time residents and fellows in ACGME-accredited programs | 162,644 |
| Number of physicians who are residents or fellows in the US | 1 in 7 |

In postgraduate medical education, the majority of DIOs are stationed at medical schools appointed as assistant deans, but many GME offices may also have an associate dean, also known as dean of GME. In any case, it will be of utmost importance that the DIO and/or dean of GME assume the responsibility of establishing a vision and mission aligned with the organization they represent that sets the pace for the general educational strategy for GME.

Nationally, the Accreditation Council for Graduate Medical Education (ACGME) sets guidelines and provides accreditation for most programs. However, some fellowship programs exist under other accreditation bodies, such as State Medical Boards or Specialty organizations. In the United States, there are 146 distinct ACGME-accredited specialties and subspecialties and a total of 13,293 ACGME-accredited programs. These programs have 162,644 active full- and part-time trainees, which comprise 1 of 7 physicians in the United States. They exist under the auspices of 905 sponsoring institutions [1] (Table 15.1). The 2023–2024 ACGME Data Resource book reported that there were 121,189 active core physician faculty in GME programs; of those, only 8316 or 7% were LHS+. Even though the Hispanic population is the largest racial or ethnic minority in the United States, it is not the most represented minority in GME programs or its leadership [4]. ACGME has included in their institutional accreditation standards expectations about the institutions and programs' ability to recruit and retain a diverse workforce that can contribute to a safe, inclusive, and equitable learning environment where all trainees are welcomed and mentored [5].

As LHS+ academic professionals progress in their professional fields, they will be presented with opportunities that can serve as developmental milestones to acquire higher appointments. This chapter aims to describe the landscape of GME in the United States and give pathways for LHS+ academicians who aspire to become GME leaders. It also describes specific challenges that LHS+ face when aspiring to have leadership in GME, along with potential actions to overcome these challenges.

## Landscape of Medical School LHS+ Faculty and GME Leadership in the United States

Although the medical schools' student and resident bodies have become more diverse, the diversity of medical school faculty has minimally increased [6]. The AAMC reports that in 2022, 8.3% (10,060) of the MD residents enrolled in ACGME-accredited programs identified as Hispanic/Latino, while 5.1% of DO residents identified as Hispanic/Latino [7]. The majority of medical school faculty, in terms of race/ethnicity, identify as White (60.0%) or Asian 21.6% [8]. In 2024, only 6.3% of full-time allopathic medical school faculty identified as LHS+, 4% as Black/African-American, and <0.1 as Native American/Alaskan Native/Native Hawaiian or Other Pacific Islander [8]. There is significant research showing that proportionately, women and underrepresented in medicine (URiM) numbers continue to decrease as one progresses to the highest ranks and in tenure status [8–14].

According to the American Association of Medical Colleges (AAMC), in 2024, 19% of all the Deans at US Medical Schools belonged to a URiM group [9]. This is despite over 30% of the US population belonging to a minoritized group [15].

This underrepresentation of LHS+ in academic positions may contribute to overlooking diverse perspectives that end up affecting [15, 16]:

- Innovation
- Research
- Teaching methodologies
- Mentoring
- Educational curriculum
- Institutional policies
- Shaping of educational experiences

In Puerto Rico (PR), graduate medical education opens opportunities for local physicians to stay in their communities, develop professionally at a higher level of education, and, as they do that, incorporate the Hispanic cultural component into their professional practice. This has a triggering effect on the retention of physicians in the island, and based on AAMC data, in Puerto Rico this can be as high as 72%.

## GME Roles

GME is focused on advancing the training and development of physicians who will serve our communities and nation through the oversight of strong and high-quality CLEs and training programs. Like every complex project, it demands a team with a wide set of skills who can support the dean of GME or DIO to carry out different roles and responsibilities in the CLE when supervising the implementation of the educational curriculum. These many roles (Table 15.2)

**Table 15.2** GME roles and development pathways

| Role | Responsibilities | Developmental pathway |
|---|---|---|
| Core faculty, faculty advisor | Teach residents and fellows on clinical and academic activities<br>Provide direct clinical care and bedside teaching<br>Role model professional behaviors<br>Teach and mentor the more junior faculty | Participate in the Clinical Competency Committee and Program Evaluation Committee<br>Showcase LHS+ values and influence ideas about the educational curriculum that addresses multicultural aspects of minorities that affect residents and patients |
| Course director for clinical clerkship | Assist in developing clinical rotations and clerkships for medical students<br>Grade students and provide mid- and final-clerkship feedback<br>Participate in the selection and recruitment of trainees into GME programs<br>Innovate on learning experiences of the population served | Participate in the design, implementation, and evaluation of the educational curriculum and the application of accreditation standards in the learning environment<br>Identify clerkship sites where underrepresented LHS+ are treated or where LHS+ successful physicians practice<br>Cultivate a network that leads to professional growth |
| GME participating site directors and liaisons | Assist in coaching, mentoring, and guiding residents during clinical rotations at the participating clinical sites<br>Represent the program director (PD) in managing concerns or situations elevated by trainees at participating sites<br>Collaborate in interfacility research projects<br>Model LHS+ multicultural approach to clinical care | Learn the role of a PD in overseeing the educational experience of trainees<br>Expand networking, serving as liaisons between institutions, the faculty, and the trainee<br>Assume advocacy role in addressing barriers to care |

(continued)

**Table 15.2** (continued)

| Role | Responsibilities | Developmental pathway |
|---|---|---|
| Assistant and associate program directors (APDs) or program director (PD) | Set the vision, mission, and program's educational goals<br>Lead the recruitment and retention of trainees<br>Design and deliver the educational curriculum<br>Provide mentorship to residents and faculty<br>Complete resident's evaluation and make recommendation about promotions and remediation plans<br>Oversee compliance with program accreditation standards<br>Support trainees' preparation for examinations and board examinations<br>Practice administrative skills and coach faculty on related competencies<br>Set expectations about addressing underrepresented minority groups | Embrace leadership roles<br>Collaborate with DIO and other PD in creating a culture that fosters a respectful learning environment and promotes excellence in patient care<br>Practice political savviness and expand professional networking that allows assuming higher complex roles<br>Work closely with their service chiefs in aligning operational and educational goals with their GME mission<br>Learn healthcare administration skills and expand on competencies related to managing people, addressing minorities, and advocating on operational decisions that create systemic barriers for LHS+ individuals who are seeking ways to grow in their careers |
| Graduate Medical Education Committee (GMEC) member | Serves as forum to join faculty, residents, and administrative personnel.<br>Establishes collaborative opportunity to learn from other services and concurrently create awareness about cross-cultural differences when teaming in GME.<br>Raises awareness about the role of mentoring and of pairing trainees with like-minded or relatable faculty. | Create perspective about underrepresented minorities when discussing accreditation topics such as wellness, fatigue mitigation, patient safety, and population health, among others, and how established programs must consider inclusive solutions.<br>Manage multiple accreditation procedures, including the evaluation of residents, promotions, grievances, and onboarding, among others. The LHS+ leader can use this |
| Vice chair for education (VCE) at a department | Harmonize training programs perspectives and needs within that clinical department<br>Learn about organizational decision-making mindset and how to influence institutional policies, inclusion opportunities, grievance procedures, and others | Expand and learn about higher executive functions and how to align programmatic and institutional goals<br>Networking opportunity to facilitate becoming a sponsor of another LHS+ clinician who is emerging as a leader |
| Designated institutional official (DIO) | Hold the authority and responsibility for the oversight and administration of its programs | Networking opportunity for higher organizational roles |

(ACGME 2025) interact with the dean of GME at medical schools and can help advance the career of LHS+ clinicians through the acquisition of knowledge and skills in graduate medical education issues, in developing mentoring skills, and in developing leadership and management skills. However, none of the following roles should be seen as absolutely necessary for becoming a dean of GME or DIO [18].

1. The DIO communicates with accreditation agencies and reports on behalf of the sponsoring institution. The DIO also assists with mentorship and guidance of all program leadership and faculty development. At times, large institutions have assistant or associate DIOs. The role of the DIO is an opportunity to expand networking across multiple clinical specialties and external academic partners, practice problem-solving, manage budgets, create coalitions, and manage conflict and mediation. DIOs have the opportunity to create and align the GME mission with the organizational goals and communicate expectations to their executives that advocate for LHS+ inclusion opportunities within their strategic plans [17]. DIOs must describe how their work of the DIO interfaces with other GME leaders, learners, faculty, executives, and regional and national organizations, requiring from the DIO a set of attitudes that model cultural humility and competence. DIOs with LHS+ lived experiences have the opportunity to model the behaviors of cultural competence and emotional intelligence, and by standing in their leadership role, they achieve the construction of structures that, through inclusiveness, recruit and retain a diverse workforce.
2. Other institutional educational roles: Depending on the size and complexity of an institution, there might be other roles that relate to GME, such as those dealing with recruitment and retention, diversity, equity and inclusion (DEI), wellness, quality and safety, innovation, etc. Partnering with these allies, the DIO can create awareness about LHS+ clinicians and trainees and provoke activities that take into consideration multicultural differences.
3. Regional/national/international GME roles:
   - Service and leadership through medical society educational roles, such as the Council of Residency Directors
   - Service in a specialty board role, such as item writing and oral board examiner
   - Leadership in medical education groups, such as the National Resident Matching Program (NRMP), National Board of Medical Examiners (NBME), National Hispanic Medical Association (NHMA), Latino Medical Student Association (LMSA), and Faculty/Physician Advisory Council (FPAC) Specialty Sections
   - Service in specialty society educational committees
   - Participation and leadership in international educational medical organizations, such as the Education Commission for Foreign Medical Graduates (ECFMG) and Accreditation Council for Graduate Medical Education–International (ACGME-I)

## GME Leaders in Setting the Climate and Culture

When LHS+ physicians aspire to become a dean of GME or DIO, they must consider that they will be exposed to an amazing opportunity to set up the climate and influence postgraduate medical education culture as leaders, academicians, mentors, and advocates for equity within the field. There are multiple responsibilities associated with the role, but the most important role that the DIO/dean of GME will have is promoting a clinical learning environment at the participating site that ensures that trainees receive role modeling, education, and clinical experiences that allow them to comply with their specialty requirements and attain the best preparation to practice independently [19]. There are skills and attitudes necessary to embrace diversity, and when considering the LHS+ identity, just one identity dimension, cultural competence will be an essential skill. Cultural competence in a health practitioner can be defined as having the knowledge, skill, behavior, and attitude to provide the best available care to individuals with backgrounds different from one's own [20]. Similarly, DIO/deans of GME must have the skills, knowledge, and attitudes to lead and oversee programs that are ready to recruit, teach, and train the next generation of physicians in a culturally competent way, and support the development of clinical faculty who will directly supervise the CLE where trainees are developing.

There are specific requirements for the role of the DIO, which are very similar to the role of the dean of GME, and these are formally delineated by the ACGME as part of the Institutional Requirements [21]. The ability to demonstrate the execution of these requirements can be observed through activities that include the following:

*Establishing the mission, vision, and institutional strategy for GME*: The DIO/dean of GME helps craft the institutional GME mission and vision, and this ramifies into each individual program's mission and vision. From this mission and vision, institutional GME strategies are then developed and prioritized [22]. All DIOs must report to a governing body, and this provides an opportunity for LHS+ DIO to advocate for organizational strategies that address underrepresented minorities.

*Assisting with individual program functions*: As a subject matter expert in institutional accreditation requirements, the DIO must provide guidance to GME office staff and program coordinators with knowledge, expertise, resources, and centralized data necessary for:

- Program accreditation activities
- Trainee recruitment and retention
- Onboarding
- Promotion and graduation
- Outcomes measurement
- Special reviews of underperforming programs
- Due process
- Program director development
- Program coordinator development

When setting the GME climate, the LHS+ DIO can coach their administrative team to explore connections through their work that embrace diversity and empower them to want to advocate for the faculty and trainees they serve.

*Accreditation and compliance of GME programs*: The dean of GME oversees and guides any issues regarding accreditation and compliance of all GME programs sponsored by the institution. One particular ACGME institutional requirement is the expectation for institutions to develop strategies to recruit and retain a diverse workforce. As a LHS+ leader, the DIO will have the opportunity to advocate to their executive leadership and GME programs for policies and systems that facilitate a diverse workforce, including LHS+ clinicians and trainees. The retention of a diverse workforce strengthens the GME culture, and this will be observed in the CLE.

*Assist with the creation of new programs*: The dean of GME and/or DIO will be responsible for approving the expansion of existing programs or the creation of new programs. This entails assessing the existing resources and ensuring that this decision does not compromise the existing programs and/or clinical learning environment. When exploring the creation of new programs, the LHS+ DIO can advocate that these programs be opened at alternate underserved locations where disadvantaged populations exist and that contribute to expanding the learning opportunities about population health.

*Due process*: This involves the creation and enforcement of all institutional policies that will address corrective actions, evaluations and promotions, performance improvement plans (PIPs) from probations and dismissals, and grievance processes. Programs always handle these in conjunction with the GME office, the office of legal affairs, and others. There are systemic barriers that minorities encounter at organizations that negatively affect grievance procedures, fair resolution of conflict, and the ability to be promoted. The LHS+ DIO has an opportunity to identify barriers and work collaboratively with stakeholders to create actions that go from creating awareness and conversations to advocacy in policy change [23].

*Program director (PD) and program coordinator (PC) development*: These activities include ensuring approval of new PDs, protected time for PDs, and the correct number of PCs for the size of each program. These individuals need to have continued education that is related to their specific educational roles. Faculty development is an institutional requirement where the LHS+ DIO can incorporate topics not only associated with teaching methodologies but also about cultural humility and competence and the role that this holds in providing trainees with developmental feedback and practicing patient-centered connections.

*Overall educational faculty development*: Teaching faculty must be knowledgeable of the educational objectives of their program. They must also receive education on issues such as teaching, providing developmental feedback, completing assessments, the role of communication, wellness and burnout, and supervision. Faculty development efforts are good opportunities to strengthen the GME culture and work on succession planning efforts for GME leaders.

*Accreditation of the sponsoring institution*: The GME office must maintain all accreditation and reporting requirements for the sponsoring institution [21].

*Financial oversight*: In some places, the dean of GME is also tasked with maintaining the internal budget, billing, contracts, and finances of the office of GME.

## Preparation to Become a GME Dean

There are several components for career planning if one desires a pathway in GME leadership. Emerging LHS+ physician leaders must know that advocating for the expansion of LHS+ representation in academic roles and higher responsibilities conveys getting involved, creating alliances, and being strategic of the opportunities encountered. Strategies and professional development opportunities are reviewed in this section.

First is to commit to developing *leadership skills*. This can be done through multiple tracks. At the program level, the clinician can aspire to become a core faculty member, a course director, or part of the program leadership. Another approach to becoming involved in medical education leadership is by fulfilling the role of a vice chair for education or becoming a member of the Graduate Medical Education Committee (GMEC). There are multiple opportunities external to academic programs that offer ways to continue leadership growth, and on many occasions, through the hands of mentors. These include state, regional, national, or international organizations of medical educators. Leadership can also be through service in governing bodies of medical education organizations, such as the Association of American Medical Colleges (AAMC), American Association of Colleges of Osteopathic Medicine (AACOM), the National Resident Matching Program (NRMP), and the National Board of Medical Examiners (NBME).

Second, consider obtaining a*dditional education through degrees or certificate programs*. There are opportunities to advance your knowledge in education and administration, such as a Master's in Education (MEd), a Master's in Public Health (MPH), or a Master's in Business Administration (MBA). The AAMC sponsors and conducts a GME Leadership Development program that is very useful for those wanting to obtain institutional GME leadership positions [24].

Third, obtain additional experience (and networking) through *attendance at courses* and other GME-specific educational opportunities. The AAMC has many courses geared toward GME leadership, such as at the National Learning Community of Sponsoring Institutions annual meeting. The ACGME conducts DIO training sessions at its annual meeting.

Fourth, get involved in *nonclinical service activities*. Nonclinical service activities are opportunities to expand on experiences, build professional confidence, gain the necessary skills to manage others, and lead people. These activities can include serving on editorial boards, reviewing scholarship for journals and national conferences, workgroups, committees, and moderating and adjudicating, to name a few examples. These activities can start at the local level but eventually must provide you with a footprint or sphere of influence well beyond your institution. As an aside, these activities matter when seeking to meet professorial promotion criteria on most tracks.

Moreover, focus on *finding mentors, sponsors, coaches, advisors, and allies*. These individuals might not be in the same specialty, but they may carefully nurture key relationships. We have met other people who have been seminal in our career development at major medical meetings, especially those geared to medical education. Also, career development courses, certificate courses, and, if pursuing an additional degree, classes. We have also engaged in coaching, and executive coaches were very important in helping me find a career path and overcome hurdles, such as impostor syndrome, life balance, goal setting, etc. They might change over time, and you might not need all these individuals, but these individuals are crucial to individualizing your professional development and success.

Finally, when reflecting on personal traits and behavioral tendencies, there are several to consider embodying to nurture the personal network, engage in quality exchanges, and grow an academic leadership career.

- *Stay curious and motivated*: Find areas of work that keep you interested and motivated. Develop yourself in areas that are newer or emerging.
- *Accept praise and take credit for work well done*: At all times, measure outcomes of all your professional activities. Communicate your success through presentations and publications. When possible, secure grants and other revenue streams that support your educational and professional activities.
- *Collaborate and network*: Find opportunities to collaborate with others with similar interests, both within and outside of your institution. Find opportunities through professional organizations. Find the thought leaders and see how you can connect with them.
- *Knowing your limits and boundaries* is crucial. You must learn when to say yes and when to say no. Overextending yourself and overcommitting can lead to burnout and unhappiness. It also makes you miss deadlines and not be able to fulfill commitments. This hampers your promotability. However, saying "no" too much is also problematic, as you might get labeled as noncollaborative. Always try to avoid contentious or heated exchanges. Fights and overt confrontation do not allow you to achieve agreement.
- *Avoid oversharing*. You must find a close group of trusted advisors and confidants. Sharing too much can lead to gossip and erode the trust that leaders must retain.
- *Overconfidence* is problematic in everyone, particularly in a leader. Leaders must know when to ask for help and guidance and learn to be agile, such as by incorporating the opinions of others in their decision-making.
- Develop your knowledge and skills in the topics of cultural humility and cultural competence. Cultural competence is the respect and understanding of diverse cultural values and practices, while cultural humility is the commitment to self-reflection, an acknowledgement of knowledge limitations, and a commitment to

partner with patients and others around us. As URiM, you are in a unique position to provide wisdom and perspective [25].
- Develop communication skills, especially as it relates to conflict management and navigating difficult conversations. Understand the importance of emotional intelligence and positive intelligence in leading diverse groups [26].
- *Understand the glass ceiling*: The glass ceiling (which is also described as a "sticky floor" at times) is an unofficially acknowledged barrier to advancement in a profession [27]. In most places, however, leadership will recognize and value excellence. When given the opportunity, your past experiences, including those in the DEI space, will create additional leadership opportunities.

## Puerto Rico: A Unique Landscape for GME and the DIO Role

Unlike medical education in the states, the four medical schools in Puerto Rico (PR) afford a bilingual experience, in medical English and medical Spanish, and collectively are the largest producer of LCME-accredited bilingual providers in the United States. Approximately 70% of graduates remain in Puerto Rico for residency, and 30% pursue opportunities in the mainland United States. GME in PR has had a trajectory of 75 years, starting in the 1950s with the opening of the University of Puerto Rico School of Medicine and eventually expanding to four bilingual LCME-accredited medical schools after the 1970s. The initial clinical workshops for medical students and residents were located at the San Juan City Hospital and the Veteran's Administration (VA) hospital, and eventually, these expanded to other hospital centers located at the Medical Sciences Campus. PR had a unique healthcare system design that provided healthcare services to anybody who needed it at the government-sponsored healthcare sites. Medical schools had access to sending their trainees to these government primary and tertiary centers located all across Puerto Rico. This co-dependent model of education exposed trainees to different systems of care while it increased the number of clinicians who could take care of patients in disadvantaged communities. The system benefited both the government and the GME programs. The clinical faculty who supervised medical students and residents worked at these clinical centers, and many of them simultaneously had academic appointments at the school of medicine. The model was a huge hit until the the 1990s when most of these government centers were sold to private entities, leading to new challenges for DIOs to reassess ways to continue the GME mission [28].

For many decades, two main institutions were sponsoring GME in PR, the University of PR, sponsored by the local government, and the VA Hospital, sponsored by the federal government. The former was and remains the largest sponsor of GME in PR, and the latter is unique, in a sense, because the VA in PR was and remains one of the only two remaining VA hospitals in the United States that still sponsors GME programs. By 2024, the number of sponsoring institutions in PR grew to 12, incorporating programs sponsored by nonprofit and for-profit private institutions, which combined now sponsor over 900 trainees in primary and subspecialty programs [28]. LHS+ DIO's have held a critical role in the growth and sustainment of these programs in PR. With the corporatization of healthcare, DIOs have been driven to master various skills, including negotiation skills, managing finances and budget, getting involved in government politics, mastering public speaking and advocacy, and becominge project managers, among some. Some of the challenges experienced by DIOs in PR include include:

- Justifying and defending GME funds to the government of PR every fiscal year for the sustainment of programs that are sponsored by the government university
- Advocating for the continuity of VA-sponsored legacy programs in PR who serve within a particular social context and demographics
- Collaborating in the design of a healthcare infrastructure that finds value in investing in GME programs, both in government- and privately sponsored programs
- Educating executives about the GME mission, how to incorporate the education mission into the private/government clinical practice, and the boundaries of collaboration
- Creating faculty development programs that compete with the expected protected time to facilitate their growth as teachers and mentors
- Managing the expanding institutional and programmatic accreditation requirements
- Collaborating with the PR Health Department in identifying strategies that ameliorate the exodus of physicians from PR
- Promoting and protecting a clinical learning environment that, although established within a modern healthcare world, still values the spirit of humanity in medicine
- Others

As physicians, LHS+ DIOs in PR have played a role that is little spoken of, and this is how their leadership in GME ends up serving the population of PR, a territory of the United States geographically isolated from the mainland and fully dependent on the healthcare professionals cultivated in-house. LHS+ values are observed in these leaders who, while performing the GME mission, embrace a respectful competition between sponsoring institutions while appreciating the power of collaboration that permits programs to excel in what they do.

## Special Paths for LHS+

There are some unique opportunities, positions, and roles that LHS+ might be uniquely positioned to undertake. Developmental pathways for LHS+ could start as early as college, and progressively through the GME pathway; an example includes the National Hispanic Medical Association's Hispanic Leadership Development Fellowship. There are some caveats and ideas for this path:

- *Genuine vs. performative reasons*
- You might be asked to serve on DEI initiatives for genuine reasons, as the institution wants to develop programs. It is important to have a seat at the table, and those opportunities serve as a platform for leadership opportunities that can culminate in deanship. However, at times, the participation is requested for performative reasons ("tokenism"). Whatever the underlying reason for the inclusion of URiM in positions of influence, you can use them to advance the DEI principles. Do not, however, allow any role to compromise your integrity and professional value system.
- *Institutional commitment to diversity*
  All institutions must have a commitment to DEI. Mission and vision statements are an important start, but programs that put the mission and vision into action are necessary. At every recruitment level, this commitment must continue and be deliberate. Specific actions include: (a) creating a strong pathway ("pipeline") by investments in the local student communities at all levels; (b) building the next generation of LHS+ GME trainees in all training programs, with a special focus on those specialties that have significant gaps in LHS+ applicants and matriculants; (c) prioritizing LHS+ inclusion in academic medicine; (d) being deliberate about research and scholarship opportunities for LHS+ residents and faculty; (e) including Latino culture and overall requiring cultural competency training for al GME trainees and their supervising faculty; (f) sponsoring initiatives that encourage diversity (such as sponsoring clerkships for URiM); and (g) active participation and collaboration with LHS+ medical organizations [29, 30].
- *The role of sponsoring institutions*
  Sponsoring institutions often care for many historically marginalized individuals. They set research agendas and help disseminate medical knowledge. They also train the next generation of physicians and other healthcare workers. Ultimately, institutions need sustained, comprehensive, and systematic implementation of programs that provide an environment that embraces and values DEI [23]. These must be present at every level and perhaps are most important at the GME level, where professional identities are being formed but also challenged [31, 32].

## The Role of Mentors and a Call for Action

It is foundational to find allies and sponsors who can serve as your advocate or sponsor. There might not necessarily be other LHS+ leaders at your institution, but you can find people who are more advanced in their career and who are willing and have the availability to advise or mentor you, regardless of their ethnic background.

Clinicians who belong to groups that have been historically underrepresented in medicine and who are in *any* positions of leadership and influence must open doors for others. This can be done at the program, institutional, regional, and national levels [30, 32]. There is a need for LHS+ in GME at every level, and current leaders must insist that institutions are deliberate about valuing and advancing diversity every step of the way [32].

## Conclusion

LHS+ physicians have the opportunity to influence the culture of graduate medical education, one that embraces the contributions of underrepresented minorities such as LHS+ trainees, clinicians, and faculty/staff. The role modeling of GME officers can set the tone for all of the above, creating expectations and mentoring those who need an experienced mind to guide them in their professional growth. The journey of LHS+ GME Officers has been full of roadblocks that question their abilities and commitment just because they embody unique lived experiences. Those who aspire to follow this career path must prepare cognitively and emotionally to not only survive but thrive and commit to a humbling process of continuous reflection that facilitates being mentored. We all hold a responsibility of paying it forward, and that should never be forgotten.

## Personal Narratives

**Larissa Velez, MD**
I was born and raised in Puerto Rico. From an early age, I wanted to be a doctor. Emergency Medicine, however, was not in my aspirations, as it was, at that time, rather unknown (and a new specialty). However, the first day I spent in the ER, I was in love. My husband and I met in medical school and were married 1 month before graduation. We *couples matched* into emergency medicine, also at the University of Puerto Rico, where I served as one of two chief residents during my senior year of training. After residency, we both were looking for jobs on the Island, only to find that jobs were not that easy to find. I wanted to have a career in academic emergency medicine, and the new residency program in PR did not have any jobs. In a fortuitous turn of events, someone from Dallas called, announcing they were opening a toxicology fellowship. After a few phone calls, both my husband and I were flying to interview in Dallas; him for an EMS fellowship, and I for the toxicology program. Though neither of us wanted to become part of the "brain drain," we thought this was a great opportunity to bring additional knowledge and skills to the Island. We both accepted the positions and moved to Dallas.

Two years later, we again tried to look for jobs in Puerto Rico, only to face the same hurdles as before. We decided to accept the offers to stay at UT Southwestern Medical Center (UTSWMC), with plans for a new and expanding Division of Emergency Medicine. My passion for education and educational leadership led me to seek out leadership positions as assistant and associate program director, with my ultimate goal of becoming the program director (PD). During that time, I also became vice chair for education. In this role, I helped with the development and accreditation of all programs in the Department of Emergency Medicine. Clinically, I worked at Parkland Health, one of the largest public hospitals and the busiest emergency department in the nation. The population we serve at Parkland is very diverse. There are many LHS+ patients in our population, so I speak Spanish for a good portion of my clinical shifts.

In 2019, I was appointed to serve as the associate dean for graduate medical education. I did not envision this career path, and I struggled for a long time with impostor syndrome. However, during my 25 years at UTSWMC, I have interacted and collaborated with many individuals. These professional collaborations allowed me to develop, at times informally and other times through courses, leadership skills, and organizational visibility.

Currently, my professional time is divided between my functions in the Department of Emergency Medicine and my time leading the Office of Graduate Medical Education. The GME office at UTSWMC oversees more than 200 GME programs with a total of over 1700 trainees. I am continually committed to excellence in GME, alignment with our clinical learning sites, and fostering an environment where trainees feel that we care about their well-being and wellness as much as we care about the rigor of their GME training.

As a woman in medicine and a mother, balancing my professional commitments while finding quality, undisrupted time for myself and my family has been the most difficult task, and one that I don't think is discussed enough.

**Maricarmen Cruz, MD, FAAPMR**
I am a first-generation physician born and raised in Puerto Rico by middle-class parents who valued education as the most important treasure parents could give to their kids. Both my parents were raised in rural zones, but under two different circumstances; one was privileged, and the other was not. The circumstances of their upbringing defined the values of the family where I was raised, and the same principles have guided my life: discipline, respect for authority, hard work, serving the vulnerable, and love for God. My altruistic spirit comes from both my parents, who embraced serving their communities and who made us participate in activities as children that exposed us to the reality of disadvantaged populations in PR and the responsibility we have in using any level of privilege that can lead to advocacy and voluntarism. On the other hand, my leadership skills come from strong women in my life, including my grandmother, mom, and other women mentors. They taught me about faith, being loyal to myself, integrity, public speaking, advocacy, and fighting for good causes. All these lessons became fundamental as I climbed the professional ladder and had to demonstrate that as LHS+ woman physician, I was not only skilled but had the character to assume more complex responsibilities.

I got involved in graduate medical education (GME) just from the moment I graduated as a Physical Medicine and Rehabilitation (PMR) specialist from the PMR program sponsored by the Veteran Affairs Hospital in PR. During the residency years, I discovered how much I enjoyed teaching, so upon graduation, I volunteered at my medical school, Universidad Central del Caribe School of Medicine, to offer musculoskeletal workshops to third-year medical students. In 2000, I returned to the VA Caribbean Healthcare System PMR residency program as an attending physician, and I got immediately involved as associate director and later as residency program director. These roles provided me opportunities to learn more about residency program accreditation requirements, creating educational curriculum, resident's supervision and evaluations, managing conflict, and so many others. I had mentors who served as sponsors to my career, who introduced me to research, guided me through the process of scholarly work publications, and facilitated the expansion of my professional network in and out of the VA. In 2006, I was accepted to the role of DIO at the VA, and looking back, this became a life-changing moment in my professional career, putting all my skills to the test. As DIO, I was expected to oversee accreditation requirements, but personally, what was most important to me was setting the bar to the way I wanted my training program directors to treat each other, since they were the first role models our trainees observed. Breaking and creating a culture was a complex task, and I devoted years of my career as DIO to do that, transitioning our programs from patronizing authority to nourishing a psychologically safe clinical learning environment. This eventually led to national recognition with the DeWitt C. Baldwin Jr. Award, presented by the ACGME and the Arnold P. Gold Foundation in 2016, for being a sponsoring institution that stands for promoting a humanistic and respectful clinical learning environment. This recognition only challenged me to continue cultivating humanistic attitudes into our residency programs' educational curriculum, getting involved in national collaboratives about healthcare disparities, and expanding institutional efforts on learning activities where residents felt psychologically safe to reflect on their emotionally vulnerable clinical experiences when caring for our patients. Making lemonade out of lemons, we took advantage of the COVID-19 pandemic to get involved in VA outreach events in the community where residents participated in mass vaccination efforts, visited patients at their homes, and had the opportunity to experience the social challenges our patients experienced in their communities. Combining altruism with adversity served the cause of teaching residents about the responsibility that we physicians hold in advocating for our patients when wanting to eliminate barriers to care. The circumstances facilitated teaching about equity attitudes, humanism, and leadership, and all of these values only reaffirmed the mission that, as DIO, I played to heal the hidden curriculum and inspire the behaviors I wanted to cultivate in GME.

I never stopped practicing in my clinical field, and I never stopped teaching my PMR residents as I led as DIO. When looking back, I have to say that I owe everything to my parents and my lifelong mentors. They cultivated in me the desire to dream of a better world, and I know that all those lessons became fundamental to deeply understand that our role as leaders should not be limited to the task but to inspire others to become the better version of themselves. As an LHS+ DIO, I used the privilege of the role to inspire a cultural change where values, tolerance to differences, and appreciation of our vulnerabilities as humans were embraced. As an LHS+ woman I hope I have inspired young physicians to discover their own strengths, to put dreams into work, and to affirm that their values can make a difference in the world.

# References

1. ACGME. About us [cited 2023, April 20]. Available from: https://www.acgme.org/about-us/overview/#:~:text=Graduate%20medical%20education%20(GME)%20refers,fellowship%20programs%20in%20the%20US
2. ACGME. Institutional requirements [cited 2025, March 9]. Available from: https://www.acgme.org/globalassets/pfassets/programrequirements/2025-reformatted-requirements/institutionalrequirements_2025_reformatted.pdf
3. ACGME. CLER pathway to excellence [cited 2024, February 27]. Available from CLER pathways to excellence. Version 3.0. ACGME 2024. acgme-cler-2024-pte3.pdf. ACGME public reports 2024. https://apps.acgme.org/ads/Public/Reports/ReportRun
4. ACGME. GME Data resource book 2023 2024 [cited 2025, February 23]. https://www.acgme.org/globalassets/pfassets/publicationsbooks/dataresourcebook2023-2024.pdf
5. ACGME. Diversity, equity, and inclusion. https://www.acgme.org/initiatives/diversity-equity-and-inclusion/. Accessed on 5 July 2025.
6. Nivet MA. Minorities in academic medicine: review of the literature. J Vasc Surg. 2010;51(4 Suppl):53S–8S.
7. AAMC. Data reports—residents executive summary. https://www.aamc.org/data-reports/students-residents/data/report-residents/2022/executive-summary. Accessed 18 May 2023.
8. AAMC. Faculty Roster: U.S. medical school faculty 2024. https://www.google.com/url?q=https://www.aamc.org/data-reports/faculty-institutions/report/faculty-roster-us-medical-school-faculty&sa=D&source=docs&ust=1752090602165935&usg=AOvVaw2pcVJzv1ScyCGxuJnVohOE. Accessed on 5 July 2025.
9. AAMC. U.S. medical school deans by dean type and race/ethnicity (URiM vs. non-URiM). https://www.aamc.org/data-reports/faculty-institutions/data/us-medical-school-deans-trends-type-and-race-ethnicity. Accessed on 5 July 2025.
10. AAMC. Diversity in medicine: facts and figures 2019. Figure 17. Percentage of full-time U.S. medical school faculty by sex, race/ethnicity, and rank, 2018. 2019 [cited 2023, April 25]. Available from: https://www.aamc.org/data-reports/workforce/data/figure-17-percentage-full-time-us-medical-school-faculty-sex-race/ethnicity-and-rank-2018
11. Choubey AP, et al. Ethnic and racial diversity among surgeon and non-surgeon deans of allopathic medical schools. Am Surg. 2022;89:31348221117036.
12. Xierali IM, et al. Recent trends in faculty promotion in U.S. medical schools: implications for recruitment, retention, and diversity and inclusion. Acad Med. 2021;96(10):1441–8.
13. Xierali IM, Nivet MA, Rayburn WF. Diversity of department chairs in family medicine at US medical schools. J Am Board Fam Med. 2022;35(1):152–7.
14. Yu PT, et al. Minorities struggle to advance in academic medicine: a 12-y review of diversity at the highest levels of America's teaching institutions. J Surg Res. 2013;182(2):212–8.
15. U.S. census quick facts. https://www.census.gov/quickfacts/fact/table/US/PST04522. Accessed on 18 May 2023.
16. Bibbins-Domingo K, Helman A, editors. Improving representation in clinical trials and research: building research equity for women and underrepresented groups. Washington, DC: National Academies Press (US); 2022. Why diverse representation in clinical research matters and the current state of representation within the clinical research ecosystem. Available from: https://www.ncbi.nlm.nih.gov/books/NBK584396/
17. Bonifacino E, Ufomata EO, Farkas AH, Turner R, Corbelli JA. Mentorship of underrepresented physicians and trainees in academic medicine: a systematic review. J Gen Intern Med. 2021;36(4):1023–34. https://doi.org/10.1007/s11606-020-06478-7. Epub 2021 Feb 2. PMID: 33532959; PMCID: PMC7852467.
18. Accreditation Council for Graduate Medical Education. Glossary of terms. 2024, June 3. https://www.acgme.org/globalassets/pfassets/programrequirements/800_institutionalrequirements_2022.pdf. Accessed on 5 July 2025.

19. Berns JS, Goldstein JL, Hartmann DM, Simons K, Opas L. The expanding role of designated institutional officials in graduate medical education. Acad Med. 2025;100(2):131–6. https://doi.org/10.1097/ACM.0000000000005922.
20. Hanyok LA, Smith KW, Lindeman B, Best JA. The DIO needs a cabinet: identifying and supporting designated institutional "others" in graduate medical education. J Grad Med Educ. 2024;16(1):7–10. https://doi.org/10.4300/JGME-D-23-00351.1.
21. Oxford Review Dictionary. Cultural competence—definition and explanation—The Oxford Review—or briefings.
22. ACGME. Institutional program requirements. 2025.
23. Nivet MA. A diversity 3.0 update: are we moving the needle enough? Acad Med. 2015;90(12):1591–3.
24. GME leadership development certificate program. https://www.aamc.org/career-development/leadership-development/gme-leadership-development-certificate-program. Accessed on 7 June 2025.
25. Stubbe DE. Practicing cultural competence and cultural humility in the care of diverse patients. Focus (Am Psychiatr Publ). 2020;18(1):49–51. https://doi.org/10.1176/appi.focus.20190041. Epub 2020 Jan 24. PMID: 32047398; PMCID: PMC7011228.
26. Hargett CW, Doty JP, Hauck JN, Webb AM, Cook SH, Tsipis NE, et al. Developing a model for effective leadership in healthcare: a concept mapping approach. J Healthc Leadersh. 2017;9:69–78.
27. Shah C, et al. Sticky floor and glass ceilings in academic medicine: analysis of race and gender. Cureus. 2022;14(4):e24080.
28. Recinto Online. Evolución Histórica del Sistema de Salud en Puerto Rico. 2019-12-18 11:17:2.
29. Flores KA, Dominguez B. University of California, San Francisco, Fresno Latino Center for medical education and research health professions pipeline program. Acad Med. 2006;81(6 Suppl):S36–40.
30. Sanchez JP, Poll-Hunter NI, Acosta D. Advancing the Latino physician workforce-population trends, persistent challenges, and new directions. Acad Med. 2015;90(7):849–53.
31. Blanchard AK, et al. Reflect and reset: black academic voices call the graduate medical education community to action. Acad Med. 2022;97(7):967–72.
32. Butler PD, et al. A blueprint for increasing ethnic and racial diversity in U.S. residency training programs. Acad Med. 2022;97(11):1632–6.

**Open Access** This chapter is licensed under the terms of the Creative Commons Attribution 4.0 International License (http://creativecommons.org/licenses/by/4.0/), which permits use, sharing, adaptation, distribution and reproduction in any medium or format, as long as you give appropriate credit to the original author(s) and the source, provide a link to the Creative Commons license and indicate if changes were made.

The images or other third party material in this chapter are included in the chapter's Creative Commons license, unless indicated otherwise in a credit line to the material. If material is not included in the chapter's Creative Commons license and your intended use is not permitted by statutory regulation or exceeds the permitted use, you will need to obtain permission directly from the copyright holder.

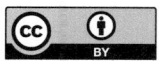

# Chapter 16
# Striving to Become a Dean of Admissions

Sunny Nakae

> **Learning Objectives**
> - Describe the functions of the Office of Admissions
> - Describe leadership competencies that are associated with various roles within the Office of Admissions
> - Identify opportunities for engagement in the Office of Admissions, with a specific focus on how LHS+ leaders can be effective at advocating for inclusion in processes and outcomes

## Introduction

Full participation from all communities in academic medicine requires increasing representation in leadership roles from students of Latina/o/x/e, Hispanic, and Spanish origin, plus intersecting identities (LHS+). Admissions is a critical function at every institution, and the faculty members involved in the process have a significant influence in shaping mission alignment. For example, schools focused on providing care for underserved communities have different emphases than schools centered on research. Selection factors must align with mission elements throughout the process. This chapter contains a comprehensive overview of admissions and the associated roles and responsibilities and will: (1) describe the functions of the Office of Admissions, (2) describe leadership competencies that are associated with various roles within the Office of Admissions, and (3) identify opportunities for engagement in the Office of Admissions, with a specific focus on how LHS+ leaders can be effective at advocating for inclusion in processes and outcomes. At the end

S. Nakae (✉)
California University of Science and Medicine, Colton, CA, USA

© The Author(s) 2026
J. P. Sánchez et al. (eds.), *Advancing Latino, Hispanic, or of Spanish Origin+ Leadership in Academic Medicine*,
https://doi.org/10.1007/978-3-032-07570-3_16

of this chapter, readers will have foundational knowledge to contribute to admissions and continue their development toward greater engagement and service in medical school selection processes.

## Key Terms and Definitions

**Admissions** Admissions includes the policies and practices of recruiting, evaluating, selecting, and matriculating a cohort of learners to an academic program to fulfill the program's institutional mission. Admissions deans oversee recruitment and outreach related to encouraging and assisting applicants throughout the process. Deans are responsible for committees that are tasked with reviewing and evaluating candidates at each phase of a process. While there is wide variability across processes, every school effectuates a process that includes screening, interviewing candidates, providing offers, managing offers, and matriculating a class on an annual basis.

**Pathway Programs** Pathway programs include structured resources for students preparing for entry to medical school. They may have specific aims to increase representation from groups historically underestimated or excluded. There are many pathway initiatives specifically focused on LHS+ students that are sponsored through medical schools, undergraduate institutions, national organizations, student organizations, nonprofits, and federal organizations. Pathway programs may include in-person or remote learning and may provide exposure to medicine as a career. Instruction about preparation, developmental coaching, and supportive mentoring may also be offered through pathway resources [2].

**Holistic Practice** Holistic practice is defined by the Association of American Medical Colleges (AAMC) as: "a flexible, mission-driven approach to recruit and assess an individual's competencies by considering their experiences, attributes, and academic metrics in order to select applicants who will best contribute to the program's unique goals, learning environment, and the practice of medicine." Holistic practices allow admissions committees to consider the whole applicant, rather than disproportionately focusing on any one factor [2]. Core principles of holistic practice as defined by the AAMC are:

Selection criteria are aligned with the program's curriculum, mission, community health needs, and the needs of the physician workforce. These criteria, including competencies and other characteristics, are assessed and supported by each applicant's experiences, attributes, and metrics. Selection criteria are:

1. Clearly defined and transparently communicated to applicants and advisors as well as faculty, staff, and leadership
2. Equitably applied and appropriately tailored for each stage of selection to create a qualified, broadly diverse, mission-aligned candidate pool
3. Defined, evaluated, and informed by performance data, educational expectations, and available support services to ensure success

Programs consider the context of each applicant to understand how their unique educational opportunities, financial resources, communities, and lived experiences may contribute to the program and the practice of medicine.

Programs review interviewed applicants to select/rank a cohort of learners encompassing the complementary experiences, qualities, and characteristics needed to achieve their institutional and program mission and goals. While programs may not make selection decisions based on protected applicant characteristics (e.g., race, sex, and disability), schools can consider an applicant's discussion of any personal experience—even those related to race, sex, or other protected characteristics—to illustrate examples of mission-aligned experiences or qualities sought by the program.

At the conclusion of each selection cycle, programs review, evaluate, and refine recruitment, screening, application review, interview, selection, and entry policies, processes, and practices to ensure they are equitable, effective, and valid.

Holistic practices also include alignment of the enrollment management and student support elements of a school, such as financial aid and well-being services, once students are enrolled. Grieco et al. have outlined student-centered, holistic support in their 2022 article, which is beyond the scope of this chapter [3].

## Beginning with Mission

Admissions are critical to the mission of the institution. Clarity of purpose can underscore the need for recruiting and graduating LHS+ students who bring lived experience, cultural acumen, language skills, community insight, and systems navigation expertise to medicine. All admissions processes must begin with identifying the mission and defining the values of the institution. Characteristics and attributes aligned with achieving the mission are designated by faculty leadership. The admissions dean must then identify stakeholders in defining and aligning the mission (faculty, community members, students, educators, patients, alumni, etc.) to operationalize selection criteria. Stakeholders define the qualities and characteristics of ideal candidates and establish evaluation and selection tools using evidence-based, mission-aligned factors within the application and application process.

Leaders in academic medicine admissions roles work directly with prospective students and applicants during the ongoing process. Admissions offices may provide seminars, workshops, or conference sessions to help students gain knowledge and skills for preparation and application. Support from the office of admissions may also include advising, mentoring, or partnering with undergraduate institutions. Very often, current medical students are involved in supporting pathways programs, recruitment activities, and admissions processes. Students may fill roles on the admissions committee as tour guides, ambassadors, interviewers, reviewers, hosts, or even voting members of the selection committee (Fig. 16.1).

# Office of Admissions: Engagement and Leadership Opportunities for Medical Students

**Sunny Nakae**, PhD, MSW, senior associate dean for equity, inclusion, diversity, and partnership, Department of Medical Education, California University of Science and Medicine; **Walter P. Parrish**, MSEd, director of diversity and inclusion, New York University Grossman School of Medicine; and **John Paul Sánchez**, MD, MPH, president, Building the Next Generation of Academic Physicians (BNGAP)

According to the 2018 AAMC Medical School Year Two Questionnaire,[1] approximately 23% of medical students plan to participate in medical school administration during their career. The office of admissions at a medical school serves as one avenue for medical students to become engaged and develop competencies to serve as future administrative leaders.

**Role of the Office of Admissions:**
To design, improve, and execute a selection process by which well-prepared students aligned with a school's mission are selected through a faculty-led process that often includes students. The process must be equitable, consistently applied, and involve multiple stakeholders and decision makers.

**Relevance of Medical Students Being Engaged in Admissions:**
Students provide critical, diverse perspectives to faculty and applicants in the admissions process. Medical students are especially adept at helping candidates explore institutional fit, particularly for those underrepresented in medicine. Engagement in admissions provides the opportunity to learn important aspects of policies and procedures as well as to develop leadership competencies.

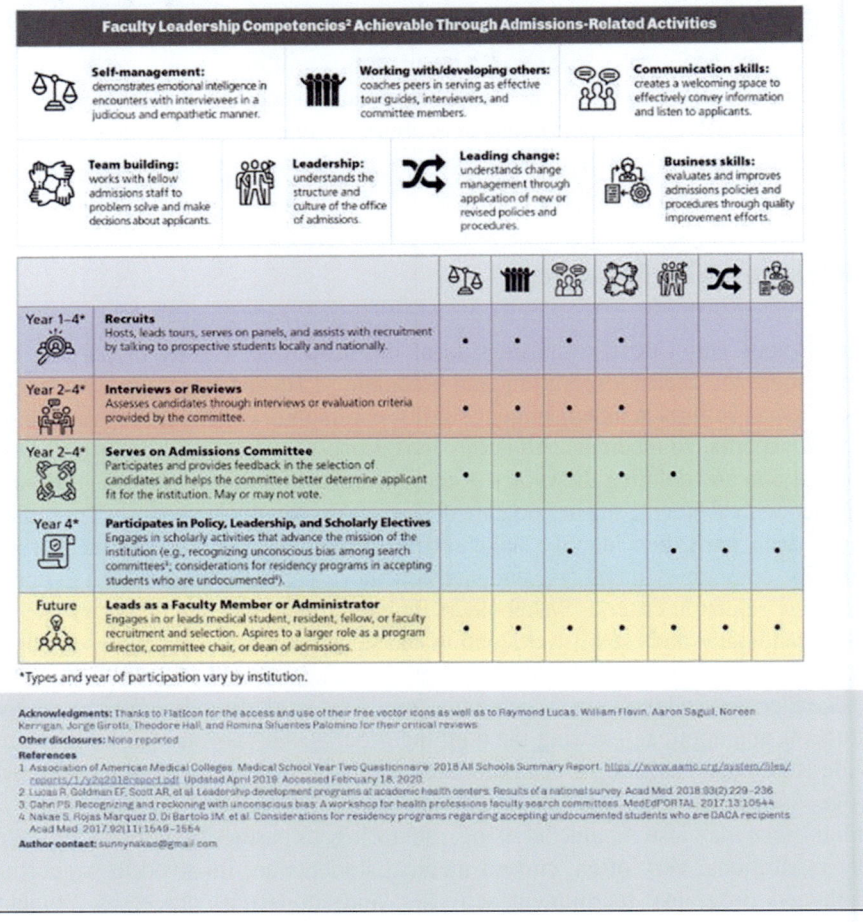

*Types and year of participation vary by institution.

Acknowledgments: Thanks to FlatIcon for the access and use of their free vector icons as well as to Raymond Lucas, William Flavin, Aaron Saguil, Noreen Kerrigan, Jorge Girotti, Theodore Hall, and Homira Sifuentes Palomino for their critical reviews.
Other disclosures: None reported

References
1. Association of American Medical Colleges. Medical School Year Two Questionnaire. 2018 All Schools Summary Report. https://www.aamc.org/system/files/reports/1/y2q2018report.pdf. Updated April 2019. Accessed February 18, 2020.
2. Lucas R, Goldman EF, Scott AR, et al. Leadership development programs at academic health centers: Results of a national survey. Acad Med. 2018;93(2):229–236
3. Cahn PS. Recognizing and reckoning with unconscious bias: A workshop for health professions faculty search committees. MedEdPORTAL. 2017;13:10544
4. Nakae S, Rojas Marquez D, Di Bartolo IM, et al. Considerations for residency programs regarding accepting undocumented students who are DACA recipients. Acad Med. 2017;92(11):1549–1554

Author contact: sunnynakae@gmail.com

**Fig. 16.1** Medical student engagement in admissions activities is critical to early career development of leadership competencies that are central to roles in academic medicine

LHS+ representation, participation, and leadership are paramount to equitable representation and practice. LHS+-focused pathway programs and partnerships can provide robust access for students to prepare and thrive in medicine, while also affirming identity, a sense of belonging, and commitment to LHS+ communities.

Admissions deans are charged with shaping each medical school class and may also collaborate with other institutional leaders in evaluating program effectiveness across the continuum. Many schools survey residency programs where their students match to get a sense of how their graduates are performing in comparison to graduates from other schools. Institutional effectiveness may also include evaluating course performance, identifying support needs, and analyzing student surveys from matriculation to graduation.

## Leadership Roles and Structures

The leadership roles and structures for admissions offices vary across institutions [4]. Admissions may be part of an enrollment management suite, integrated with student affairs, or it may be freestanding. Health sciences universities may have a combined delivery model for MD programs with other health professions programs, such as physical therapy or pharmacy. There is a combination of administrators, faculty, and staff members that comprises the team that operates the admissions process. Each medical school must have, by virtue of its accreditation process with the LCME, admissions bylaws of which the faculty approves [1]. There must also be evidence of training materials and sufficient processes in place to ensure a process free from outside influences and bias. The dean or provost of the medical school may oversee the faculty appointment process and the selection of members for the admissions committee(s), including the chair. Committee members may also be elected through faculty governance structures such as senates or councils. Length of terms or term limits varies by school.

### *The Committee Chair*

The chair of the admissions committee is usually a faculty member in the school of medicine. Schools may have co-chair structures, such as a basic science faculty member and a clinical faculty member. The chair may be a compensated role or strictly volunteer as part of professional service expected under a faculty appointment. Service on committees, such as the admissions committee, is customarily essential in demonstrating contributions to the institution in the rank, promotions, and tenure process for faculty. Admissions committee chairs are not expected to be procedural or technical experts but rather effectuate leadership and accountability among their faculty colleagues to facilitate the process and ensure that it is carried out according to the standards set forth by the faculty. The chair works closely with the dean and admissions professional staff over the course of the cycle, which takes 12–15 months.

## The Dean for Admissions

The role of the admissions dean may be at any level—assistant, associate, senior, vice, etc., depending on institutional structures and personnel of the school. The role can be held by a clinician or nonclinician. It may be the equivalent of full-time, or the person may have other duties such as teaching, research, or patient care in addition to the dean role. The admissions dean works closely with staff to oversee the admissions process. Typically, faculty members gain experience in administrative roles through committee service. Participating in admissions committees provides an in-depth experience that allows faculty to learn the process and tools.

## Professional Staff Support

The day-to-day duties in admissions are carried out by skilled professional staff. The process is generally led by a full-time administrator at the director level or above. Admissions staff members may have a wide array of educational backgrounds and skill sets. Staff roles in admissions teams may be managers, directors, counselors, recruiters, data analysts, engagement specialists, advisors, scheduling coordinators, IT managers, administrative assistants, marketing specialists, etc. The professional staff are the vital engine behind any admissions process as they attend to tools, committee processes, questions from applicants and stakeholders, and fidelity throughout the admissions cycle.

# Roles and Responsibilities of the Admissions Dean

The admissions dean is responsible for ensuring compliance with all LCME requirements related to admission, which are standards 10.1–10.9 [1]. The dean, most typically, is the primary author of these areas for an accreditation preparation document for the institution. The accreditation data include tracking of target groups identified as underrepresented by the school of medicine across pathways, applications, interviews, offers, matriculation, and graduation, as defined under standard 3 [1]. The admissions dean provides updated bylaws, training materials, committee rosters, and supplemental tools and materials describing the process during accreditation review.

The dean works with faculty to establish selection criteria aligned with the school's mission. Using the common application (AMCAS, AACOMAS, or TMDSAS), the dean identifies areas of focus and works with professional staff to design tools that are both holistic and mission-aligned [5–8]. Some common elements of eligibility criteria are immigration status, state residency, premedical coursework, criminal history, institutional action, and degree completion. Screening criteria may include prerequisite courses, course performance (GPA), MCAT performance, service contributions, shadowing and career exposure, leadership experiences, employment, and clinical experiences. Selection criteria may include achievements in leadership, research, service, community advocacy, community service, distance traveled, scholarly activity, lived experience, etc.

Deans must be familiar with the literature and best practices within the field of medical school admissions. They regularly consult the literature to maintain knowledge of the practices of peer institutions. Deans must also be skilled at analyzing data and identifying bias, trends, opportunities, and losses within their admissions processes. Innovation and process change are also competency areas for an admissions dean. They may be asked to implement or explore new selection tools or modalities or design pilots for new aspects of a process, such as incorporating a situational judgment test or a values exercise into selection.

The admissions dean oversees the process of constructing and designing the phases of admissions from start to finish. This includes selecting and maintaining an application and enrollment management software for applicants, staff, and committee members. Typically, a software system serves applicants and evaluators while providing a master platform for professional staff to track all components. Deans need to know the basics of data management and security in order to guide the team when using information technology services. At each phase, the dean must attend to question or interview design, scoring scales and tools, evaluation rubrics and descriptive elements, and cumulative data aggregation and reporting.

Although there is no set committee structure across all schools, all deans must establish committee(s) for the work of selecting students. Training materials, such as those related to bias mitigation, conflicts of interest, rater consistency, and school information, must be curated and designed by the admissions team. When faculty have clear tools and robust training, an admissions process can be well situated to operate equitably and effectively.

## Admissions Practice for the Inclusion of LHS+ Students

LHS+ applicants are incredibly diverse as a group, and there are some key data and practices that admissions deans may utilize to increase consideration for LHS+ applicants in admissions practice. Not all LHS+ students were considered underrepresented in medicine until 2004, when the AAMC stopped defining underrepresented nationally and opted for schools to define it locally. The AAMC's decision followed the US Supreme Court's decision in Grutter, where the court upheld holistic review but struck down practices that awarded admissions advantage based on race alone [9]. This led to an expansion of the designation of underrepresented at most medical schools to all LHS+ groups from Mexico, Central America, and South America, rather than only Mexican American and Mainland Puerto Rican. The consistent attacks on holistic practice in admissions, framed by opponents as affirmative action, have created setbacks for pathway programs and recruitment efforts in increasing LHS+ representation. According to the Medical School Admission Requirements (MSAR) 2021 data, of the 154 schools represented, just 28 (18%) enrolled a class that year that had at least 17% of their students identifying as all or part LHS+ [10]. The enrollment of the four medical schools in Puerto Rico is equal to the enrollment of the next 62 schools when sorted by LHS+ enrollment [10]. While there has been progress, significant enrollment gaps remain for LHS+ students in medicine.

The intersection of immigration status and LHS+ identity is another important consideration for admissions practitioners. The largest proportion of DACA (Deferred Action for Childhood Arrivals) recipients applying to medical school are LHS+, followed closely by students from Asia and India [11, 12]. Schools focusing on meeting the needs of underserved communities can increase their talent pool by including DACA recipients and undocumented students in their admissions eligibility criteria. Many students have achieved strong levels of preparation for medical school and can complete their training and licensure if they have work authorization and access to private funds or nonfederal loans. Even individuals without current immigration relief and no form of work authorization can bring critical talent, perspectives, and promise to medicine.

Promising practices for ensuring the inclusion of LHS+ students in an admissions process are:

Ensure that screening parameters consider postbacc and graduate GPAs as separate from the cumulative undergraduate totals. LHS+ students have high enrollment in postbacc education [13].
Consider students from a wide array of MCAT scores, with calibration of averages appropriate for your school's mission. Examine the average scores for test takers identifying as LHS+ in the annual MCAT guide before establishing ranges and guidelines [14]. Avoid cutoffs, if possible.
Focus pathway efforts on community colleges and more accessible/affordable four-year institutions, as LHS+ enrollment at these institutions is high [13].
Form admissions pathways and partnerships with institutions that provide high LHS+ enrollment and/or applications to medical school [11].
Identify community organizations that serve LHS+ groups and establish relationships and partnerships with them.
Elevate Spanish language skills as a plus factor, especially for advanced and native Spanish speakers. These are specifically designated on the application and can be used to prioritize and elevate LHS+ students while also elevating students with Spanish language skills to serve LHS+ communities.

Elevate service, leadership, and mentoring experiences as a plus factor. Evaluate experiences in the primary application and include essays in your supplemental materials that ask about service to underserved communities, lived experiences, cultural insights, etc.

Highlight programming and supportive structures at your institution in your recruitment efforts, such as the Latino Medical Student Association, medical Spanish curricula, career mentoring, and consideration for undocumented students.

Consider intersectionality and the diversity of LHS+ applicants as a group with a wide range of socioeconomic status, immigration histories, work experiences, volunteer experiences, and additional identities.

Leaders in academic medicine must cultivate LHS+ representation to ensure that admissions practices and procedures are inclusive, excellent, and adaptive to ensure better health and healthcare for all groups. LHS+ currently account for almost 19% of the US population in 2024 and are projected to be 25% by 2045 [15]. Knowing core areas of preparation and practice can provide a guiding framework for intentional career decisions that facilitate preparation, participation, and thriving from LHS+ students and leaders.

## Reflection Questions

What qualities and characteristics are important for a physician to possess and demonstrate? What preparation activities and experiences might provide evidence of these qualities and characteristics?

Why is mission alignment critical to admissions practice?

How can institutions ensure they train providers prepared to care for LHS+ communities?

What activities during medical school or residency could help an individual prepare to be an admissions dean?

Consider current practices in medical school admissions. What changes might be possible? How might practices be improved?

What are the skills, qualities, and characteristics necessary for leadership roles within admissions? How can leadership influence the inclusion of LHS+?

## Resources

- BNGAP module on admissions: https://www.mededportal.org/doi/10.15766/mep_2374-8265.11018
- Bias breaks training. https://www.mededportal.org/doi/10.15766/mep_2374-8265.11285

- Reducing gender bias in letters of recommendation. https://www.mededportal.org/doi/10.15766/mep_2374-8265.11419
- Reducing virtual interviews bias. https://www.mededportal.org/doi/10.15766/mep_2374-8265.11416
- Enrollment management and holistic review. https://pubmed.ncbi.nlm.nih.gov/33298697/
- Holistic review site of resources (AAMC site). https://www.aamc.org/services/member-capacity-building/holistic-review
- AAMC data site for applications and matriculants. https://www.aamc.org/data-reports/students-residents/report/facts
- Using MCAT tools guide. https://www.aamc.org/services/mcat-admissions-officers/resources
- AM last page graphic on admissions engagement. https://journals.lww.com/academicmedicine/fulltext/2022/03000/office_of_admissions__engagement_and_leadership.36.aspx

## Skill Set Group Mixer

For this group learning activity, please download Appendix D from the BNGAP admissions module, *Office of Admissions: Engagement and Leadership Opportunities for Trainees* at: https://www.mededportal.org/doi/10.15766/mep_2374-8265.11018. This group activity will provide an opportunity for students to identify the skills and experiences among the group that apply to leadership within admissions. Each participant needs a printed grid handout and a pen or pencil. provide an opportunity for students to identify the skills and experiences among the group that apply to leadership within admissions. Each participant needs a printed grid handout and a pen or pencil. The time required for the activity is about 10-15 minutes.

Ask attendees to mingle and find individuals in the room who have experience in one of the areas on the leadership skills mingle sheet. Participants sign the box where they have the experience. For example, if a student has helped to change a policy during their undergraduate years or in medical school, they would sign their name in that box. Ask participants to fill their sheets as quickly as possible. Limit duplicate signatures according to group size. There are 25 boxes. For example, if there are 16 participants, limit each participant to signing three boxes on any one participant's sheet to encourage interaction.

When time is up, reconvene the group for discussion.

## Discussion

How did the group do? How many experiences are covered?

What activities during medical school or residency, or early career could help further develop these skills?

How might these skills have previously manifested in the group's experience/involvement with admissions?

## Personal Narrative

### Sunny Nakae, MSW, PhD

I started my career in pathways programs as an outreach coordinator at a medical school more than 20 years ago. Since then, I have become progressively more involved in understanding student preparation journeys and designing and implementing admissions tools and processes. My personal and professional mission is to increase access and equity in medical education and healthcare. I have been involved in supporting LHS+ faculty, students, communities, and leaders from the beginning of my career. I am a woman of color of Japanese and European descent. My ancestors, citizens and legal immigrants, were incarcerated for 3 years by the War Authority of the United States during World War II. The injustice in my own family's history fuels my passion for equity and inclusion in medicine and compels me to join in solidarity with my colleagues who are also from groups that have been excluded, marginalized, minoritized, divested, and underestimated.

Early in my career, the institution I was part of endured a state audit aimed at discrediting all non-white and non-male students admitted by the medical school. The complaint from a high-ranking representative kicked off more than a year of audits and terrible press that fueled racism and exclusionary deficit rhetoric both within the school and in the surrounding community. I witnessed the pain that students of color and women students endured, having their place, hard-earned and rightfully deserved, questioned and threatened. This early experience was the start of my passion to understand admissions and a drastic realization of the power of admissions to shape the identity and culture of an entire institution.

As I grew my career, I continued to advise, educate, and share the journeys of premedical students who were from historically and presently excluded groups. Students trusted me and afforded me the opportunity to learn through their experiences the aspects of the admissions process that are unjust, inaccessible, inequitable, and opaque. I joined the admissions committee as a reviewer and interviewer at my next institution. Through committee service, I was able to understand how application elements were utilized and interpreted by decision makers, which improved the guidance I offered to advisees. In my role as a director of diversity, I continued to learn from LHS+ students about unique aspects of their experiences in medical education. For my doctoral dissertation, I studied the backgrounds of applicants to allopathic medicine and examined stratification and inequality in admissions outcomes. My goal was to build a skill set for advancing policy for equity and inclusion in medicine.

In year 14 of my career, I accepted a role as assistant dean of admissions, recruitment, and student life. It was an opportunity to design and retool the admissions process, implementing mission alignment and holistic practice principles. This provided an opportunity to explore tools and boldly structure inclusion into the admissions process. Working with faculty to effectuate a process was rewarding and challenging. While at the helm of an admissions process, intentional recruitment for LHS+ students meant specific outreach to DACA recipients, undocumented students, postbacc students, community college students, limited-income students, and first-generation students. I also focused on elevating students who spoke a language in addition to English and/or were not born in the United States. Following matriculation, it was critical to ensure support structures for LHS+ students to continue to thrive in medical school, such as an institutionally funded LMSA chapter, a medical Spanish elective, and transparent/accessible resources for performance and well-being.

Over the course of my career, I have served as a leader and consultant across the medical education continuum in admissions and selection practices, learner support, institutional equity practice and skill building, representation and talent management, and mission alignment. I believe that every faculty member and leader in academic medicine should understand how critical equitable, mission-aligned admissions practice is in ensuring that medicine thrives. I remain passionate about advocating for innovative tools and greater access to medicine for LHS+ students and their underestimated peers.

## References

1. Liaison Committee on Medical Education. Standards, publications, & notification forms. n.d. Retrieved February 5, 2025, from https://lcme.org/publications/
2. Association of American Medical Colleges. Holistic review. n.d. Retrieved February 12, 2025, from https://www.aamc.org/services/member-capacity-building/holistic-review
3. Grieco CA, Currence P, Teraguchi DH, Monroe A, Palermo A-GS. Integrated holistic student affairs: a personalized, equitable, student-centered approach to student affairs. Acad Med. 2022;97(10):1441–6. https://doi.org/10.1097/ACM.0000000000004757.
4. Nakae S, Parrish WP, Sánchez JP. Office of admissions: engagement and leadership opportunities for medical students. Acad Med. 2022;97(3):471. https://doi.org/10.1097/ACM.0000000000004439.
5. TMDSAS. Application guide: coursework. TMDSAS website. University of Texas System. https://www.tmdsas.com/application-guide/coursework.html
6. Association of American Medical Colleges. Using MCAT data in 2024 medical student selection. 2023. https://www.aamc.org/media/18901/download
7. Association of American Medical Colleges. Undergraduate institutions supplying 10 or more Hispanic, Latino, or of Spanish origin applicants to U.S. medical schools, 2024–2025. 2024a. https://www.aamc.org/media/79786/download?attachment
8. Association of American Medical Colleges. Applicants, acceptees, and matriculants with Deferred Action for Childhood Arrivals (DACA) status to U.S. MD-granting medical schools, 2018–2019 through 2024–2025. 2024b. https://www.aamc.org/media/79906/download?attachment

9. Grutter v. Bollinger, 539 U.S. 306. 2003. https://supreme.justia.com/cases/federal/us/539/306/
10. Association of American Medical Colleges. Medical school admissions requirements. 2021. Retrieved January 8, 2022, from https://students-residents.aamc.org/medical-school-admission-requirements/medical-school-admission-requirements-msar-applicants
11. Association of American Medical Colleges. 2024 facts: applicants and matriculants data. AAMC. https://www.aamc.org/data-reports/students-residents/data/facts-applicants-and-matriculants.
12. U.S. Citizenship and Immigration Services. Consideration of Deferred Action for Childhood Arrivals (DACA). n.d. Retrieved February 9, 2025, from https://www.uscis.gov/DACA
13. Postsecondary National Policy Institute. Latino students in higher education. 2022. https://pnpi.org/wp-content/uploads/2022/09/LatinoStudentsFactSheet_September_2022.pdf
14. Association of American Medical Colleges. Using MCAT® data in 2024 medical student selection. Washington, DC: AAMC; 2023.
15. U.S. Census. New estimates highlight differences in growth between the U.S. Hispanic and Non-Hispanic populations. 2024. Retrieved April 8, 2025, from https://www.census.gov/newsroom/press-releases/2024/population-estimates-characteristics.html

**Open Access** This chapter is licensed under the terms of the Creative Commons Attribution 4.0 International License (http://creativecommons.org/licenses/by/4.0/), which permits use, sharing, adaptation, distribution and reproduction in any medium or format, as long as you give appropriate credit to the original author(s) and the source, provide a link to the Creative Commons license and indicate if changes were made.

The images or other third party material in this chapter are included in the chapter's Creative Commons license, unless indicated otherwise in a credit line to the material. If material is not included in the chapter's Creative Commons license and your intended use is not permitted by statutory regulation or exceeds the permitted use, you will need to obtain permission directly from the copyright holder.

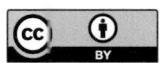

# Chapter 17
# Striving to Become a Dean of Faculty Affairs and Development

**Beatriz Tapia and Guadalupe Federico-Martinez**

> **Learning Objectives**
> - Distinguish the unique advantages and persisting challenges for individuals identifying as LHS+ considering the role of Dean of Faculty Affairs and Development.
> - Describe the roles and responsibilities of a Dean of Faculty Affairs and Development.
> - Review the opportunities and potential obstacles related to the core functions.

## Introduction

Have you paused to think about how you got where you are now and the role models, advisors, mentors, sponsors, and faculty leaders that have, perhaps serendipitously, contributed to your professional life? Do you enjoy advocating for others? Are aspects of recruiting faculty interesting to you? Do you want to make a difference in how faculty experience each stage of their career in academic life? Then a role in Faculty Affairs and Development (from this point forward, referred to as, FAD) might be a rewarding pathway for you!

---

B. Tapia (✉)
Past Chair – Planning Committee for AAMC Group on Faculty Affairs (2024–25), Harlingen, TX, USA

G. Federico-Martinez
DLM Coaching, Consulting & Wellness LLC, Paradise Valley, AZ, USA

© The Author(s) 2026
J. P. Sánchez et al. (eds.), *Advancing Latino, Hispanic, or of Spanish Origin+ Leadership in Academic Medicine*,
https://doi.org/10.1007/978-3-032-07570-3_17

What an honorable opportunity to one day lead from behind with department chairs, an academic medical center's most valuable asset to high-quality teaching, research, and patient care: the faculty [1]. This chapter will introduce you to what an Office of Faculty Affairs and Development (OFAD) means to an academic medicine center and its partnering clinical sites. Unlike other deanships, the roles and responsibilities of a dean of faculty affairs and development (DOFAD) may be one position or (at a minority of schools) be separated into two positions [2]. Sonnino et al. seminal work on the evolution of centralized OFADs notes a variation of office names that aligns with the dean role [2]. Those variations that one could expect are "office of faculty affairs," "faculty affairs and development, "faculty administrative services," "office of faculty success," or "academic affairs" with "faculty affairs" serving as the predominant title at 80% of academic medical centers at the time [2]. Our lived experiences as deans of faculty affairs and development align with Sonnino et al.'s finding that "centralized faculty affairs offices and departments now appear to share responsibility for career planning and mentoring programs," (p. 1370) and are wholeheartedly true [2]. As such, you should expect the role of DOFAD to be one position with a bicameral structure. We distinguish between *faculty affairs* and *development* functions for a more nuanced understanding of the responsibilities and the inherent bidirectional relationship between the two concepts.

Moreover, as you may know, while progress has been made in increasing equity, diversity, and inclusion (EDI) in academic medicine in general, there is still work to be done to achieve equitable representation of LHS+ individuals specifically at the level of executive leadership roles within medical schools. By observation, we tend to see executive leaders of minoritized groups in EDI positions. Or we tend to think that EDI "positions" are our mainstay for us, a path toward leadership of least resistance and where we could potentially contribute our energy, knowledge, and experience the most. Instead, our chapter challenges you to reframe how you (a) contemplate the role of DOFAD, (b) can leverage your LHS+ identity to improve your self-efficacy in achieving such a position, and (c) once in the position, capitalize on your unique positionality to advance meaningful inclusivity initiatives that deeply impact the faculty you serve and penetrates your partnering hospital cultures. This chapter will sensitize you to the position of DOFAD and the preparation needed to assume the leadership responsibilities.

Before exploring the role of DOFAD, we review three broad but important concepts that come with multiple definitions and, thus, multiple understandings among seasoned academicians.

## Review of Key Terms and Basic Information

In this chapter, we articulate below the scope and specific meaning we assign to three core concepts you will need clarification on to successfully operate within the realm of centralized OFADs.

## Key Terms

*Faculty Affairs*: What it is not! Although they work closely, the concept and functions of the leadership position are *not* a duplication of Human Resources for faculty. Instead, we are faculty advocates who work closely with Human Resources. Recruitment, initial appointment, promotion, orientation/onboarding, shared governance, and ombudsman make up the day-to-day support of current faculty members and prospective recruits [2].

*Faculty Career Development*: Learning activities designed to assist faculty members in developing and enhancing their skills, knowledge, and competencies in areas such as teaching, research, leadership, and professional and individual growth [3, 4]. Findings from a systematic review in *Academic Medicine* show an expansion in the scope and nuanced meanings of the term *faculty development* over the last decade that are important to acknowledge. As such, we rely on Leslie et al.'s explanation of the new nature and scope of faculty development which includes specific terms for the multiple domains of development. These are (a) instructional and curricular development, (b) research and scholarly development, (c) career development, (d) organizational and administrative development, (e) social and cultural integration development, and (f) personal/well-being development [5].

*Promotion*: The process of advancing a faculty member to meet the criteria of the next professional rank in the academic hierarchy.

## Being a Dean of Faculty Affairs and Development Who Identifies as LHS+: ¡Si, Se Puede!

As a DOFAD who identifies as LHS+, you may face both unique obstacles and advantages in your role. Historically, LHS+ individuals have been underrepresented in leadership positions within medical schools and academic medicine [6–8]. This underrepresentation extends to roles such as deans, department chairs, and other administrative positions [9, 10]. We also know that the representation of LHS+ faculty members in medical schools is lower compared to other racial and ethnic groups [11]. This underrepresentation at the faculty level impacts the pool of potential candidates for leadership positions, including deanships [12]. Moreover, despite some improvement in the representation of those identifying as women, and minoritized groups throughout the continuum, stagnation continues within the highest levels of medical school leadership positions such as FAD deanships. Factors that continue to constrain opportunity for such achievement continue to be a combination of limited access to mentorship, insufficient social network, bias and discrimination, microaggressions, poor morale, and low self-efficacy that contributes to a limited pool of interested LHS+ applicants for executive leadership [9]. However, it is not all doom and gloom! We celebrate the considerable efforts to address the obstacles and promote diversity that can help create a more inclusive and supportive environment for faculty members from diverse backgrounds. Medical schools and national organizations like AAMC, Insight into Diversity, and Building the Next Generation of Academic Physicians (BNGAP) have recognized the importance of diversity and inclusion in leadership roles that touch on *all aspects of the medical education continuum*. They have implemented development programs with specific attention to the LHS+ identity (e.g., Healthcare Executive Diversity and Inclusion Certificate, Minority Leadership Development Program, BNGAP Leadership and Academic Medicine Seminar: Opportunities for Diverse Medical Students and Residents), awards (e.g., Higher Education Excellence in Diversity—HEED), and national positions to elevate EDI by specifically cultivating expectations and opportunities among multiple affinity groups, other organizations, and schools that cultivate collaboration and inclusion of EDI dimension into Faculty Affairs, Graduate Medical Education, Student Affairs, and the like.

Additionally, the Latino Medical Student Association (LMSA) has been actively working to advance EDI in academic medicine. LMSA LIDEReS (LHS+ Identity, Development, Empowerment, and Resources Seminar—https://fpac.lmsa.net/center/lideres/) is a 2-day seminar that brings together faculty members, physicians, senior staff members, and advisors from across the USA, providing participants with inspirational and practical guidance and tools for pursuing career advancement in academic medicine. The seminar helps participants develop key professional competencies that build self-efficacy, communication skills, and leadership while expanding their network of colleagues, role models, advisors, and champions.

All in all, the lesson garnered from these collective initiatives is: ¡*Veras, si se puede cambiar el subjecto si no te gusta!* If you do not like the narrative, change it and then build on it. As LHS+ scholars, physicians, role models, colleagues, and friends, we are at a critical juncture in time where we can more potently impact patient care for an evolving community by reshaping the medical education experience by improving the leadership representation at our academic medical centers. We must strongly consider, where else and how else we can influence the academic organizational culture if we are going to make further inroads in patient care. It is all connected. We are not saying it will be easy or welcoming, but recall that within our LHS+ culture, one of the distinguishing cultural factors is that we tend to lead *con cariño* [13]. This is almost the antithesis of academic and medical hierarchical culture. Ceasing executive leadership opportunities like in FAD is paramount. It will allow us to flex that style in sincere hopes of cultivating a greater extent of collaboration, inclusivity, and accepting work culture for the faculty and the rest of the dean's cabinet.

## Overview of Roles and Responsibilities of Dean of Faculty Affairs and Development

In tandem with the department chairs, and mentors, the DOFAD provides continuous education and guidance to faculty at all stages of their career: This includes recruits, onboarding, ongoing engagement and development to late-stage career through retirement and emeritus. This is commonly referred to as the *faculty life cycle* or *Career Management Life Cycle Model* as coined by Viggiano and Strobel [14]. A DOFAD is expected to understand, thoroughly, the faculty life cycle and, thus, oversee the supporting mechanism for faculty vitality within a school of medicine. Before presenting the typical duties associated with the role, it is critical to remember that responsibilities will vary across institutions and can be influenced by factors such as the size of the faculty, institutional culture, academic disciplines involved, and employment and compensation plans. Despite the variations and uniqueness of how OFADs are matrixed within their respective institutions, the AAMC Group of Faculty Affairs (GFA) is the premier guide that sets the national guardrails for the role that search firms and institutions often turn to when recruiting and conceptualizing. The GFA is a professional network within the AAMC that focuses on faculty affairs and development. They offer resources, conferences, webinars, and networking opportunities specifically tailored to faculty affairs professionals. The GFA website provides access to valuable information and resources related to faculty development, leadership, and career advancement. Of particular interest will be the online text, GFA Leadership Guide for Faculty Affairs Professionals (2022) [15] which serves as a collection of essays offering information, strategy, and advice as written by deans of faculty affairs and development about the role and functions [16].

According to the GFA 2023 Steering Committee leadership, the core responsibilities traditionally seen in an office of faculty affairs are recited verbatim below. This list of responsibilities and duties was greatly influenced by the work of Sonnino et al. [2] (Table 17.1).

As you can see from this list, the faculty affairs dean plays a critical role in supporting faculty in their career progression and their professional development. Given the extensive list of responsibilities, in the next section, we focus the discussion on what we consider to be the most poignant, impactful, and rewarding aspects of the role and in the context of LHS+ identity. Simultaneously, while there are aspects of the role that can greatly benefit from your ability to influence, there is a reality and dimensions to the role that can be particularly challenging given the changing landscape of medical education today.

**Table 17.1** Responsibilities and duties of office of faculty affairs [2, 17]

| |
|---|
| Manage appointment, promotion, and tenure |
| Provide programs to develop leadership skills |
| Plan for leadership and succession |
| Ensure the incorporation of diversity, equity, and inclusion |
| Advocate for faculty well-being and vitality |
| Provide teaching, research, and clinical skills |
| Assist in faculty retention |
| Provide and organize faculty onboarding and orientation |
| Support faculty governance |
| Manage the annual faculty evaluation process |
| Initiate faculty reviews (post-tenure, department chair reviews, administrative reviews) |
| Collaborate with human resources |
| Assist faculty in applying for awards, scholarships, fellowships, and other recognition |
| Provide counseling and mentoring (mentorship programs) |
| Development of faculty handbooks, bylaws |
| Collaborate with department chairs and directors to develop and standardize faculty offer letters |
| Represent faculty affairs/faculty development at the institutional level |
| Collaborate with the Title IX office |
| Assist with faculty leave and accommodations |
| Aid faculty across the faculty career life cycle |
| Review faculty policies |
| Assist with clinical faculty credentialing |
| Participate in institutional committees |
| Assist in the faculty licensing process |
| Participating in the grievance/ombudsman process |
| Connecting resources to address faculty assessments |
| Conduct research and assess faculty, professional, and leadership programs in a scholarly way |
| Uphold LCME accreditation standards for the faculty workforce |
| Representation on a national level for the AAMC's Group on Faculty Affairs |

## The Opportunities and Potential Obstacles Inherent to the Faculty Affairs and Development Core Functions

Based on our lived experiences, we review the most critical functions of the role. We also place what we know about the role into the LHS+ context.

## The Opportunities: The Faculty Affairs Aspect

***Promotion*** The Dean of Faculty Affairs helps faculty members navigate the professorial promotion process successfully through education, guidance, support, and broad oversight. There are multiple tracks available now that include nontenure and traditional tenure tracks that better capture what all the different subgroups of faculty contribute to the institution, such that each has a pathway to promotion. You should pay particular attention to the evolving definition of the value (monetary and philosophical) of tenure for physicians and nonphysicians at your medical school

[18]. These are defined, valued, and assigned differently across the nation with monetary values being communicated by your dean of the medical school or university provost of faculty affairs as set by the university's board of regents or trustees. Philosophically, the value is set by you internally through introspection, and what your organizational culture is signaling through behaviors and traditions. As a result, knowing the nuanced values of each track will improve your ability to articulate promotion motivators and criteria as you prioritize your educational workshops and sessions across the departments [19].

LHS+ identity, we think, could bring a heightened awareness of the importance of monitoring dashboards that might be available for leaders at your school to reference when examining several faculty rates such as (a) time to promotion, (b) retention stratified by key demographics, and (c) rank composition [20]. Through targeted outreach and robust development programs, mentors can help faculty with career goal setting. Having timely and accurate information about the promotion criteria and appropriate track placement at the time of onboarding is important to setting faculty up for success. Moreover, remember to extend educational sessions about careers in academic medicine and the idea of promotion and advancement to future physician trainees at the medical school and Graduate Medical Education (GME) level. It is a critical aspect for DOFAD to participate in educating throughout the continuum to invest and reach those in premedical school bridge and early pipeline programming [21, 22]. We know that LHS+ barriers to promotion are learning the rules of the promotion game. Previous literature reveals that LHS+ tend to receive inaccurate or late information, being on a track that does not align with goals and misaligned with workload time allocations, and expectations, and getting such information late into the early-career stage [23]. Naturally, as dean, we are in the perfect position to make timely education, monitoring, and influencing, that can remove the barriers, a top priority.

***Shared Governance/Committees*** As the DOFAD, you have close collaboration with the general faculty body and the dean of the medical school to ensure and execute shared governance processes such as ballot building for the elected and appointed positions for the school's standing committees. In unison with the dean's cabinet, these campus committees provide significant input and influence over policies and practices and help set the tone of organizational behaviors, traditions, and values. These policies cover a wide range of areas, including faculty workload expectations, evaluation criteria, academic governance, and leave policies. Collaboration with relevant stakeholders helps ensure that policies are fair, transparent, and aligned with the institution's mission and values, particularly strategic plans around inclusivity. Given the nature of elected and appointed positions for these influential committee roles, DOFAD deans can positively influence the composition of these important committees by keeping valued national, institutional, and office goals in mind when advocating and persistently communicating open opportunities to faculty. Such actions can increase visibility and provide capital to faculty such that they gain recognition as a campus leader when on such committees.

***Recruitment*** In most institutions, the DOFAD is deeply involved in executive recruitment, for example, filling open dean positions such as GME, Clinical Affairs, and Student Affairs. These posts compose the dean of the school's leadership cabinet along with the department chairs. This is a highly influential and powerful role! Think of all the impact you can make in terms of moving cultural norms, behaviors, traditions, and shared goals by being in the position of educating and collaborating with the dean, internal search committee members, and corporate search firms (when and if utilized). As a DOFAD, the lived experiences and in-depth knowledge you have about practices and organizational cultures may uniquely position you. You may have a first-hand understanding of what it means to belong to an organization. You may have special insight into what behaviors may give rise to fertile and hospitable experiences for faculty. As a result, this could profoundly shape your institution's leadership recruitment policies and practices. This could include an advertisement strategy wherein you can ensure that appropriate pools of diverse candidates are built. Another is setting the tone for special training that shares national and institutional data that reviews hiring trends and sets the tone for the search committees involved.

## The Opportunities: Faculty Development Aspect

As the DOFAD at a medical school, it is important to navigate the overwhelming nature of the field and effectively identify the needs of your faculty. There are many strategies and considerations to help prioritize and create a faculty development program. For example, the go-to exercise of a DOFAD leader early in their assumptions of duties and then every 5 years is the engagement in a Faculty Needs Assessment Survey. Conducting an annual faculty needs assessment survey is a common practice to gather feedback from faculty members. This survey can help you understand their specific development needs and preferences. A recommendation would be to gather your development committee with the department chairs and colleagues in the offices of EDI, research, GME, and Continuing Medical Education (CME) to collaborate and capture multiple dimensions. Ultimately, existing enduring materials online, mentoring, leadership, well-being, and other specialized cohort-based programs, and home-grown content should be offered in different modalities such as face-to-face interactions, web-based platforms, asynchronous training, and podcasts. Incentives like certificates, membership into a formalized community of practice that participants can note on the curriculum vitae or CME credits can help encourage attendance and engagement.

Nationally, what is known as The AAMC Standpoint Survey, can provide valuable insights to you by comparing your institution's training and development needs with those of other medical schools. This survey can be individualized to the unique factors at your institution that drive faculty engagement and inform your faculty development initiatives.

## Potential Obstacles: Faculty Affairs and Development

As more universities are partnering with health systems, there is a more complex matrixed relationship that, depending on the cultures and contractual terms between the partnering entities, can be a potential obstacle for the role. As a result of this complexity, one significant issue at the forefront for FA professionals today is, who exactly employs the faculty that you are directly and indirectly overseeing. Again, depending on your context, the employment of faculty may be based on the health system and not the university that you represent [24]. This factor may keep the role distanced from effectively influencing division/departmental actions. When the faculty you represent and advocate for are direct reports or employees of the academic institution but are employees of the hospital, it is much more difficult to exert influence. It is possible but much more challenging. To this notion, there are several core areas that you should be cognizant about. First, hiring will have implications on the composition of faculty and likely shared institutional goals. So just as we mentioned recruitment is an area of opportunity, likewise, it can also be an obstacle. In centralized models as discussed earlier, the office is usually charged with assisting the dean's office with the recruitment of executive-level positions as opposed to managing faculty hiring within the departments and faculty who are, instead, employed by the partnering health systems. In the same vein, if search firms are utilized at your site, your influence will largely depend on the depth of familiarity and shared values between your school and the firm's main recruiter. This relationship is important and will take persistence to convey goals and values, particularly around inclusivity. Much of what we know from the literature and lived experience is new territory for firms. Educating search firms about the challenges faced by LHS+ applicants and the desire to ensure a diverse applicant pool is important to achieving recruitment goals. We encourage investing considerable effort to remain connected to the department chairs and physician executives, hospital strategy teams, and search firm leads to stay relevant and ahead of the curve.

Next, faculty orientation and onboarding are impacted. Onboarding provides new faculty with essential information about the institution, its policies, resources, and expectations. This longitudinal experience provides essential information about the institution's culture, policies, resources, and expectations, helping new faculty integrate smoothly into their roles and the academic community. The benefit of LHS+ identity is how we are keenly aware of the challenges and desired style of integrating and learning [25]. We must make it a point to incorporate this into the blended cultures of the hospital systems and academic institutions.

Additionally, it is the area of compensation. Many offices work closely with their main campus' provost's office to establish compensation guidelines and conduct salary equity analysis. Developing frameworks and regular analysis to promote fair and equitable compensation for faculty members and considering factors such as experience, qualifications, and workload can be difficult when these exercises get divided by separate employers. Other times, the faculty solely employed by their hospital systems are not subject to these analysis and compensation plans which can complicate the experience and not align with the academic goals of recognition and equity [26, 27].

Finally, and similar to the compensation complexity, the grievance process within FA will depend on the employer. When they are managed within FA, the expectation for deans is to ensure the development of fair and transparent procedures that address the issues impartially and are resolved in a timely and equitable manner.

## Reflection Exercise

To examine your interest and reflect upon our readiness for the role in faculty affairs and career development, below is a series of e-journal prompts that we suggest you explore. The spirit of the prompt questions is to help you explore the fundamental functions of the role, so you can assess its fit for your career vision and identify areas of personal development that you can build upon. Once you identify these areas, make it a point to incorporate these as goals for professional growth in your annual performance review. Along with discussing these professional goals with your supervisor (e.g., chair, chief), we encourage you to share your aspirations of having a leading role in faculty affairs and development with mentors and sponsors. Consider a steppingstone position (i.e., vice chair for development; vice of faculty affairs) or offer up leading an internal project like leading faculty mentoring programs or development committee work within your department or division.

The below prompts are many and are derived from our personal career paths and experiences. Take your time contemplating each one and connecting these to your annual and broader professional goals (Table 17.2).

**Table 17.2** Preparing to become a faculty affairs leader

| Reflection prompt | Who and/or what resource can help me? (*Additional hints from the authors*) | Action item I will take: Approximately when would this be appropriate? |
|---|---|---|
| 1. How knowledgeable am I about the faculty life cycle in academic medicine? | | |
| 2. How well do I understand the interplay and model (centralized/decentralized) between the school and departments? | *Business administrators or department chair can tell you the model, which will clue you into the extent of your sphere of influence and the optimal method for communicating and supporting departments/faculty learning* | |
| 3. How knowledgeable am I about the policies and handbooks for faculty as set by the broader university? | *Check your university's provost for faculty affairs office for handbooks and policies that might heavily influence your school's parameters* | |
| 4. How might the worlds of human resources, academic affairs, and research (clinical and education) overlap or complement my vision for the office? | | |
| 5. How familiar am I with my School's professorial promotion criteria for all available tracks? | *Go to your home institution's faculty affairs website and read each track's description and requirements* | |
| 6. When I think of the following: approachable, trustworthy, knowledgeable, accessible, reliable—which traits do I excel in, and which might I need help developing? *These are soft but important attributes to embody since the expectation is that you will serve as an advocate, advisor, talent recruiter, and scholar* | | |

(continued)

**Table 17.2** (continued)

| Reflection prompt | Who and/or what resource can help me? (*Additional hints from the authors*) | Action item I will take: Approximately when would this be appropriate? |
|---|---|---|
| 7. Given the combination of my LHS+ positionality, experiences, and background, what unique value-added do I bring to the school if I were to lead people in this role? | *Consider drafting a personal argument or "value proposition" about yourself. Consider it a sophisticated elevator pitch!* | |
| 8. Do I know the many subgroups of faculty that contribute to the school's missions? (i.e., private, community, traditional tenured) | *Socialize with the division chief, chair, directors of faculty affairs offices, or human resources to uncover the scope of your context. Each subgroup views and engages academic medicine uniquely* | |
| 9. Since I would play a key role in executive recruitment, how familiar am I with national search firms' reputations and processes for engaging them? | *If you have not been hired through a search firm before, read Chap. 1 of this book!* | |
| 10. Since I would play a key role in advising chairs and deans on faculty retention, how familiar am I with national/industry funding opportunities focused on faculty retention and development (i.e., NIH-R25s; NIH-U54s)? | *Engage your research office for access to calls from national or federal entities Consider searching for educational research grants from the Josiah Macy Jr. Foundation, the American Medical Association (AMA), Alfred P. Sloan, the Robert Wood Johnson Foundation, and the Society of Academic Continuing Medical Education (SACME). These groups often consider small grant awards for faculty development and recruitment* | |
| 11. Do I have a basic understanding of the philosophical and monetary value of tenure for nonphysicians and physicians? | *Multiple academic articles discuss the recent changes in the value of tenure in higher education in general. What is important is how it is contextualized on your site. This will be a series of discussions and negotiations with your university's provost, dean, and department chair and may not be easy to bring up* | |
| 12. For offers, retention, and general advice-giving, do I know where to find the AAMC Salary Tables for my region online or within the Business or Dean's Office? | *If not readily available to you, table information can be purchased on the AAMC website.* | |

Original worksheet authored by Beatrice Tapia and Guadalupe Federico-Martinez (2023).

## Skills-Based Exercise

The purpose of this exercise is packaged into a short-term mini project to get you into the habit of monitoring national faculty trends and gaining trust among colleagues. As mentioned in our chapter, you must have an annual understanding of trends related to faculty composition (e.g., ranks, gender identity, ethnicity), retention, promotion, and compensation compared to your local context for effective advocacy and persuasion in the role of faculty affairs and development dean. Treat this mini project as an opportunity that could potentially gain you increased positive visibility.

*Instructions* Go to the AAMC Data Reports—Faculty Trends section by the last two most recent academic years posted and/or decade. Review the demographic breakdowns.

*Exercise* Depending on your current role and levels of access/privileges to similar faculty information for your division/department, work with an administrative support staff and supervisor to access such faculty information for your division/department through raw data or dashboard summary. Compare the two data sets to gauge, firsthand, how your home site measures up to the national landscape. Maybe pose some interesting, specific questions by LHS+ identity: For example, there are more Black women than men faculty. What does gender representation look like for LHS+ men and women across assistant, associate, and full professor ranks? Draft an executive summary for your intended audience of leaders (e.g., supervisor, chair, chief, residency program director, WIMS director) that covers the most salient faculty points of interest for them. Focus your end goal on making a case for a change or implementation of a new program, process, or departmental value that should be embedded in the local strategic plan for faculty success. You should first approach your supervisor with this exercise and complete any sensitive information training that might be required. Access to data is an important first step in advocacy but, at times, can be the most difficult to get! Start practicing persistence for access now.

## Additional Resources to Assist with Decision-Making and Advancement

To support your pursuit of a position as a Dean of Faculty Affairs and Development, there are organizations, annual scholarly meetings, and text resources below that you can refer to for nuanced guidance and networking.

### Societies/Organizations
1. The International Association of Medical Science Educators (IAMSE) is an organization dedicated to advancing the field of health professions education.

They offer conferences, webinars, workshops, and publications that cover various aspects of faculty development, including teaching methodologies, assessment, curriculum design, and educational scholarship. https://www.iamse.org/
2. BNGAP is an organization committed to the career development of students, residents, fellows, and early-career physician-faculty to learn about the academic career options available to them. Participation in leading career seminars and guest speaking will provide you with appropriate exposure to the day to day of what one could expect from the faculty affairs role. https://bngap.org/
3. ElevateMD is an organization that provides financial support and mentorship to future physicians. Its goal is to increase the diversity within the physician workforce, improve cultural competence, and reduce health disparities in the USA. https://www.elevatemed.org/who-we-are
4. LMSA is an organization dedicated to supporting LHS+ medical students and professionals. While primarily focused on students, LMSA can be a valuable resource for networking and connecting with LHS+ professionals in the medical field. They may provide guidance and support as you pursue a leadership position in faculty affairs and development. https://national.lmsa.net/
5. NHMA (National Hispanic Medical Association): NHMA is an organization dedicated to improving the health of Hispanics and underrepresented populations by providing leadership and advocacy in health care. While primarily focused on medical professionals, NHMA offers opportunities for networking, mentorship, and professional development that can support your career growth and goals. https://www.nhmamd.org/

## *Book Reads*

Roberts, L. W. (Ed.). (2019). Roberts Academic Medicine Handbook: A Guide to Achievement and Fulfillment for Academic Faculty. Springer Nature.
Lane, P. H. (2015). The Promotion Game: Your Guide to Success in the Academic Medical Center. BookBaby.

## *National Scholarly Meetings*

AAMC Group on Faculty Affairs Annual Scholarly Meeting (typically over the summer months). If you attend this meeting, you will have the opportunity to join the group's Mentoring Circles cohort for specialized mentoring with a seasoned faculty affairs leader within the USA. You can expect to have meet and greets with directors, assistant deans, associate deans, and provosts for faculty affairs in academic medicine. If you are engaging in educational research, you have the potential to have your poster abstract or podium presentation of your original findings on this national platform for other deans of faculty affairs to consume. Every other year, the group conducts a joint conference proceeding with another AAMC affinity group like the Group on Diversity and Inclusion or the Group on Women in Medicine. As a result, you double your social network web and account for the complex intersectionality of the faculty that you seek to lead. This forum is a must if you are serious!

## Nos Despedimos

As concluding advice for this chapter, we offer the following sentiments: First, in addition to the aforementioned organizations, it is important to stay updated on relevant literature and research in the field of faculty affairs and development. Regularly reading journals and publications such as Medical Education, Academic Medicine, The Journal of Graduate Medical Education, MedEdPORTAL for teaching and learner assessment materials, and The Journal of Faculty Development can help you stay informed about current trends, best practices, and innovative approaches in faculty development.

Finally, prioritizing networking with colleagues in your field, attending relevant conferences and workshops, and seeking mentorship opportunities can also contribute to your professional growth and help you navigate the path to becoming a Dean of Faculty Affairs and Development. Early on heavily explore opportunities for professional development within your institution as well. Your current colleagues and administrators will likely be able to provide guidance and support as you seek to advance your career in faculty affairs and development. As such, make it a point to visit your home institution's Faculty Affairs website, introduce yourself to your faculty affairs dean, and familiarize yourself with promotion criteria at a minimum of three different sites so you can compare the commonalities and differences. This last one is a "two-for-one" that will not only give your perspective on promotion but will aid you with planning your advancement. You will have the advantage of knowing the rules of the game!

## Personal Narrative

### Beatriz Tapia, MD, EdD, MPH
*A Journey from Translator to Dean of Faculty Affairs*

As a first-generation Mexican American, born and raised in Chicago until I was 12, my path in health care began far earlier than most. At just 8, I was thrust into the role of translator and, though I didn't know it at the time, a *patient navigator* within the complex US healthcare system. My father, then only 35, started experiencing severe muscle spasms and numbness—symptoms that, despite his persistence in his job as an airplane motor technician, would ultimately force him to stop working. Diagnosed with myotonic dystrophy, a genetic disorder, he faced countless appointments and therapies that needed interpretation and explanation. With each medical encounter, I sensed the limitations of our knowledge and resources but also a desire to help beyond what I could do at that young age.

Returning to my parents' homeland in Mexico soon after, I pursued an MD, determined to make a difference in the lives of underserved communities like those of my childhood. Yet, even as a practicing healthcare provider, I felt drawn back to my roots and the communities in Chicago where health disparities were stark and ever-present. To better understand these disparities, I pursued an MPH in epidemiology, with a focus on health inequities and occupational and environmental medicine. My journey into medicine, from that young girl translating in hospitals to a physician, remains intertwined with a vision of creating change for the Hispanic community. It is what fueled my journey and purpose in returning to academic medicine.

I entered academia in the late 1990s, unexpectedly finding joy in teaching health education. During my first academic position in Texas, I encountered Hispanic physicians in leadership roles for the first time—deans and leaders who reflected my background and shared my experiences. Inspired by these trailblazers, I committed myself to a career that would open doors for others. The opportunity to complete a doctorate in Education for Health Science Educators was transformative, further refining my commitment to serve and educate.

In 2015, despite my lack of formal experience in faculty development, I was given the opportunity to become the assistant dean of faculty development at a new medical school. At the time, the senior associate dean of faculty affairs saw something in me—motivation, passion, and a desire to teach. This belief empowered me to step into an entirely new field, and it's a reminder to take a chance when someone believes in you, even if you haven't done it before. That chance allowed me to participate in the AAMC Group on Faculty Affairs (GFA), where I found a community and an opportunity to contribute. Through the GFA, I embraced leadership, eventually becoming the chair of the program planning committee. My connection with these colleagues and the mentorship within these circles instilled a deep sense of belonging and purpose.

These experiences prepared me for my current role as the Associate Dean of Faculty Affairs. Over the years, I also had the honor of cofounding and leading the Texas Consortium for Faculty Success (TCFS), a network dedicated to supporting faculty development in Texas' academic health institutions. This consortium has brought together like-minded leaders to promote the success of faculty in Texas. Additionally, I was recognized as an AMA Health Systems Science Scholar, which allowed me to delve deeper into research areas close to my heart, including border health, environmental medicine, and faculty development. Currently, I am the chair of the AAMC GFA Program Planning Committee 2024–2025.

Today, as I live in the US-Mexico border, my journey feels both full-circle and ever-evolving. Whether enjoying the beach at South Padre Island or traveling with my family to the Midwest and Mexico, I am reminded of the communities that shaped my journey. Each step of this path, from a young interpreter for my father to a dean guiding faculty affairs, is built on a commitment to inclusivity, equity, and perseverance. I hope our chapter continues to inspire others to pursue transformative work in academic medicine and faculty affairs. *Sí, se puede.*

**Guadalupe Federico-Martinez, PhD**

As a nonphysician Latina faculty member, I started my professional journey and found a home in academic medicine over a decade ago. While serving as a graduate medical education residency manager, I was also working on my doctoral studies in higher education. The study of higher education is about investigating how certain sectors within university systems operate.

My home clinical department of internal medicine valued studying the social science aspect of medical education and the social construct that is academic medicine. Given my studies at the time, physician-educators and senior leaders in the department were interested in using educational theory and investigatory approaches common to the sociology of education to better understand the needs of trainees, faculty, and administrators learning and working within. It was made explicitly clear to me that leadership saw the potential benefits of having a relatively "nontraditional" faculty member in a clinical department, being a different lens toward understanding organizational culture, and the training and socialization of physicians we groom to work inside and outside of academic medicine. I think I was very fortunate to have forward thinking leaders who took a risk, invested resources, understood the value of education specialists, and trusted in my developing expertise. Family, these leaders, colleagues, former professors, mentors, sponsors, and role models in my life merged to form a constellation of support. Some of these actors shared similar backgrounds with me, while most of them, however, shared very little in common with me in terms of upbringing, educational pathway, and demographics. It is not lost on me that we, particularly those underrepresented in medicine and leadership, need to surround ourselves with experts and people who think and look different than ourselves. My trusted group of advisers functioned as my "cabinet," if you will, for mentorship and talking out options.

Upon diving into educational research projects and managing the education department, progressive leadership opportunities present themselves. I assisted physician-faculty members with their educational research ideas, teaching techniques, and making sense of career progression at the institution. My current position still includes identifying as a faculty member. Until recently, I also served in two administrative roles: one at the local level within my institution and another at the national level for the AAMC. At my institution, I served as the assistant of faculty affairs and career development, and for the AAMC, I served 1 year as the national chair-elect of the Group on Faculty Affairs. It pains me to say that we are still experiencing "first Latina" moments in 2024; however, I was the first Latina to serve in both roles. I found these opportunities intimidating at first, but upon long and hard reflection, they aligned with my strength: advocacy. I had to muzzle the inner critic and listen to what others saw in me and believe in my decisions. This has taken me years of practice to manage and is a continued effort.

Most recently, I transitioned out of the Assistant Dean of Faculty Affairs and Career Development. I made the scariest decision of my life as I am the breadwinner of my family and have responsibilities to my son and husband. This decision included me accepting the inner call to challenge myself more and risk evolving. I decided to get additional training in coaching and counseling, so I can operate within what social posts are now calling, "privademics." I saw an opportunity to transition from academic leadership to business leadership. I wanted to address a gap in availability and services that I often criticized institutions about, lack of mentorship and individualized faculty development. I pulled the trigger on my vision. I retained a volunteer faculty, switched tracks from *Educator Scholar* to *Professor of Practitioner*, and started my own career coaching and consulting company for physicians. I find deep satisfaction in serving as the founder and CEO of my own space within the academic career development stratosphere. I very much enjoy CV reviews and strategizing with faculty, of all walks, about their career (and life) planning and progression. I simply believe that an individualized tailoring of professional development, and truly available mentorship, as we tend to operate in time poverty in academics, is the future. I see serious gaps in how our institutions attempt to provide individualized career services and advocacy to faculty that are untenable in the higher education culture, I want to change that now that I have seen internal operations from the D-suite.

I hope this chapter provides overt and clear guidance on how to prepare yourself for a career as an advocate for your medical school's faculty. If people tell you, "Thank you for having my back," or if you have thought, "I wish I could influence policies that improve the education faculty receive about how to get promoted," or "I want to help my colleague work through the grievance process," then, you are in the right place for some answers!

## References

1. Whitcomb ME. The medical school's faculty is its most important asset. Acad Med. 2003;78(2):117–8.
2. Sonnino RE, Reznik V, Thorndyke LA, Chatterjee A, Ríos-Bedoya CF, Mylona E, et al. Evolution of faculty affairs and faculty development offices in US medical schools: a 10-year follow-up survey. Acad Med. 2013;88(9):1368–75.
3. McLean M, Cilliers F, Van Wyk JM. Faculty development: yesterday, today and tomorrow. Med Teach. 2008;30(6):555–84.
4. Khan N, Khan MS, Dasgupta P, Ahmed K. The surgeon as educator: fundamentals of faculty training in surgical specialties. BJU Int. 2013;111(1):171–8.
5. Leslie K, Baker L, Egan-Lee E, Esdaile M, Reeves S. Advancing faculty development in medical education: a systematic review. Acad Med. 2013;88(7):1038–45.
6. AAMC data report diversity in medicine: facts and figures 2019. https://www.aamc.org/data-reports/workforce/data/figure-15-percentage-full-time-us-medical-school-faculty-race/ethnicity-2018#:~:text=Diversity%20in%20Medicine%3A%20Facts%20and%20Figures%202019,-Diversity%20in%20Medicine&text=The%20largest%20proportions%20of%20faculty,with%20another%20race%2Fethnicity.
7. Contreras F. Latino Faculty in Hispanic-Serving Institutions: Where Is the Diversity? Association of Mexican American Educators Journal, v11 n3 p223–250 2017. EISSN-2377-9187.
8. Geiger G, Kiel L, Horiguchi M, Martinez-Aceves C, Meza K, Christophers B, et al. Latinas in medicine: evaluating and understanding the experience of Latinas in medical education: a cross-sectional survey. BMC Med Educ. 2024;24(1):4.

9. AAMC data report US medical school deans trends by race and ethnicity. 2023. https://www.aamc.org/data-reports/faculty-institutions/data/us-medical-school-deans-trends-type-and-race-ethnicity
10. Nobles A, Martin BA, Casimir J, Schmitt S, Broadbent G. Stalled progress: medical school dean demographics. J Am Board Fam Med. 2022;35(1):163–8.
11. Kaplan SE, Raj A, Carr PL, Terrin N, Breeze JL, Freund KM. Race/ethnicity and success in academic medicine: findings from a longitudinal multi-institutional study. Acad Med. 2018;93(4):616–22.
12. Saxena MR, Ling AY, Carrillo E, Alvarez AA, Yiadom MYA, Bennett CL, Gallegos M. Trends of academic faculty identifying as Hispanic at US medical schools, 1990-2021. J Grad Med Educ. 2023;15(2):175–9.
13. Eordas J. The power of Latino leadership: culture, inclusion, and contribution. Berrett-Koehler Publishers; 2013.
14. Viggiano TR, Strobel HW. The career management life cycle: a model for supporting and sustaining faculty vitality and wellness. In: Faculty health in academic medicine: physicians, scientists, and the pressures of success; 2009. p. 73–81. https://doi.org/10.1007/978-1-60327-451-7_6.
15. GFA Leadership Guide for Faculty Affairs Professionals. https://www.aamc.org/career-development/affinity-groups/gfa/leadership-guide-faculty-affairs-professionals. Accessed 5 July 2025.
16. Gibson J, Freeman E, Ripley B, Hill J, Brazeau C, Rowland M, Best B, Love J, Runge C, editors. Association of American Medical Colleges (AAMC), Group on Faculty Affairs (GFA). Leadership Guide; 2025. https://www.aamc.org/career-development/affinity-groups/gfa/leadership-guide-faculty-affairs-professionals
17. Lucas R, Brutus N, Federico-Martinez G, Soremekun C, Gemeda M, Rodriguez J, Townsend J, Callahan E, Sánchez JP. Academic career exploration: learner opportunities through the Office of Faculty Affairs. MedEdPORTAL. 2024;20:11460. https://doi.org/10.15766/mep_2374-8265.11460.
18. Balch B. Tenure is declining in U.S. medical schools. Could this threaten academic freedom? AAMC News. 2024. https://www.aamc.org/news/tenure-declining-us-medical-schools-could-threaten-academic-freedom
19. Martinez G and Knox K. Precepting medical students in the clinical setting: Its time, not money. Medical Education. 2022;56(7):698–700. https://doi.org/10.1111/medu.14815.
20. Yoo A, Auinger P, Tolbert J, Paul D, Lyness JM, George BP. Institutional variability in representation of women and racial and ethnic minority groups among medical school faculty. JAMA Netw Open. 2022;5(12):e2247640.
21. Sánchez JP, Castillo-Page L, Spencer DJ, Yehia B, Peters L, Freeman BK, Lee-Rey E. Commentary: the building the next generation of academic physicians initiative: engaging medical students and residents. Acad Med. 2011;86(8):928–31.
22. Lee R, Lucas R, Dickerman J, Day LW, Guzman D, Kothari P, et al. Designing pre-faculty competencies for diverse learners through a modified Delphi process. JAMA Netw Open. 2024;7(7):e2424003.
23. Sotto-Santiago S, Moreno F. LHS+ faculty development and advancement. In: Latino, Hispanic, or of Spanish origin+ identified student leaders in medicine: recognizing more than 50 years of presence, activism, and leadership. Cham: Springer; 2023. p. 209–19.
24. Ricardo, Azziz. What Is the Value and Role of Academic Medicine in the Life of Its University? Academic Medicine. 2014;89(2):208–11. https://doi.org/10.1097/ACM.0000000000000095.
25. Torres V, Martinez S, Wallace LD, Medrano CI, Robledo AL, Hernandez E. The connections between Latino ethnic identity and adult experiences. Adult Educ Q. 2012;62(1):3–18.
26. Sánchez JP, Peters L, Lee-Rey E, Strelnick H, Garrison G, Zhang K, Castillo-Page L. Racial and ethnic minority medical students' perceptions of and interest in careers in academic medicine. Acad Med. 2013;88(9):1299–307.
27. Abraído-Lanza AF, Echeverria SE, Flórez KR, Mendoza-Grey S. Latina women in academia: challenges and opportunities. Front Public Health. 2022;10:876161.

**Open Access**  This chapter is licensed under the terms of the Creative Commons Attribution 4.0 International License (http://creativecommons.org/licenses/by/4.0/), which permits use, sharing, adaptation, distribution and reproduction in any medium or format, as long as you give appropriate credit to the original author(s) and the source, provide a link to the Creative Commons license and indicate if changes were made.

The images or other third party material in this chapter are included in the chapter's Creative Commons license, unless indicated otherwise in a credit line to the material. If material is not included in the chapter's Creative Commons license and your intended use is not permitted by statutory regulation or exceeds the permitted use, you will need to obtain permission directly from the copyright holder.

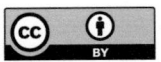

# Chapter 18
# Striving to Become a Dean for Student Affairs

**Leonor Corsino and Luis Alzate-Duque**

> **Learning Objectives**
> - Describe the role of the Dean of Student Affairs.
> - Describe how the Dean of Student Affairs role helps advance educational equity.
> - Share the lived experiences and professional recommendations of two LHS+ identified Deans of Student Affairs.

## Introduction

The Dean for Students Affairs in medical schools represents an important, critical, and extremely valuable role within the medical school leadership suites. Deans for Students Affairs work closely with the students, leaders, and faculty to ensure students' success in medical school and beyond. The Deans for Students Affairs are responsible for fostering and supporting an environment where all students strive. By advising, supporting, advocating, and working closely with the students and other members of medical schools, the Dean for Students Affairs is, in some instances, the glue that keeps all going. Without diminishing the importance of other roles in the School of Medicine, this role plays a significant role in medical schools. Deans for Students Affairs are usually embedded in all aspects of medical education by collaborating closely with medical schools' offices of curriculum, admissions office, and office of financial support, among many more. The role of the Deans for

L. Corsino (✉)
Duke School of Medicine, Durham, NC, USA

L. Alzate-Duque
Rutgers New Jersey Medical School, Newark, NJ, USA
e-mail: alzatelf@njms.rutgers.edu

Students Affair comes with significant responsibility that might include significant workload and burden. However, the role also comes with various rewards and significantly impacts medical education beyond students. The impact of the Dean for Students Affairs is invaluable and is one of the most rewarding aspects of the job. In this chapter, we share with the reader the roles and responsibilities of the Dean for Students Affairs, the rewarding and challenging aspects of this role, suggestions, and resources for those contemplating this career path.

## Dean for Students Affairs

### *What Is a Dean for Students Affairs?*

The Dean for Students Affairs is a leader within the medical school who works closely with students to support their medical education journey [1, 2]. In addition, the Dean for Students Affairs might provide oversight and coordinate student-related events. Additional responsibilities might differ from one institution to another.

## Roles and Responsibilities as Dean for Student Affairs

The role and responsibilities of the Dean for Students Affairs might vary depending on the medical school and institution. However, the Dean for Students Affairs' main role and responsibility include supporting students academically and personally to ensure successful completion of medical school and transition to postgraduate roles [3].

Table 18.1 A brief list of roles and responsibilities of the Dean for Students Affairs (Fig. 18.1).

**Table 18.1** Dean for Students Affairs role and responsibilities[a]

| Dean for Students Affairs role and responsibilities |
|---|
| Leadership role within the medical school |
| Oversight students advising career, academic, personal, and professional |
| Oversight students' academic progress |
| Oversight of academic events, including orientation, white coat ceremony, match day, and graduation |
| Work collaboratively with other leaders/staff/faculty within the school of medicine |
| Serve as the primary contact for students |
| Serve as the liaison between students and available institutional and external resources |
| Oversight of the match process |
| Participate in School of Medicine committees |

[a]Responsibilities might vary from institution to institution

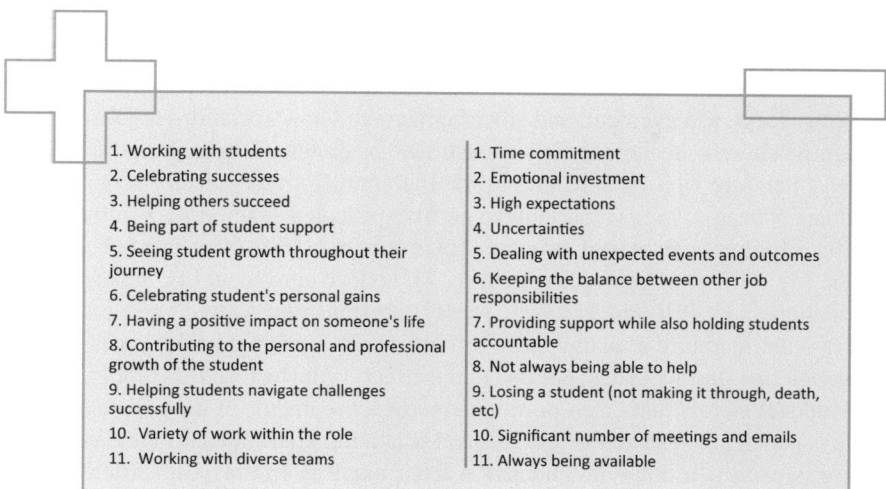

**Fig. 18.1** The most rewarding and challenging aspects of the Associate Dean for Student Affairs role

## The Role of the Dean of Student Affairs Through an Educational Equity Lens

In the conversations of health equity, a major driving concept is the topic of health disparities as influenced by social drivers of health. It is imperative to highlight that these differences in health outcomes are *preventable*. Additionally, they are not explained through physiologic processes but rather are attributable to the *disproportionate allocation of resources* grounded in social constructs of race, ethnicity, gender, or other identities [3, 4]. Moreover, these disparities in health are influenced by drivers of health such as social determinants of health (SDoH), adverse childhood experiences (ACEs), and mitigated by social connectedness and increased social capital, among others [5]. Unfortunately, Black and Brown communities are disproportionately burdened by these drivers of health, resulting in worse health outcomes—as observed in increased rates of asthma, disparities in diabetes control, higher rates of coronary artery disease morbidity and mortality, disparities in colorectal cancer screening and cancer survivorship, higher rates of infant and maternal mortality (on and on), and all impacting mortality as a whole [3]. It is imperative to highlight, as to avoid the stigmatization of minority populations, that differences in health outcomes are *not due to minority status* rather due to the disproportionate burden of *inequity* in drivers of health within minority communities (the disproportionate allocation of resources—wealth, income, education, access to care, etc.) [3].

Is there space for Deans of Student Affairs in the Health Equity conversation? Parallels exist between health equity, as defined by the World Health Organization (WHO) as "the absence of avoidable or remediable differences among groups of people, whether those groups are defined socially, economically, demographically or geographically" and educational equity—as the absence of avoidable or remediable educational differences among groups of people, whether those groups are defined socially, economically, demographically, or geographically.

In their roles, Deans of Student Affairs should be aware of disparities in academic success, achievement, and advancement, and how social driving forces play a significant role in the existing educational inequities. Disparities in academic achievement are well documented in the literature from elementary school [4] to graduate education [5] as it pertains to underrepresented or minority groups experiencing differences in rates of academic achievement [4], pre-K to high school graduation [5], STEM program placement [6, 7], college enrolment [8], undergraduate graduation rates [9], and graduate school attrition rates with SDoH as driving forces—the literature explains these differences in academic achievement are not grounded on minority status, but due to the effects of factors such as SDoH, ACE's, and societal factors that disproportionately impact segments of the population. Yet, there is paucity of research within medical education in this area. There continue to exist disparities in delay of graduation from medical school [10], differences in match rates to "highly competitive" specialties [11], and differences in match rates to preferred specialty in the URM experience [12]. Again, it is important to circle back to the drivers of health, SDoH (conditions where we are born, grow, eat, play, live, GO TO SCHOOL, age and the forces that shape these conditions), rooted in inequitable distribution of resources as drivers of these disparities [13]. Hence, it is reasonable to hypothesize that factors such as SDoH, ACEs, social capital, and connectedness continue to influence academic achievement; that these differences are preventable; that they affect all medical students; and that they disproportionately impact URM students in medical education [14].

Anecdotally, in a survey of the medical student body at a large Northeast Allopathic Medical School, we have observed higher rates of food insecurity [15], housing insecurity, financial concerns, etc., disproportionately affecting URM students. Deans of Student Affairs are tasked with incorporating student-centered approaches that are applicable broadly to student bodies and are grounded in frameworks that facilitate educational equity. The URM experience, specifically the LHS+ experience, should be holistically explored within the context of SDoH, ACEs, and others to better understand how these may impact academic achievement while paying special attention to factors prevalent in URM students such as impostor syndrome [16], the impact of first-generation advance degree achievement (when applicable) [17, 18], intersectionality of identity, and need for mentorship. The use of these frameworks and the use of social connectedness/social capital analysis may help inform mitigating factors and help build stronger networks of support via early identification of relevant societal factors resulting in timely referral to student services [3], improved multidisciplinary collaboration, improved sense of belonging, and improved social connectedness to address educational disparities. Importantly, these frameworks can be applied broadly, help support *ALL students* through student-centered approaches, and are especially well suited to aid URM students mitigate preventable differences in academic achievement and strive for educational equity.

## Steps to Consider

An important initial step is to self-reflect if a Dean for Students Affairs role is the right path for you. By self-reflecting, you will better understand how this role aligns with your values and strengths and how it will provide you with the personal and professional satisfaction we all strive to achieve. Taking the time to do this also fosters a unique opportunity to determine a path to this job. It is also important to remember to be open to change and take opportunities when they come. You should consider how taking smaller roles within your school will allow you to acquire the life and hands-on experience that will prepare you for a larger role as Associate Dean for Students Affairs. For example, you can start advising students within student organizations at your school or taking roles in school committees that will give your insight into how a school of medicine works. Also, take advantage of professional development opportunities within your school, professional organizations, or the Association of American Medical Colleges (AAMC). These professional development opportunities are extremely valuable, because they serve as entryways to leadership in medical education, networking with leaders in similar roles, identifying role models, increasing your awareness of existing resources, and getting insight into role expectations and emerging innovation and change (Tables 18.2 and 18.3).

**Table 18.2** Reflection exercise 1

| Value | Description of how the value aligns with a role as Dean for Student Affairs |
|---|---|
| 1. Service | The role of the Dean for Students Affairs focuses closely on serving others to achieve their goal |
| 2. Honesty | In this role, it is essential to be honest and transparent with students to build and maintain trust |
| 3. | |
| 4. | |
| 5. | |

Write down your top five personal values and describe how these align with the role of a Dean for Students Affairs. Examples below

**Table 18.3** Skill-based exercise 2

| Strength | Likely to contribute | Potential impact |
|---|---|---|
| 1. Communication | Critical to be able to work with students, faculty, and administrators | Facilitate respectful and bidirectional collaborations |
| 2. Resourceful | Important to be able to tap into resources that will help you guide the students and provide the best advice | Increase your ability to tap into resources beyond your school of medicine and institution |
| 3. | | |
| 4. | | |
| 5. | | |

Write down your top five strengths. How are your strengths likely to contribute to a role as Dean for Students Affairs? How might these strengths impact your function? Examples below

## Resources

For those considering this as a future role, there is no straightforward plan to do this. However, as mentioned previously, getting engaged and pursuing opportunities for professional development will help.

Below are some professional development opportunities you should consider.

*Formal mentoring training*
For example, formal mentoring training offered by the Center for the Improvement of Mentored Experiences in Research Although geared towards research this type of training will be valuable while working with students as a Students Affairs Dean.

*Leadership training opportunities*
The Association of American Medical Colleges offers many opportunities throughout the year. Also, consider offering at your institution via your Office of Faculty Development and your Department.

*Get a mentor*
A mentor in medical education can help you navigate the medical education path and will help you identify resources to prepare you for this role further.

*Attend meetings*
Participate in the Association of American Medical Colleges (AAMC) annual meeting or your regional AAMC meetings.

## Personal Narratives

### Leonor Corsino MD

Oh, the places you'll go if you start thinking about how your professional path aligns with your values and strengths. Perhaps I can begin this chapter by sharing how, despite derailments, I finally ended up in a place of joy and honest content. But, before I start sharing my journey, I want to be clear that the path to making it here was not easy and all rosey; it required significant growth, acceptance, reflection, losses, and sacrifices.

My journey in academia started with the intention to be a physician-scientist working toward ameliorating health disparities with a particular focus on Hispanics/Latinos; growing up and witnessing my father's struggles with diabetes motivated me to pursue a path to find ways to help patients impacted by this disease that disproportionately affects people of Hispanic/Latino heritage; this began with a laser-focused strategic plan that included where I pursued my fellowship training and my first faculty role. Being a physician-scientist remains part of my current journey, but aspects of this path do not closely align with my strengths, e.g., writing.

During my 7th year as faculty, I experienced a significant loss in my personal life that required an intentional reassessment of my life and what it meant to be in a privileged role to help others succeed. In addition, an opportunity emerged that allowed me to engage more in health professions education. Teaching, mentoring, and advising have been part of my life while pursuing my traditional physician-scientist path. At the time, I worked closely with students who did not have people like them as role models in medicine or higher education. I was the first and only person some knew who looked like them in academia. Reflecting on my core values and strengths, I realized that working with students and others in the early stages of their careers by helping them achieve their goals, dreams, and full potential was how I saw myself further contributing to health care and medicine beyond research and patient care. This transition was risky, because it required completely changing my path from the world of grants applications and intense manuscript publications to advising, mentoring, curriculum development, and health professional education. For some, this transition was not the best move, considering that I was on an upward trajectory with my research; however, sacrifices and risk are always in line to achieve your happy place. Through this journey, I also realized that being an Associate Dean for Students Affairs was my dream role, because it allows me to help others succeed and impact the lives of many that will go beyond my own. If you are someone that finds happiness in service, helping others achieve, supporting others during challenging times, celebrating successes, being a people person, and love to talk, this might be the path for you. A path that will have no boundaries regarding the impact you can make in health care.

**Luis Alzate-Duque MD**
The joy of student affairs for me is the application of health equity frameworks within the medical school experience. As we progress toward inclusion of under-represented groups to have a seat at the table, in all facets of the rung of the ladder—or the educational continuum—we must remain vigilant of disparities and the effects of social determinants of health (SDoH), adverse childhood experiences, and socially constructed/influenced factors that contribute to inequity—whether in health outcomes or educational outcomes. We must stay resolute in our ability to mitigate these through social connectedness [4], increased social capital (especially well-suited for the role of student affairs!), and in the improved sense of belonging. These should be holistically and systemically ingrained within medical education—just as disparities continue to systematically impact minority populations and must be continuously addressed.

Written by a privileged, formerly undocumented, English as a second language, first-generation college graduate, impacted by SDoH, impostor syndrome, blessed by a strong network, who overcame through the social connectedness/capital of mentorship and support from trailblazers along the way, (and of course grit), to become a Latino physician and Assistant Dean in Student Affairs whose goal is to *serve all* patients and students *holistically* and *equitably*.

# References

1. My Career Path. Students Affairs Dean (2). Association of American Colleges (AAMC). https://careersinmedicine.aamc.org/explore-options/my-career-path-student-affairs-dean-2?check_logged_in=1. Accessed 4 Sept 2023.
2. Nakae S, Haywood Y, Love LJ, Kothari P, Saldaña F, Sánchez JP. Office of student affairs: engagement and leadership opportunities for medical students, residents, and fellows. MedEdPORTAL. 2021;17:11093. https://doi.org/10.15766/mep_2374-8265.11093.
3. Holt-Lunstad J. Social connection as a public health issue: the evidence and a systemic framework for prioritizing the "social" in social determinants of health. Annu Rev Public Health. 2022;43:193–213. https://doi.org/10.1146/annurev-publhealth-052020-110732.
4. Paschall KW, Gershoff ET, Kuhfeld M. A two-decade examination of historical race/ethnicity disparities in academic achievement by poverty status. J Youth Adolesc. 2018;47(6):1164–77. https://doi.org/10.1007/s10964-017-0800-7.
5. Peterson JW, Loeb S, Chamberlain LJ. The intersection of health and education to address school readiness of all children. Pediatrics. 2018;142(5):e20181126. https://doi.org/10.1542/peds.2018-1126.
6. Bowman NA, Logel C, LaCosse J, Jarratt L, Canning EA, Emerson KTU, Murphy MC. Gender representation and academic achievement among STEM-interested students in college STEM courses. J Res Sci Teach. 2022;59(10):1876–900. https://doi.org/10.1002/tea.21778.
7. Rozek CS, Ramirez G, Fine RD, Beilock SL. Reducing socioeconomic disparities in the STEM pipeline through student emotion regulation. Proc Natl Acad Sci. 2019;116(5):1553–8. https://doi.org/10.1073/pnas.1808589116.
8. Villalobos AD. College-going in the era of high expectations: racial/ethnic disparities in college enrollment, 2006 to 2015. Socius. 2021;7:Article 23780231211009994. https://doi.org/10.1177/23780231211009994.
9. National Center for Education Statistics. National Center for Education Statistics (NCES) home page. U.S. Department of Education. n.d. https://nces.ed.gov/
10. Jones AC, Nichols AC, McNicholas CM, Stanford FC. Admissions is not enough: the racial achievement gap in medical education. Acad Med. 2021;96(2):176–81. https://doi.org/10.1097/ACM.0000000000003837.
11. Harris AB, Vankara A, McDaniel C, Badin D, Laporte D, Aiyer A. Match rates among underrepresented minority and female applicants to orthopaedic surgery residency programs from 2011 to 2021: how are we doing? JBJS Open Access. 2023;8(3):e23.00049. https://doi.org/10.2106/JBJS.OA.23.00049.
12. National Resident Matching Program. Applicant demographics and the transition to residency: it's time for change. 2023. https://www.nrmp.org/wp-content/uploads/2023/02/Demographic-data-perspectives-paper_FINAL.pdf
13. Centers for Disease Control and Prevention. Social determinants of health. n.d. https://www.cdc.gov/public-health-gateway/php/about/social-determinants-of-health.html
14. Nguyen M, Chaudhry SI, Desai MM, et al. Association of Sociodemographic Characteristics With US Medical Student Attrition. JAMA Intern Med. 2022;182(9):917–924. https://doi.org/10.1001/jamainternmed.2022.2194
15. Payne-Sturges DC, Tjaden A, Caldeira KM, Vincent KB, Arria AM. Student hunger on campus: food insecurity among college students and implications for academic institutions. Am J Health Promot. 2018;32(2):349–54. https://doi.org/10.1177/0890117117719620.
16. Bravata DM, Watts SA, Keefer AL, Madhusudhan DK, Taylor KT, Clark DM, Nelson RS, Cokley KO, Hagg HK. Prevalence, predictors, and treatment of impostor syndrome: a systematic review. J Gen Intern Med. 2020;35(4):1252–75. https://doi.org/10.1007/s11606-019-05364-1.

17. Alves-Bradford J. Supporting first-generation medical students—improving learning environments for all. JAMA Netw Open. 2023;6(12):e2347475. https://doi.org/10.1001/jamanetworkopen.2023.47475.
18. Delgado AC, Dowling S, Sanchez-Guzman M, Sebok-Syer SS, Gisondi MA. Belongingness among first-generation students at Stanford School of Medicine. MedEdPublish. 2023;13:288. https://doi.org/10.12688/mep.19912.1.

**Open Access** This chapter is licensed under the terms of the Creative Commons Attribution 4.0 International License (http://creativecommons.org/licenses/by/4.0/), which permits use, sharing, adaptation, distribution and reproduction in any medium or format, as long as you give appropriate credit to the original author(s) and the source, provide a link to the Creative Commons license and indicate if changes were made.

The images or other third party material in this chapter are included in the chapter's Creative Commons license, unless indicated otherwise in a credit line to the material. If material is not included in the chapter's Creative Commons license and your intended use is not permitted by statutory regulation or exceeds the permitted use, you will need to obtain permission directly from the copyright holder.

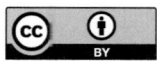

# Chapter 19
# *MedEdPORTAL*: Publishing Educational Innovations

Hannah Turner, Débora Silva, Pilar Ortega, and Sara Hunt

> **Learning Objectives**
> - Describe principles of educational scholarship.
> - Identify strategies for framing educational activities to enhance their publishability.
> - Showcase *MedEdPORTAL* publications that highlight the work of the LHS+ community that can be used to generate ideas of future publications to enhance equitable care of LHS+ patients and communities.

## Introduction

Most institutions uphold the trifold mantra of academia: research, teaching, and service. These core tenets, in their right balance, determine success in higher education. However, not long ago, the definition of scholarship was limited to traditional discipline-specific research. In 1990, Ernest Boyer, then president of the Carnegie Foundation for the Advancement of Teaching, challenged what it meant to be a well-rounded scholar [1]. He argued that knowledge is acquired not just through traditional discovery but also through integration, engagement, and teaching [1]. Boyer developed a model that redefines and clarifies the different domains

---

H. Turner (✉) · S. Hunt
AAMC (Association of American Medical Colleges), Washington, DC, USA
e-mail: hturner@aamc.org

D. Silva
University of Puerto Rico, San Juan, Puerto Rico

P. Ortega
University of Illinois College of Medicine, Chicago, IL, USA

National Association of Medical Spanish, Chicago, IL, USA

© The Author(s) 2026
J. F. Sánchez et al. (eds.), *Advancing Latino, Hispanic, or of Spanish Origin+ Leadership in Academic Medicine*,
https://doi.org/10.1007/978-3-032-07570-3_19

**Table 19.1** Boyer's expanded model of scholarship [1]

| Domain | Knowledge acquired by |
|---|---|
| Scholarship of discovery | Traditional research |
| Scholarship of integration | Interdisciplinary connection-building |
| Scholarship of application | Practical problem-solving |
| Scholarship of teaching | New and innovative approaches in the presence of learners |

of scholarship, showing how different facets of academic life contribute to the inclusivity of knowledge acquisition (Table 19.1). Scholars have further built upon this framework, invoking additional components of academic medicine that have not been sufficiently captured by the three core tenets. For example, Roberts proposes a five-mission model for academic medicine, adding two additional dimensions to the trifecta of research, education, and clinical service: collaboration with communities and a commitment to professionalism, ethics, and justice [2]. The expansion of the mission of academic medicine has important implications for how scholarship is defined, potentially allowing for a growing number of innovative scholarly products to be published that may not have fit more traditional definitions of scholarship. It also has implications regarding who is qualified and well positioned to generate scholarship that addresses the multiple facets of academic medicine. For example, individuals who have been historically excluded from academic discourse, such as LHS+ scholars and those marginalized by race, ethnicity, gender identity, language, religion, disability, or other factors, may play a particularly important role in generating robust educational innovations that can be published as scholarship.

## Educational Scholarship

The scholarship of teaching and learning, also known as educational scholarship, is distinct from scholarly teaching. Scholarly teaching is an effective and purposeful approach designed to maximize learning. An example of scholarly teaching is the refinement of an established instructional method or a teaching strategy that improves learner outcomes.

Educational scholarship extends beyond what is taught. It encompasses a comprehensive and rigorous research process, drawing from the literature and employing a scholarly lens to explore how learners comprehend information and how teaching practices impact this cognitive process [3]. An example of educational scholarship is the publication of an innovative, tested instructional method in a peer-reviewed journal.

It is important to note that scholarship is not a casual endeavor or based on subjective factors. The work must be successfully peer-reviewed based on established standards of scholarly development, made public through dissemination, and available through a platform that others can build on [4].

Boyer's model revolutionized the definition of a successful faculty member, leading institutions to recognize the value of educational scholarship in promotion and tenure decisions.

## *MedEdPORTAL*: The Evolution of a Journal

Recognizing the increasing demand for acknowledging teaching and learning as a valid scholarly pursuit, the Association of American Medical Colleges (AAMC) identified an opportunity to support the academic medicine community by providing a platform for peer review and dissemination of educational works. In 2005, *MedEdPORTAL* was launched as a peer-reviewed, online repository, enabling educators to freely publish and share educational resources worldwide while receiving scholarly credit and recognition to support their career advancement.

Funded by the AAMC, *MedEdPORTAL* has experienced significant growth over the past two decades, culminating in several key milestones. In 2018, *MedEdPORTAL: The Journal of Teaching and Learning Resources* achieved official MEDLINE indexing, making it searchable through the PubMed database. The journal also joined the Directory of Open Access Journals and fully adhered to the International Committee of Medical Journal Editors' Recommendations for the Conduct, Reporting, Editing, and Publication of Scholarly Work in Medical Journals (https://www.icmje.org/recommendations/). These achievements solidified *MedEdPORTAL's* position as a premier journal in health professions education, showcasing its commitment to excellence in teaching and learning.

In 2020, *MedEdPORTAL* formally expanded its mission to encompass author development, further reinforcing its commitment to increasing access for all scholars, including those historically underrepresented in medicine and publishing. Additionally, the journal maintains its dedication to the *MedEdPORTAL* Author Development Program (https://www.mededportal.org/author-development). This program, composed of trained volunteers who are experienced authors themselves, offers guidance and support to faculty seeking to submit their work to the journal, assisting them in their journey toward successful publication.

## Journal Overview

*MedEdPORTAL* publishes stand-alone, complete teaching or learning innovations that have been implemented and evaluated with medical trainees or practitioners. All publications are turnkey, meaning they are ready for immediate download and implementation without requiring significant customization. Types of publications include faculty development workshops, team-based learning sessions, standardized patient and simulation cases, and more. All *MedEdPORTAL* publications are open access and thus free for anyone to view and use.

While the most current submission instructions and author guidelines are available on the *MedEdPORTAL* website (https://www.mededportal.org/author), the following general characteristics apply to all submissions.

*The learner population is within the journal's scope.*
The educational innovation must be designed for and implemented with training or practicing physicians (e.g., medical school, residency, fellowship, faculty development, continuing professional development) and may also include trainees or practitioners across the health professions. Even though interprofessional learners are welcome, the primary audience must represent those within the medical education continuum.

*The educational objectives and the evaluation are appropriate and aligned.*
All objectives should be learner-centered and SMART (specific, measurable, action-oriented, realistic, timely) [5]. Objectives should be aligned with the instructional method and level of evaluation, whether in knowledge, skills, attitudes, or some combination of these. Bloom's taxonomy may be helpful in identifying the appropriate extent of the objectives [6]. See the *Skills Exercise* at the end of the chapter to learn more.

*The submission contains an Educational Summary Report (ESR) that is comprehensive, scholarly, and appropriate to the pedagogy used.*
The ESR is a required element for all submissions and serves as a succinct and scholarly expression of the educational activity. It is similar to a traditional journal article in that it should adhere to a structured format with the following sections: Introduction, Methods, Results, and Discussion. *MedEdPORTAL* provides templates to help authors ensure their ESRs are complete and properly formatted. Templates are based on the pedagogy used in the implementation of the educational activity; while most submissions use the standard template, there are specific requirements and templates for activities involving standardized patients, simulation, team-based learning, or assessment.

*All key materials needed to implement the educational activity are provided.*
Each submission needs to include all the files, referred to as appendices, needed to implement the activity (e.g., facilitator preparation, learner prework, handouts, discussion guides, evaluations). The submission should feature an activity that can be easily adapted to other settings and files in commonly accessible formats. All appendices are peer-reviewed as part of the submission and considered key scholarly elements of the publication.

*All third-party content (e.g., images, videos, charts) included in the submission is appropriately attributed and permitted for online publication.*
Unlike most journals where authors transfer the copyright of the words, figures, and tables they publish, *MedEdPORTAL* authors maintain ownership of their publica-

tions via a Creative Commons license. Upon submission, all files will be checked by staff to ensure the authors either own the copyright on all components or have properly attributed the original creators and provided any necessary citation or permission to include those third-party materials in their submission.

All authors should upload their complete submission (the ESR plus all appendices) via the submission form in Editorial Manager (https://www.editorialmanager.com/mededportal/default2.aspx). The submission form asks for information regarding author details, ethical approval, and prior dissemination. Each submission is initially reviewed by editorial staff for formatting and copyright concerns, and edits may be required. Once the authors have addressed these initial concerns, an associate editor and external peer reviewers review the submission. The editor-in-chief makes the final editorial decision and always requests the authors address recommended revisions by the reviewers prior to acceptance. The journal's official acceptance rate is 19%, but it increases to 70% for submissions that adhere to the journal's submission standards and make into peer review.

## Characteristics of a Successful Submission

Submissions to *MedEdPORTAL* are reviewed according to established standards of scholarship. All submissions must be generalizable and demonstrate value for a broad audience of health professions educators. Additionally, all submissions should be innovative and address an important problem that advances teaching and learning of the topic or pedagogy used. Finally, the work must be delivered through a scholarly lens. As noted earlier in this chapter, both the ESR and the appendices should systematically present the activity, using established criteria (Glassick et al. 1997) found in the associated self-evaluation exercise (Table 19.2). This evaluation exercise, adapted from the *MedEdPORTAL* Educational Scholarship Guide (2008), helps users in assessing educational materials based on established criteria for scholarship, enabling them to determine the readiness of these materials for dissemination [7]. As a reflection exercise, while reading the Educational Scholarship Self-Evaluation (Table 19.2), choose an educational activity you think may be transformed into scholarship and decide if it meets all of the criteria.

While *MedEdPORTAL* supports a variety of pedagogies and activity types, there are a few key principles that authors should consider when determining which of their teaching activities will be successful submissions.

**Table 19.2** Educational scholarship self-evaluation (2008) [7]

| |
|---|
| Define your innovative educational activity (i.e., workshop, simulation, assessment, module): |
| *Clear goals*: The scholar explicitly defines the purposes for the work with realistic and achievable objectives for desired goals and outcomes. Important questions regarding teaching and learning methods have been taken into account |
| *Adequate preparation*: The scholar has a solid understanding of existing scholarship relevant to the endeavor (generic and discipline-specific) as well as adequate skills and resources drawn from this research and from prior experience to advance this specific project |
| *Appropriate methods*: In conjunction with the material and the teaching/learning context, the scholar's selections of educational methods fit the goals and are used effectively; the methods are modified as necessary to accommodate situational changes |
| *Significant results*: The scholar achieves or exceeds the original goals; the scholar's work contributes substantially to others (e.g., learners and colleagues) and to the field; the scholar's work is open to further exploration (e.g., by self, by others, collaboratively with others) |
| *Effective presentation*: The appropriate style and methods of presentation are used, and the resulting communication to the intended audience is clear and unambiguous |
| *Reflective critique*: The scholar thoughtfully assesses the work and uses the resulting perceptions along with reviews and critique from others, to refine, enhance, or expand the original concept |

## *Active Learning*

Following best practices in adult learning theory, most submissions include active learning strategies that appeal to the visual, auditory, and/or kinesthetic learner and incorporate one or more of the following elements: case discussions, small- or large-group work, simulation cases, standardized patients, role-play, intermittent assessment, and/or debriefings [9]. A workshop or module may include some didactic elements interspersed with interactive elements, but a purely lecture-based submission will likely not be successful. This is because lecture-based formats tend to be passive, requiring less engagement from learners, and thus are less effective in promoting deep learning and skill development. By contrast, active learning strategies encourage learners to engage directly with the material, fostering better critical thinking and application of knowledge in practical settings. Innovative strategies for active learning beyond the elements described here can also be considered, as long as they meet the overall definition of active learning and other criteria with regard to replicability and generalizability. For example, some authors have published educational innovations such as the use of games [10], narrative medicine [11], and graphic medicine as pedagogical approaches [12].

## Appropriate Size

Since all elements of an activity need to be submitted, peer-reviewed, and usable by others, the overall size of the educational innovation—such as the number and size of files and the number of curricular hours required—should be considered. Discrete activities, such as workshops, focused small-group sessions, or simulation cases, are more likely to move through peer review and be implemented by others looking to supplement their programs. Multisession curricula or longitudinal courses tend to be too large for peer review and are less generalizable for readers to implement at their institutions due to curricular variability and space. Authors implementing a longitudinal or multisession curriculum should consider evaluating and submitting one or more smaller, stand-alone components. For example, a longitudinal medical Spanish course involving 80 h and multiple sessions is too unwieldy for a single *MedEdPORTAL* publication, but stand-alone modules focused on specific clinical encounters, such as conducting a patient history interview or discussing treatment options in Spanish, have been successfully published.

## Sufficient Evidence

The learning activity should have been implemented with and evaluated by enough learners to garner generalizable results. The activity should build on existing evidence or published scholarship in its content and/or format and also in its evaluation (e.g., learner type, Kirkpatrick level [13], pre-/posttest significant difference). The submission of assessment tools requires validity evidence. For instance, a 1-h workshop on Deferred Action for Childhood Arrivals (DACA) for 112 medical students, where a comparison of average pre- and posttest results revealed a significant knowledge increase, would meet this criterion [14].

## Uniqueness

The submitted activity should not already be widely disseminated online or in the literature. Similarly, the core material should be original to the submitting authors. Activities such as journal clubs that primarily rely on learners accessing preexisting (e.g., articles, videos, podcasts) do not demonstrate a unique contribution by the authors. Prospective authors should search the existing literature to ensure that their submission would represent a unique contribution to *MedEdPORTAL* and the broader medical education literature. Table 19.3 lists specific examples of more successful and less successful submission types.

**Table 19.3** Educational activities potential in *MedEdPORTAL* peer review—do any of your teaching activities meet the criteria for success?

| More successful in peer review | |
|---|---|
| Activity | Reason |
| Discrete workshops | Reasonable size<br>Active learning elements<br>Concrete learning objectives |
| Simulation cases (SP or manikin) | Templates are available<br>Content is scriptable |
| Interactive modules | Exportable for local use<br>Easy to distribute |
| Less successful in peer review | |
| Activity | Reason |
| Lectures | Tend to be passive<br>Tend to be less unique |
| Assessment tools | Requires several sources of validity evidence |
| Longitudinal courses | Excessive number of appendices<br>Sheer size hinders peer review and usability |

## Writing the ESR

Once authors choose an appropriate activity for submission to *MedEdPORTAL*, they will need to describe the activity and its scholarly contribution via the ESR. As mentioned above, the ESR includes the traditional sections (Introduction, Methods, Results, Discussion) as well as a section listing educational objectives. Both the ESR and the appendix files, which include the actual activity, together form a comprehensive submission to *MedEdPORTAL*. Each component undergoes a detailed peer review process.

*MedEdPORTAL* provides ESR templates in its author instructions (https://www.mededportal.org/author) to help outline the key points of each ESR section. Most submissions follow the standard ESR template. The pedagogy-specific templates include additional detail and case schemas that authors should utilize for successful submission.

The following sections outline key considerations for writing each section of the ESR based on the content of the ESR workshop [15].

## Educational Objectives

The educational objectives must follow the SMART format [5], with verbs selected according to Bloom's taxonomy [6]. Most submissions include three to five educational objectives that are supported by the evidence reported in the results section. A *Skills Exercise* at the end of this chapter provides practice writing SMART objectives.

## Introduction

The introduction is where the authors engage the reader (or editor) in the significance of the submission. Using Lingard's (2015) problem/gap/hook framework, authors can consider a simpler problem/gap/purpose outline for structuring this session [16]. At least one paragraph dedicated to each element:

- Problem: Define the clinical or educational problem addressed (e.g., mental health in Puerto Ricans post-hurricane María, nonalcoholic hepatitis in LHS+ patients) or the gap in existing education (e.g., teaching medical students to work with qualified interpreters during history-taking with a Spanish-speaking patient).
- Gap: Describe the gap in the existing literature that this activity and the related evidence aim to fill. Authors should show familiarity with medical education literature, including prior *MedEdPORTAL* publications and/or other relevant publications, to convince the editors/peer reviewers that their work adds value.
- Purpose: Outline the goal of implementing the educational activity for the target learners.

## Methods

The methods section should cover the who, what, where, and how of the educational activity, with specifics down to room setup, timing queues, and references to each appendix file in order of implementation. Assessment methods should also be described. Additional guidance can be found in ESR templates on the *MedEdPORTAL* website (https://www.mededportal.org/author).

## Results

The results section includes such details as the number of participants, the number of respondents to surveys or assessment tools, and a summary of the analysis of the data collected to demonstrate the authors achieved the educational objectives through their activity. Authors may include illustrative tables and figures where appropriate.

## Discussion

The discussion section has a suggested five-paragraph structure:

*Summary.* Provide a high-level summary of what was taught and/or discovered.

*Results Analysis.* Analyze the results, describing three key findings and why each occurred.

*Lessons Learned.* Discuss lessons learned from implementation (e.g., change in group sizes for more robust discussion, leadership buy-in, adaptations from passive to active learning or from in-person to virtual formats).

*Limitations.* Address any limitations, often focusing on evaluation methods (e.g., self-report surveys or knowledge gain assessments rather than patient outcomes) and the extent to which the activity met stated educational objectives.

*Implications and Future Directions of the work.* Cover the implications of the findings, potential for future work, or expansion to new audiences or instructional methods (e.g., how the authors have advanced the science of teaching and learning, policy implications, potential audiences or instructional methods for expanding results).

## Collections

*MedEdPORTAL* publications are searchable by keyword and, at the time of writing, were organized into collections on the website. Collections curate publications around emerging areas in health professions education. The journal has identified two areas that represent a long-term focus: *Interprofessional Education* (established 2018 in partnership with Interprofessional Education Collaborative) and *Diversity, Equity, and Inclusion* (established in 2018 by Associate Editor, John P. Sánchez, MD, MPH). At the time of writing, there are also several subcollections covering timely topics, each affiliated with an active call for submissions: *Anti-racism in Medicine, Telehealth Education, and Language-Appropriate Care and Medical Language Education.*

Given that 70% of LHS+ individuals report speaking Spanish at home (Pew Research Center 2019), comprising 57% of US-born LHS+ individuals and 94% of those foreign-born, the Language-Appropriate Care and Medical Language Education is especially pertinent to the LHS+ community. Additionally, according to data from the AAMC Electronic Residency Application System, the vast majority of LHS+-identifying residency applicants report having advanced or higher skills in Spanish [17]. Hence, this collection provides a unique venue for accessing and publishing peer-reviewed content that addresses the healthcare needs of Spanish-speaking patients and may also be of particular interest to learners and physicians motivated to care for LHS+ communities and other linguistically diverse groups. Two of the three collection aims are to publish language-concordant clinical and communication skills relevant to specific populations with non-English language preferences and educational materials that will improve the knowledge and clinical skills needed to access and collaborate with medical interpreters and other healthcare team members who can enhance language-appropriate care. The call for submissions is driven by the *MedEdPORTAL* Diversity, Equity, and Inclusion Collection under the guidance of collection editors Pilar Ortega MD, MGM and Débora H. Silva MD, FAAP, MEd. Since this collection will include material in languages other than English, such as educational material to teach medical Spanish, the instructions for this collection include specific guidelines to support multilingual authors and ensure the quality of non-English language materials.

It is also important to note that the concept of addressing multiple languages in a US peer-reviewed journal represents a key innovation that recognizes linguistic diversity as a professional asset with regards to publishing. Unique elements of the language collection on *MedEdPORTAL* include the following:

- Submissions should include *more than just the use of a different language* as their sole distinguishing feature. In other words, they should not simply be translations of previously published English-language curricula. For example, submissions should consider what clinical topics are most appropriate based on the importance of patient communication and shared decision-making and the target linguistic community's unique health needs.
- In the ESR Methods section, authors must *describe the strategies used to ensure the quality of the non-English content*. One approach is to ensure that one or more authors have confirmed native or functionally native proficiency in the target language for the specific language domains (e.g., writing, speaking, reading, listening). For example, if the materials are videos, a person with native functionally or native proficiency in the speaking and listening domain will be critical. If written materials are provided, then writing and reading proficiency will be needed. Other strategies may include conducting an internal critical review by a nonauthor who has the required expertise, engaging a professional translator, or using focus groups of linguistically qualified participants to review and confirm the usability of the material.
- Authors should *be mindful of inclusive terminology* when referring to linguistically diverse groups. For example, terms like "language barrier" and "limited English proficiency (LEP)" centralize English monolingualism as the norm. Instead, terms like "language discordance" (instead of "barrier") and "language preference" (instead of LEP) reframe language as an opportunity to advance health equity through language-appropriate strategies [18].
- To facilitate usability of multilingual content, submissions must *include English translations of any non-English materials*. Additionally, authors are strongly encouraged to *recommend multilingual reviewers* and to specify the language(s) in which those individuals can provide expert review. All reviewers can indicate proficient languages in their Editorial Manager profiles.

Not all publications are featured in collections, and submission to a particular collection is not necessary; rather, authors are invited to submit any innovative and generalizable educational materials in health professions education that meet the journal's submission criteria.

## Expanding Access to Scholarly Publishing

### *Commitment to Diversity, Equity, and Inclusion*

Recognizing the essential role diverse perspectives play in enriching medical education and improving health outcomes for all, *MedEdPORTAL* has developed initiatives that provide meaningful publishing opportunities for scholars whose contributions may be underrepresented in medical education literature. Faculty often dedicate significant time to teaching, service, and mentorship, contributions that are essential but may not be fully reflected in traditional academic metrics. *MedEdPORTAL* supports scholars in translating these valuable experiences into peer-reviewed publications, amplifying their impact on medical education. For instance, in 2019, a group of three medical students and five faculty members created a module titled *Taking Care of the Puerto Rican Patient: Historical Perspectives, Health Status, and Health Care Access*. The authors were able to implement the module at seven medical schools during Hispanic Heritage Month where the team gathered evaluation data that contributed to a successful publication [19]. This project enriched the academic community with new content focused on the health of the LHS+ community and showcased mentorship, educational leadership, and regional impact, supporting the career progression of those involved.

To expand opportunities for participation, *MedEdPORTAL* collaborates with organizations like the Latino Medical Student Association (LMSA) to offer training and development. Through partnerships with the LMSA Faculty/Physician Advisory Council, *MedEdPORTAL* has led dedicated sessions at the LIDEReS (LHS+ Identity, Development, Empowerment, and Resources Seminar) and the LISTOS (LMSA Instruction, Support, Training & Orientation Session for Advisors) conferences and presented posters at the National Hispanic Medical Association (NHMA) and Medical Organization for Latino Advancement (MOLA) conferences. *MedEdPORTAL*'s editorial team has also conducted faculty development workshops at Puerto Rico's four medical schools, fostering skills and confidence in publishing among LHS+ educators and trainees.

*MedEdPORTAL*'s Author Development Program complements these outreach efforts by offering mentorship tailored to the needs of first-time authors, especially those who may lack access to traditional publishing support networks, giving them the tools and guidance needed to share their unique insights and innovations in medical education. This targeted support is a vital component of *MedEdPORTAL*'s inclusive strategy, helping scholars contribute their unique insights and innovations in medical education.

## Mentorship and Guidance for Prospective Authors

*MedEdPORTAL* is committed to providing robust support for prospective authors through various mentorship and resource opportunities designed to simplify the publishing process and foster academic growth. The *MedEdPORTAL* Author Development Program offers monthly Zoom Q&A sessions tailored to authors at all stages of the submission process. These small-group sessions create an accessible environment for participants to discuss project ideas, receive feedback, and gain insights from both experienced mentors and peers, promoting a collaborative learning experience.

In addition to live support, authors are encouraged to utilize the Author Center, a comprehensive online resource that complements *MedEdPORTAL*'s submission instructions. The Author Center provides scholarly guidance on aligning submissions with the journal's standards, offering valuable tools to ensure that authors' contributions meet publication criteria. Together, these resources aim to empower authors by enhancing their skills and confidence, ultimately broadening their access to academic publishing opportunities.

This integrated support system reflects *MedEdPORTAL*'s dedication to making scholarly publishing more inclusive and accessible. By offering structured mentorship and clear, practical guidance, *MedEdPORTAL* actively supports authors from all backgrounds, equipping them to share their unique contributions in medical education and contribute to a richer, more representative academic landscape.

## Supporting LHS+ Health Education

*MedEdPORTAL* has a long-standing history of publishing educational resources that address the unique healthcare needs of LHS+ patients and communities. The journal currently includes over 50 publications focused on LHS+ health topics, ranging from culturally responsive care practices to language-concordant communication tools, and this number continues to grow each year (Fig. 19.1). These publications not only provide critical resources for educators but also advance knowledge and skills in areas essential to improving healthcare outcomes for LHS+ populations. The vast majority of publications focused on LHS+ patient populations are written by authors who identify as part of the LHS+ community, leading to both enhanced population health and career advancement for LHS+ scholars.

*MedEdPORTAL*'s commitment to supporting LHS+ education extends across the continuum of medical education, from foundational training to advanced skills building for experienced educators. Many of these resources address specific, high-impact areas such as chronic disease management, mental health, preventive care, and language-appropriate patient communication.

Table 19.4 highlights selected publications focused on LHS+ community needs across the life span, illustrating *MedEdPORTAL*'s dedication to inclusivity in

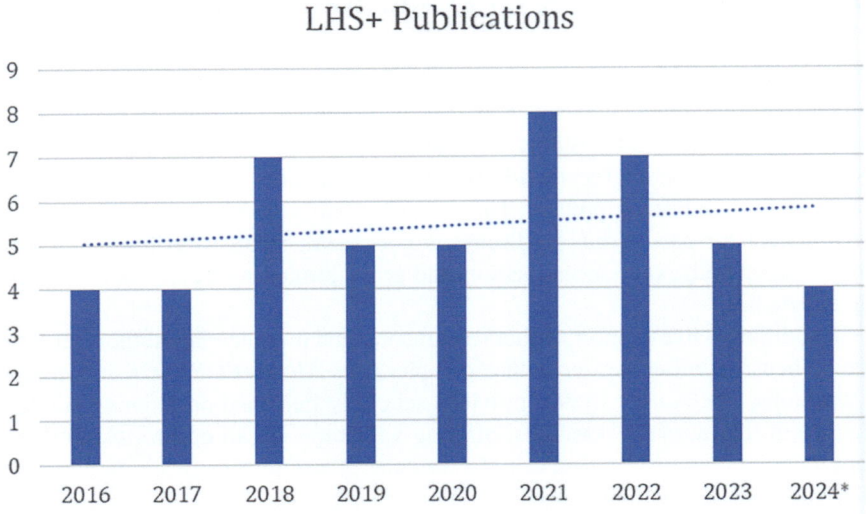

**Fig. 19.1** Quantity of *MedEdPORTAL* LHS+ publications per volume (*2024 Jan.–Oct. only)

**Table 19.4** Examples of *MedEdPORTAL* publications by and for LHS+ communities

| Publication | Brief summary |
| --- | --- |
| "Medical Spanish Endocrinology Educational Module" [18] | An 8-h medical Spanish endocrine module targeting language and cultural skills acquisition. Students practice obtaining a past medical history, obtaining a medications history, providing and explaining a diagnosis, explaining discharge instructions, and discussing sociocultural aspects of endocrine health in Spanish |
| "HIV Pre-exposure Prophylaxis Education for Clinicians Caring for Spanish-Speaking Men Who Have Sex with Men (MSM)" [20] | An education module to train clinicians to discuss pre-exposure prophylaxis (PrEP) with Spanish-speaking men who have sex with men. The module is adapted from an English module on PrEP education. It includes a Spanish-language PowerPoint slide deck with information about PrEP as well as a Spanish-language videotaped scripted clinical encounter |
| "Taking Care of the Puerto Rican Patient: Historical Perspectives, Health Status, and Health Care Access" [19] | A 60-min interactive workshop consisting of a PowerPoint presentation and case discussion aimed at increasing health care providers' knowledge and understanding of the historical perspective that led to Puerto Rican identity, health issues, and disparities, as well as the healthcare access problems of mainland and islander Puerto Ricans |
| "Caregivers Like Me: An Education Intervention for Family Caregivers of Latino Elders at End-of-Life" [21] | A bilingual (English/Spanish) education intervention that includes a video soap opera or telenovela. The video is followed by discussion of hospice, palliative care, and caregiver stress definitions and ends with an explanation of services available for caregivers (i.e., social services, support groups, adult day care, chore workers, home care with or without palliative care, and respite care under hospice) |

educational content and support for healthcare professionals committed to improving health outcomes for all. By prioritizing these resources, *MedEdPORTAL* not only enriches medical education but also plays an instrumental role in bridging healthcare gaps and promoting well-rounded, culturally competent physicians.

## Educational Scholarship Aligned to Career Mission

Aligning educational scholarship with one's career mission and goals is essential when incorporating it into a professional portfolio. LHS+ learners and scholars are often motivated to care for LHS+ and Spanish-speaking communities; incorporating this motivation and skillset into their scholarship agenda can help build a strong academic portfolio that connects personal motivation with professional advancement. Community-aligned initiatives within journals such as *MedEdPORTAL* can be key opportunities for LHS+ scholars to advance their careers.

Faculty members should assess opportunities for educational scholarship that align with their career aspirations and current responsibilities. Converting existing activities like workshops, presentations, small-group teaching discussions, and standardized patient training sessions into publishable modules demonstrates the alignment of educational scholarship with career goals. Seeking additional avenues for scholarship, such as presenting at national meetings to gather evaluations and evidence of effectiveness, can further enhance a scholarly portfolio. Reviewing journal submission guidelines before developing teaching materials ensures compliance with publishing requirements and streamlines the submission process.

Another effective strategy for building scholarship is collaboration. Inviting others to participate in the development and implementation of the teaching activity fosters multi-institutional collaboration and demonstrates the generalizability of one's work. Finding a mentor can open doors to new collaborations and create a supportive environment that builds confidence in the impact of one's contribution to the community. Mentors and collaborators can often be found by reviewing publication bylines and reaching out to authors of papers, even if those authors are outside one's own institution.

Faculty should also consider signing up to review for their target journal(s). Reading and reviewing for journals strengthens teaching and scholarship potential by highlighting best practices and common pitfalls in submissions. As a bonus, consistently providing strong reviews can position faculty as favorable candidates for editorial positions.

## Skills Exercise: Writing Learning Objectives

Learning objectives must be SMART [22]: specific, measurable, achievable, relevant, and time-bound.

*Specific*: Clearly define what you want to achieve with the educational intervention.
*Measurable*: Establish criteria to track progress and success of the educational intervention. This should guide assessment.
*Achievable*: Set realistic goals. Take into consideration available resources.
*Relevant*: Objectives are aligned to the purpose of the educational intervention.
*Time-bound*: There is a deadline for completion.

The verb of the learning objective must be measurable (Table 19.5).

When writing objectives, think of how you are going to measure their attainment. Refer to Kirkpatrick Evaluation Model [13] (Table 19.6):

Let's Practice: Think of an educational intervention you may want to implement. Think about what learners should achieve during the session. Think about the level

**Table 19.5** Measurable verbs for learning objectives

| Examples of measurable verbs | | | Examples of verbs that are not measurable | | |
|---|---|---|---|---|---|
| Define | Match | Recall | Understand | Recognize | Acknowledge |
| Describe | Explain | Identify | Reflect | Realize | Examine |
| Assign | Demonstrate | Interpret | Affirm | Think | Consider |
| Assess | Discriminate | Create | Imagine | Theorize | |

**Table 19.6** Levels of the Kirkpatrick evaluation model

| Level 1: Reaction | Assess the learners' thoughts regarding the educational intervention's relevance, engagement, and their satisfaction<br>Examples: Survey or focus groups at end of intervention |
|---|---|
| Level 2: Learning | Measure the learners' acquisition of knowledge, skills, attitudes, confidence, and commitment<br>Example: Pre- and posttests of knowledge or skills or pre- and post-questionnaires related to learners' attitude, level of confidence, or commitment |
| Level 3: Behavior | Assess that there has been a change in behavior and an implementation of what they learned<br>Example: Observations, interviews, chart reviews, months after the educational intervention |
| Level 4: Results | Measure the overall outcomes of the changed behavior or implementation of what they learned<br>Example: Improved patient satisfaction after a communication skills training of pediatric residents |

of evaluation you will need to implement to evidence successful results of the intervention. Write three SMART learning objectives. Remember to use measurable verbs.

By the end of the session, learners will be able to:
1._____
2._____
3._____

For each objective, check for SMART characteristics:

- Is the objective specific to what the learners should achieve?
- Is the objective written using a measurable verb?
- Is the objective achievable with the available educational resources?
- Is the objective relevant to what the learners should achieve?

## Personal Narratives

### Hannah Turner, MPH

Working for *MedEdPORTAL* for the last 13 years has been an incredible journey as our editorial team has worked to influence and reflect the culture shifts occurring in medical schools across the globe. While I joined the AAMC as an eager, recent pre-med college graduate, my experiences soon revealed another, albeit less direct and immediate, avenue to help improve the health of the world around me. Working as an editor for *MedEdPORTAL*, I have the honor of working with the best and the brightest every day and helping channel and uplift their expertise for the betterment of the medical education community and the patients they serve. Our editorial team prioritizes our authors and readers in every decision we make. In 2005, we began as an open access journal, published under Creative Commons licenses, in order to give our authors full copyright of the work they submit and publish in the journal. In 2016, we changed to a more formal submission format through the addition of the educational summary report, in order to uplift the scholarship our authors were creating. In 2018, we further increased the impact and credibility of our authors' work by undergoing the rigorous application process for MEDLINE indexing. In 2021, we added a CME offering for our reviewers. And today we are working on website modifications to further demonstrate the impact of each publication for its authors with fully accessible metrics for each publication. In between these major milestones, we have also made incremental changes with our community in mind. We constantly work to clarify author instructions and offer to meet with authors to elaborate on decision letters. With a culture of ongoing process improvement, we have revised workflows to improve submission processing times and created calls for submissions in important and timely topics. And in recognition of some overdue self-reflection, motivated by the murder of George Floyd, we formalized our commitment to inclusion through an inclusive language policy, a novel training on bias in editing, the addition of demographic questions to evaluate representation in our contributors, and diversifying our editorial team. Our editorial team values the development of our contributors, and the importance of helping the community see a path forward for their teaching and their career in academic medicine. We bring this mindset into every submission we review and every email we send. We hope that you feel a part of the *MedEdPORTAL* community and see us as a part of your academic journey whether as a reviewer, author, editor, or reader.

**Débora H. Silva Diaz, MD, MEd**
The journey to develop educational scholarship may be straightforward for most faculty, but some really struggle with it, even when they are very successful in other areas of academic medicine. As a Professor of Pediatric Hospital Medicine at the University of Puerto Rico School of Medicine for more than 20 years, I have been blessed with very good mentors and incredible opportunities since early in my career. For many years, I invested time and effort to develop skills as an educator and leader, which led me to important administrative positions such as curriculum office director, associate dean for academic affairs, and section chief, among others, but left very little time for research. It never occurred to me that I could use the educational materials I develop as part of my usual responsibilities and test their effectiveness with the purpose of publication, thus converting them into educational scholarship. I was familiar with *MedEdPORTAL* and had used published material for faculty development workshops but had no real knowledge of how it "worked."

In August 2019, I attended a workshop on *MedEdPORTAL* publishing where I had the privilege of listening to Dr. Grace Huang, *MedEdPORTAL* editor-in-chief and Dr. John Paul Sanchez, *MedEdPORTAL* associate editor. This workshop changed my perspective and attitude toward educational research. Drs. Huang and Sanchez not only went through the steps of how to publish in *MedEdPORTAL* but also inspired me to engage in it. At the time, I was 49 years old, had very little experience with doing educational research, and only two published articles in peer-reviewed journals. My first publication in *MedEdPORTAL* was related to taking care of Puerto Rican patients in the mainland USA. Dr. Sanchez asked if I would be willing to do an educational module on this topic. Once the module was done, Dr. Sanchez asked me if I wanted to participate in a research project to see the effectiveness of the module. Of course, I said yes, and the module was transformed into my educational research project. As part of the methodology of that project, the module was presented and evaluated at seven medical schools in New York which led to collaborations with different faculty that became coauthors of the publication.

This first *MedEdPORTAL* publication opened many doors that I never imagined were possible. First, I am a reviewer for *MedEdPORTAL* and as recommended in the chapter, being a reviewer is very important to develop the skills needed to publish in *MedEdPORTAL*. Second, after being a reviewer for 2 years, I was invited to be a Faculty Mentor, and, in this role, I have been providing guidance to others at my medical school that are interested in publishing in *MedEdPORTAL*. Although the mentoring has not resulted, yet, in submissions, I do not give up and keep at it, because I have learned that to be successful at publishing, one must be patient and keep trying. Third, I was invited to be the Coeditor of the Language-Appropriate Healthcare Medical Language Education Collection. This new endeavor is very close to my heart as it is directed to improving the health of all patients that do not have English as a first language, including patients with sensory conditions that need varied methods of communication. As a bonus, I have been invited to present the module and the topic nationally and international. So, what started as a regular task developing an educational module in a topic I am very familiar with, led to a *MedEdPORTAL* publication, and this is what I which you all to consider doing. It is never too late to start engaging in educational scholarship, and it may lead you on a career path that you never imagined.

**Pilar Ortega, MD, MGM**
My first experience with *MedEdPORTAL* was as a prospective author eager to disseminate my work in medical Spanish education. I had been designing and evaluating my medical Spanish curricular materials for years before I realized there was a journal where curricular materials could be peer reviewed and published. In discussing the challenge of publishing medical Spanish educational scholarship with colleagues, Associate Editor JP Sánchez, MD introduced me to *MedEdPORTAL* as a potential venue for publishing my work. Since my medical Spanish curricular materials were in Spanish, this possibility immediately raised interesting questions about whether and how non-English language content could be incorporated into journal submissions. I decided to embark on the journey to submit my work to *MedEdPORTAL* because the journal was open to working with me on how non-English materials could be appropriately reviewed and published within the journal's structure. In addition to the linguistic aspects, I also had other challenges, such as thinking about how my multi-modular medical Spanish course could be best represented in a *MedEdPORTAL* submission. The entire course was too big to fit into a single ESR and too overwhelming to be readily replicated at other institutions. Thus, the experience of preparing my content for a *MedEdPORTAL* submission helped me reframe and evaluate the material in standalone modules that would be more usable and replicable by others. After my first successful submission, which was a module focused on teaching musculoskeletal and dermatologic Spanish, I was then able to engage other faculty and learners in submitting another module within the medical Spanish course. This second submission was focused on endocrinology Spanish for medical students. During the time that I began to engage as a *MedEdPORTAL* author, I also began participating as a reviewer. Serving as a reviewer provided insights into the overall peer review and publication process that can contribute to reviewers' understanding of what makes a submission more or less likely to succeed. Additionally, as a multilingual medical educator and researcher, I felt that serving as a reviewer was particularly important and meaningful in the

context of the journal's expanded content involving non-English languages. Around that time, I also started informally disseminating information and tips on publishing in *MedEdPORTAL* through my educational and leadership roles, such as through the medical school where I worked as well as through the non-profits that I had founded. For example, the Medical Organization for Latino Advancement (www.chicagomola.com) is a non-profit organization that aims to improve LHS+ health equity and advance the careers of LHS+-identifying and LHS+-serving students and health professionals. I also encouraged colleagues from the National Association of Medical Spanish (NAMS, www.NAMSpanish.org) to submit their work; NAMS is an interdisciplinary group of linguists and health professionals focused on enhancing language equity and medical Spanish education and assessment throughout the medical education continuum. My more recent involvement as Collection Editor for the Language-Appropriate Healthcare and Medical Language Education collection has been the culmination of my prior work as a *MedEdPORTAL* author, reviewer, and as someone who is passionate about mentoring others to enhance their academic portfolio and disseminating knowledge and resources to improve equitable patient care. It has been wonderful to see the collection grow over time, providing evidence-based curricular content to enhance the health of a growing number of diverse populations, languages, and cultures. Continuing to participate as a Collection Editor is also a wonderful way for me to remain strongly connected to the community of medical education scholars. This connection with the academic medicine community and ability to mentor learners and faculty in publishing their medical education work greatly informs my current role as Vice President, Diversity, Equity, and Inclusion at the Accreditation Council for Graduate Medical Education. I encourage anyone interested in contributing to the collection to reach out to me with ideas and questions!

**Sara Hunt**

My mentors and experiences have taught me the importance of acknowledging the influence of others in shaping our journeys and identities. Educators like William Neblett and Carlos Hernandez emphasized the value of coalition building and consensus in community organizing during my undergraduate years. Philosophy professors Minerva San Juan and Cynthia Chance showed me the strength of collective discourse and debate in developing well-reasoned arguments. Colleagues such as Grace Huang and John Paul Sánchez taught me the grounding power of critique and feedback, while friends like Milagros Martinez and Chris Utley highlighted the necessity of true reconciliation for healing collective pain and trauma.

Through these influences, I've come to understand that we need each other to thrive and succeed. This belief aligns with the core values of *MedEdPORTAL*, where the diverse community and mentorship hold significant meaning. The journal's commitment to author development is evident in its mission, which aims to provide access to all scholars, including those historically excluded from medicine. The nationally recognized Faculty Mentor Program, with its one-on-one consultations, group sessions, and conferences, supports authors in their journey toward success. Moreover,

*MedEdPORTAL*'s 35 associate editors, diverse in demographic identities and expertise, collaborate to ensure rigorous scholarship that advances the field and is accessible to all.

*MedEdPORTAL* goes beyond traditional publishing by actively engaging in the growth, development, and success of others. By disseminating resources and tools that showcase best practices and innovations in teaching and learning, the journal not only augments the scholarship of discovery but also strengthens the scholarship of teaching and learning. This commitment to engagement and inclusivity sets *MedEdPORTAL* apart and underscores its role in fostering the growth, development, and success of diverse voices in education and publishing.

# References

1. Boyer EL. Scholarship reconsidered: priorities of the professoriate. Carnegie Foundation for the Advancement of Teaching; 1990.
2. Roberts LW. Innovation and leadership across the five missions of academic medicine. Acad Med. 2021;96(12):1623–4. https://doi.org/10.1097/ACM.0000000000004425.
3. Chick N. A scholarly approach to teaching. Vanderbilt University Center for Teaching. n.d. Retrieved August 29, 2022, from https://my.vanderbilt.edu/sotl/understanding-sotl/a-scholarly-approach-to-teaching/
4. Simpson D, Brownell AM. Educational scholarship: how do we define and acknowledge it? Association of American Medical Colleges. 2006, January 31. Retrieved August 29, 2022, from https://www.aamc.org/professional-development/affinity-groups/gfa/faculty-vitae/defining-educational-scholarship
5. Lawlor KB, Hornyak MJ. SMART goals: how the application of SMART goals can contribute to achievement of student learning outcomes. Dev Bus Simul Exp Learn. 2012;39:259–67.
6. Anderson LW, Krathwohl DR, editors. A taxonomy for learning, teaching, and assessing: a revision of Bloom's taxonomy of educational objectives. Pearson Education; 2000.
7. Glassick CE, Huber MT, Maeroff GI. Scholarship assessed: evaluation of the professoriate. Jossey-Bass; 1997.
8. MedEdPORTAL educational scholarship guide. Association of American Medical Colleges. 2008.
9. Russell SS. An overview of adult-learning processes. Urol Nurs. 2006;26(5):349–52, 370
10. Pisano TJ, Santibanez V, Hernandez M, Patel D, Osorio G. The Bloody Board Game: a game-based approach for learning high-value care principles in the setting of anemia diagnosis. MedEdPORTAL. 2020;16:Article 11057. https://doi.org/10.15766/mep_2374-8265.11057.
11. Silver M, Hussain F. A resident narrative medicine curriculum to promote professional identity development: story-based sessions grounded in narrative learning theory. MedEdPORTAL. 2024;20:Article 11446. https://doi.org/10.15766/mep_2374-8265.11446.
12. Ortega P, Cisneros R, Park YS. Medical Spanish Graphic Activity: a MeGA deliberate practice approach to reducing jargon use with spanish-speaking acute care patients. MedEdPORTAL. 2024;20:Article 11377. https://doi.org/10.15766/mep_2374-8265.11377.
13. Kirkpatrick JD, Kirkpatrick WK. Kirkpatrick's four levels of training evaluation. ATD Press; 2016.
14. Garcia A, Lapidus A, De Witt ML, et al. Deferred Action for Childhood Arrivals (DACA): maximizing impacts in medical education and health care. MedEdPORTAL. 2022;18:Article 11279. https://doi.org/10.15766/mep_2374-8265.11279.

15. Sabina RL, Woods GL, Turner H, Abali E, Simmons JM, Huang GC. The *MedEdPORTAL* infinity mirror: conducting an interactive workshop on how to develop an educational summary report for *MedEdPORTAL*. MedEdPORTAL. 2021;17:Article 11197. https://doi.org/10.15766/mep_2374-8265.11197.
16. Lingard L. Joining a conversation: the problem/gap/hook heuristic. Perspect Med Educ. 2015;4(5):252–3. https://doi.org/10.1007/s40037-015-0211-y.
17. Diamond L, Grbic D, Genoff M, Gonzalez J, Sharaf R, Mikesell C, Gany F. Non-English-language proficiency of applicants to US residency programs. JAMA. 2014;312(22):2405–7
18. Ortega P, González C, López-Hinojosa I, Park YS, Girotti JA. Medical Spanish endocrinology educational module. MedEdPORTAL. 2022;18:Article 11226. https://doi.org/10.15766/mep_2374-8265.11226.
19. Díaz DHS, Garcia G, Clare C, Su J, Friedman E, Williams R, Vazquez J, Sánchez JP. Taking care of the Puerto Rican patient: historical perspectives, health status, and health care access. MedEdPORTAL. 2020;16:Article 10984. https://doi.org/10.15766/mep_2374-8265.10984.
20. Alzate-Duque L, Sánchez JP, Marti SRM, Rosado-Rivera D, Sánchez NF. HIV pre-exposure prophylaxis education for clinicians caring for Spanish-speaking men who have sex with men (MSM). MedEdPORTAL. 2021;17:Article 11110. https://doi.org/10.15766/mep_2374-8265.11110.
21. Cruz-Oliver DM, Ellis K, Sanchez-Reilly S. Caregivers like me: an education intervention for family caregivers of Latino elders at end-of-life. MedEdPORTAL. 2016;12:Article 10448. https://doi.org/10.15766/mep_2374-8265.10448.
22. Doran GT. There's a S.M.A.R.T. way to write management's goals and objectives. Manag Rev. 1981;70(11):35–6.

**Open Access** This chapter is licensed under the terms of the Creative Commons Attribution 4.0 International License (http://creativecommons.org/licenses/by/4.0/), which permits use, sharing, adaptation, distribution and reproduction in any medium or format, as long as you give appropriate credit to the original author(s) and the source, provide a link to the Creative Commons license and indicate if changes were made.

The images or other third party material in this chapter are included in the chapter's Creative Commons license, unless indicated otherwise in a credit line to the material. If material is not included in the chapter's Creative Commons license and your intended use is not permitted by statutory regulation or exceeds the permitted use, you will need to obtain permission directly from the copyright holder.

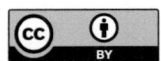

# Chapter 20
# Serving as a Reviewer, Associate Editor, or Journal Editor in Chief

Ana Nuñez, David Sklar, and José Rodríguez

**Learning Objectives**
- Describe the roles of reviewer, associate editor, and editor in chief of a journal.
- Note the steps of the review process for an article submission to a peer-reviewed journal.
- Describe the importance of LHS+ individuals participating in journal work.

## Introduction

Like in medicine in general, LHS+ voices are underrepresented in publishing in the medical literature. While many articles include LHS+ patients as research subjects, relatively few LHS+ physicians serve as editor in chief, associate editor, or reviewer roles. A recent survey of reviewers for Family Medicine reveals that less than 5% of the reviewers identify as LHS+ [1]. In this chapter, we will talk about serving in these roles, with the perspectives of three editors—Dr. Ana Nuñez, Founding Editor in Chief, *Health Equity*; Dr. José Rodríguez, Associate Editor, *Annals of Family Medicine*; and Dr. David Sklar, former Editor in Chief, *Academic Medicine*, the

---

A. Nuñez
University of Minnesota School of Medicine, Minneapolis, MN, USA

D. Sklar
Arizona State University, Phoenix, AZ, USA

J. Rodríguez (✉)
University of Utah School of Medicine, Salt Lake City, UT, USA
e-mail: jose.rodriguez@hsc.utah.edu

© The Author(s) 2026
J. P. Sánchez et al. (eds.), *Advancing Latino, Hispanic, or of Spanish Origin+ Leadership in Academic Medicine*,
https://doi.org/10.1007/978-3-032-07570-3_20

leading journal in medical education. The chapter is written in a questions and answer format with each editor.

## Ana Nuñez MD, Founding Editor in Chief, Health Equity

### How Did You Get to Be an Editor?

I had a working relationship over several decades with a cohort of other Principal Investigators who were also national Center of Excellence Directors in Women's Health collaborators. One colleague who collaborated with our group approached me after a national meeting and asked if I'd help with a presentation on an important topic, so I did. As a thank you, my colleague provided complimentary access to their national meeting, journal, and stipends, so that students could attend their conference. A few months later, the colleague said, "I have an interesting proposition for you. We want to start a new journal and would love to have you consider being the founding editor." I set up a meeting to discern details and checked in with other colleagues engaged in editorial positions to assess the pros and cons. I didn't find anyone who had spearheaded a new journal, and it sounded like an interesting and exciting new opportunity. I had plenty of reviewing experience and mentorship of junior faculty as they crafted grant applications and manuscripts. It was an eye-opening adventure in the world and business of scientific publishing.

### How and Why Did You Start Reviewing?

Fundamentally, it started with a yes. I received emails from journal editors asking me to review articles, and I started as a reviewer. At times, colleagues would ask for my help and I would assess my bandwidth in terms of time available. Early on, there were more yeses than nos. Volunteering to review is an easy way to get involved, there is a great need and far more manuscripts than reviewers. Plus, you learn a lot by reviewing articles.

### What Aspects of Your LHS+ Identity Are Useful in Reviewing, Editing, or Serving as an Editor in Chief?

I have a "soft spot" for individuals who write as they speak, which can be more loquacious than is wanted in standard academic papers. My LHS+ identity likely informs my worldview and penchant for process approaches. I gravitate to a mixed methodology of qualitative and quantitative, since the "why and how" are essential—not just "how much." I am probably more in tune with providing optimistically framed feedback. This is in reaction to what I received, on occasion, comments that landed on me as cruel and unhelpful. I enjoy helping highly motivated individuals by providing feedback for their improvement.

## What Is the Role of a Diversity, Equity, and Inclusion Editor, and If You Served as One, Please Comment

I never served as such, but I think all editors need an eye for recruiting all voices, enabling access and equity in the process and content.

## What Do You Want LHS+ Identified Individuals to Know About Reviewing, Editing, and Writing?

Engaging and being successful in academic medicine requires discrete tools and expertise. Reviewing, editing, writing are skills and have to be honed to improve. The first step is to identify what tools you have, garner new ones, practice a lot, and gain expertise. The point of doing this work is to share your excellent work and ideas with a larger audience, so that you can join the virtual "national conversation" and also learn more from others. Crafting articles and grants are core academic medicine activities. To gain skills in writing—READ! Read beyond the content and the summary. Read to analyze the format of the manuscript—what is its architecture? How could your work benefit from being presented similarly? Reduce the scope of the work covered—you can't effectively write a paper if your thesis is so expansive that it needs a book size to cover the topic. Read the citations; they may be rich with information that will help you in your work. Then, annotate them all—how does this contribute to your thoughts on the subject? Use a robust citation software that enables easy access. Spend the time watching videos to learn robust citation managers—it will pay off in the future. Easy ones are great and fast. Complex ones usually have more features and nuance, so becoming an expert is a good time investment. In addition to reading a lot, attend journal clubs even if you don't completely understand all the aspects of the article. Engagement helps you get a sense about what are the current issues, ideas, and challenges in your field. It helps you optimally frame your article. The more you attend, the more articles you read, the easier it will be to craft manuscripts.

It is important to remember that when you write a review, a human is on the other side reading what you wrote. What did the author do well? What could make it better? Write your reviews as helpful as possible and consider how you would feel receiving what you wrote. If the submission is disjointed, suggest additional readers and reorganization. If unclear, ask if what landed on your interpretation is what they were going for, and if not, how else could they clarify/refine this.

A useful technique to practice editing is to take an article, ignore the abstract, and attempt to write your own abstract based on what you read. Another method is to practice writing presentation abstracts which require concise framing due to word limits of 250 words or 500 words. It can be challenging but is a great exercise in summarizing pertinent information.

With writing, there are some schools of thought that you should write every day to refine your skills. Others are more like binge writers—they need clear space to think and write. The challenge with the latter is that the availability of this open time is rare and hard to secure. Often this results in no writing happening. The best way to write is to write regularly. Put your thoughts down and use the skill of writing to massage and clarify your ideas and messages. It can help you better crystalize your ideas even if every word doesn't result in an immediate manuscript. I am a fan of group writing, since externalizing expectations effectively forces you to write and get it done promptly. Consider when your optimal times are to write. Is it first thing in the morning? Is it in the evening when distractions seem less? Aligning efforts with the best focus is helpful. Just be aware that if you write late at night, you may not be in touch with cognitive fatigue. Cognitive fatigue can be nuanced. It is when you get tired while working, and your output or efforts become less and less, but you don't notice. Plan breaks every 20 min, and assess your progress after the break. Notice if your mind wanders more. It might be time to stop or go to sleep!

## Dr. Jose Rodríguez MD, Associate Editor, Annals of Family Medicine and Deputy Editor, Family Medicine

### *How Did You Get to Be an Associate Editor?*

I applied for the position at Annals of Family Medicine, at the insistence of a friend and mentor. I connected with the editor in chief and was hired the day after the interview. I loved working at Annals of Family Medicine, but I also knew that I would need to make a major career change if I were to ever become an editor in chief. An opportunity arose for me to become a deputy editor, and I again applied for that position. I was hired a few weeks later, but I decided to leave my associate editor job at Annals of Family Medicine because of time constraints. Family Medicine was a better fit for me and published educational research, which is most of my research publications.

### *How and Why Did You Start Reviewing?*

I was asked to review an article for Family Medicine when I submitted an article to that journal. I frequently submitted to that journal, so I was asked frequently to review. I was later asked to be on the editorial board, and part of my service in that role was to review multiple manuscripts per year. I found that I loved the work, and it became something that I did for fun.

## What Aspects of Your LHS+ Identity Are Useful in Reviewing, Editing, or Serving as an Editor?

My LHS+ identity informs much of what I do. Since the LHS+ voice is underrepresented in medical literature, I find that my voice matters in this space and that I offer a unique perspective to the medical literature. Although I do not speak for all LHS+ people, there are things that I have in common with my LHS+ community which need to be studied and published in the literature. At times, if the subject matter of the article is important for LHS+ patients or physicians, I will work more closely with the authors to help them get the paper to a publishable state.

## What Is the Role of a Diversity, Equity, and Inclusion (DEI) Editor, and If You Served as One, Please Comment?

My first editorial job was as the inaugural DEI editor at Annals of Family Medicine. I was hired in January 2021, and I had plenty of work, as multiple manuscripts on DEI were submitted on the heels of the events surrounding the murder of George Floyd. My editor, Dr. Caroline Richardson, was very selective in what she sent to me, but she never limited the articles to DEI articles, and I soon found myself editing non-DEI articles and assisting other associate editors with their papers on DEI.

At Family Medicine, however, I am not a DEI editor, but I work closely with the DEI editor, Dr. Octavia Amaechi.

## What Do You Want LHS+ Identified Individuals to Know About Reviewing, Editing, and Writing?

LHS=-identified individuals can get started in editing by becoming reviewers. Review first and review often. After reviewing, you can start writing with entry-level products like letters to the editor and personal narratives. Moving forward, you can team up with faculty to write more advanced articles, like literature reviews, and brief reports on research projects.

# David Sklar MD, Former Editor in Chief, Academic Medicine

## What Is the Purpose of Medical Journals?

Medical journals exist as a trusted source of information for health professionals and the public, and ultimately, they can have a role in improving the health of the population by providing new information and changing the behavior of health professionals and the public. For this to occur, there must be a rigorous review process of submitted articles, so that accurate, high-quality articles are identified and published. Over time, the number of published articles has multiplied, so journals must work to provide material of greatest value to readers. Thus, curating the submitted articles is a principal role of journal editors.

During the COVID-19 pandemic, in the first 20 months up until August of 2021, there were over 200,000 COVID-related publications in the medical literature [2]. Sorting these articles and making publication decisions required time, expertise, and a balancing of accuracy and timeliness of publication. Volunteer peer reviewers read the articles and submitted their recommendations to the journal editors, who decided on acceptance, revision, or rejection. During the pandemic, access to new information could be the difference between life and death for many patients suffering from the new disease. The public depended upon the peer-reviewed literature for information that might help them make critical healthcare decisions for themselves and their families.

One can follow several pathways to becoming a reviewer, such as a nomination from a current reviewer to the editor based on that person's knowledge of your expertise. Still, another standard route can occur when you submit an article you have written, and the journal may request that you become a reviewer at that time.

There are several other purposes of medical journals. Medical journals improve the quality of articles submitted through the review process. Comments, suggestions of peer reviewers, and suggestions of the editors and staff should improve the article's clarity. Reviewers examine the methods, analysis, and conclusions to identify any errors or ambiguity, which the authors can then address to make the article's message clear to readers.

Medical journals also allow authors, reviewers, and editors to communicate and share ideas and experiences through participation in the journal's activities. This loose social activity has been referred to as a community of practice recognizing the nurturing and support that often occurs for those who participate in the work of the journal at meetings for reviewers from the journal. Medical journals have an important role in the promotion process of many medical schools both through providing a good venue for publication of scholarly work for validation of the quality of the scholarship of faculty and to recognize the participation of faculty as excellent reviewers through letters to promotion committees.

For faculty who might be considering becoming a reviewer, associate editor, or editor in chief, it is important to understand the purpose of the journal and whether there is a good fit between the journal and individual's interest. Typically assistant, associate, and editor in chief positions are selected from among those who have distinguished themselves as excellent reviewers, so becoming a reviewer is the first step in the progression toward an editor role.

If a faculty member may be interested in becoming involved with a journal either as a reviewer, or at a higher level of commitment, the first step is to become competent in research and submit articles to journals that might be of future interest. Because there is a constant need for new reviewers at most journals, one source of possible of new reviewers is those who have recently had an article accepted by the journal. Many journals routinely invite those who have an article accepted to become a new reviewer. The initial invitation of a new reviewer often comes with some education about the journal's review guidelines including expected format, turn-around time, and areas of special interest or expertise. There may also be a checklist to assist the reviewer. Academic Medicine, where I served as Editor in Chief for 7 years, has a wonderful resource that includes information about the steps in reviewing an article with a checklist called the Review Criteria for Research Manuscripts [3]. By reviewing the articles submitted by others, most scholars improve their own work in the process as they look critically at every part of the article in a very close reading. Many journals rate the quality of the reviews and can provide a history of ratings and numbers and types of decisions made by reviewers. Reviewers who refuse an invitation frequently and/or do not respond to invitations risk being removed from the reviewer pool.

## *What Is the Review Process?*

Submitted articles go through a review process in which there is an initial screening process. In some cases, the screening process is done by the editor in chief or deputy editor. In other cases, more junior associate editors screen the articles. The reason the screening process is necessary is that for many journals, there are more submissions that can be sent out to reviewers and to prevent burning out reviewers with too many reviews a portion of submissions are rejected without review. For some journals, that may constitute 50% or more of the submissions.

Unfortunately, if an article is rejected without review, no explanation for the rejection accompanies the rejection letter, so that the authors do not learn what the problem with the article might be as they would if the article had been sent out to reviewers. On the other hand, the rejection without review usually happens quickly and so does not delay the submission to another journal. There is an article from Academic Medicine by Meyer et al. that provides some further information about the reject without review process at that journal [4]. In general, the factors that lead to a reject without review decision are that the article is not a good fit for the journal in terms of content or the article does not appear to add anything new to what is already known about the topic. One can avoid the fit issue by reading the several issues of the journal and making sure that topics that are related to the submission have been published in the journal. As to the second issue, one needs to read the brief literature review that usually occurs in the article's introduction to see if the submitted article fills some of the gaps in the literature.

If the submitted article survives the initial screen it gets sent out to two or three or in some cases four reviewers depending upon the journal. Often, one of the reviewers is a statistical/methodology expert who may not be familiar with the specific content of the submission and is looking at methodological and statistical issues or in a qualitative paper there may be a qualitative expert who looks at the qualitative methods. The other reviewers are generally content experts who will also look at the methods but are primarily considering whether the article is presenting novel, important information that will change thinking about a topic or fill in gaps in our knowledge. They will write comments and grade the article as accept, minor revisions, major revisions, or reject. Very few articles receive an acceptance upon first review. Minor revisions usually denote interest in the article if minor issues are addressed. Major revisions indicate a need to significantly rewrite the paper with attention to the problems identified, and there is no guarantee of acceptance even if all the problems are addressed. Reject means that the journal is not interested in seeing the article again even if all of the problems identified by the reviewers are addressed. Sometimes the comments from reviewers appear to be positive and encouraging, yet the editor's decision is to reject the article. This may occur, because in confidential comments to the editor, a reviewer raised more serious problems that were not shared in the reviews back to the authors.

When an author gets an article back from review and the decision is major or minor revisions, it is a good idea to pause and think about the comments before racing back to work on the paper. Some comments may appear to be unfair or too critical, but there is no point in fighting with reviewers. My own experience has been that even when I don't agree with the comments from reviewers, I usually find that the paper is better with the revisions that were suggested than it was without them. After sufficient time has passed, the author should create a matrix with each comment from a reviewer. Then the author should create another column about how the comment was addressed, and then another comment about where the editor can find the evidence that the author did what they said they did in the new manuscript. Every comment from reviewers should be addressed and if they are contradictory or impossible to fix that should also be addressed in the matrix and in a letter back to the editor.

The revised manuscript will then be resubmitted (in the time frame indicated), and there will then be another round of reviews and a new decision. This process may continue for several revisions. I had one of my articles go through three revisions recently, so perseverance and patience are helpful attitudes.

I have spent some time going through this process, because by and large, this makes up the major work of editors at all levels. They have to read the articles, read the reviews, make decisions, read the articles again and the revisions, and make decisions again, and all of this typically occurs late at night or on weekends when another work from one's main job is complete. If these seem like tedious tasks, the role of editor might not be a good fit, and a reviewer role might be better.

## *What Is the Role of the Editor in Chief of a Journal?*

The voice of every journal is the editor in chief (EIC). The EIC sets direction of the journal usually with an editorial board that provides input. The EIC is the final arbiter of decisions about publication, and the reviewers and associate editors are all advisory to the EIC. This is a very senior position and depending on the journal not only has responsibility for what is published in the journal but is also responsible for the review process, the choice of invited commentaries and editorials, and any political controversies raised by the content of the journal. EICs usually have had experience at the journal as a reviewer or assistant or associate editor before becoming EIC and negotiate a term if service with the organization that is financially responsible for the journal. The EIC may be paid a salary or may be voluntary and unpaid. In some cases, the financial well-being of the journal may be a partial responsibility of the EIC in conjunction with the publisher or sponsoring organizations. Some journals are provided to members of organizations as a benefit of membership and with those journals the EIC may have other roles with the sponsoring organization. The EIC appoints deputy, associate, and assistant editors as well as reviewers, and the number of these positions and their function and authority vary depending upon the journal. The diversity of the associate editors and editorial board is important, because these positions contribute to the outreach for invited articles and also can suggest special issues or concentrations that address topics of interest to diverse readers and to those in leadership positions who may be influenced by the content. EICs who appreciate the important contributions of a diverse group of associate editors and editorial board will benefit by conducting meetings in which the ideas and opinions of the editors and editorial board can be shared and may lead to editorials and other articles that are outgrowths of the discussions.

While every EIC is different in terms of what they look for in an article, I tended to look for something with new and important ideas that aligned with the interests of our readers and that would influence the thinking of our community and the public about an issue. I would like the article to tell a story which starts by explaining what the problem or issue is that authors are trying to address with the article. The problem has to be important and of interest to the readership of the journal. Then I would want to know what is already known about the topic based upon the literature that has been published, so a good literature review needs to accompany the article. As part of the description about what is known, I also want to know what the gaps are in our knowledge about the problem. Hopefully the article will address some or all of the gaps. If I am happy that the article addresses an important problem, I look at what methods were used and why were they the right methods for the problem. And then what results were found using the methods and did they answer or solve the problem. If so how. If not, why not. There should then be a discussion that explains what we have learned from the article that is new and important and what unanswered questions remain. We also should have some description of the limitations of what has been studied. The conclusion should only address what the methods have shown and succinctly tell us the take-home message from the study.

There are many opportunities for diverse faculty at all levels to participate in journals. Journals are looking for a diverse group of reviewers, editorial board members, and assistant and associate editors. Some journals have opportunities for students, residents, and junior faculty or those interested in being a fellow for a year with an EIC or senior editor to learn about the journal and the various skills needed to be a leader. It is worth exploring the fellowship option even if it is not officially offered. Sometimes, the EIC may be interested in offering a new position on the editorial board for a person who represents a new perspective that is missing at the journal. In our current environment where there is enormous change in the influence of media and technology in the healthcare system, someone with a new idea and new perspective is usually welcome to make a pitch to the EIC. It may not succeed, but it might lead to other opportunities with the journal.

Medical journals are undergoing enormous change as technology makes it possible to share new research findings prior to formal review. COVID-19 accelerated such change because of the critical need for information to understand and treat a new disease. The review process of traditional journals was too slow to provide a rapid dissemination of information, and so various online platforms and "living reviews" were published. Individuals shared information through blogs that sacrificed validity for speed and misinformation and intentional disinformation appeared side by side with legitimate research. The future role of journals and editors will be influenced by both the useful innovations in publishing and the dangers of misinformation. The role of a diverse editorial voice and leadership will be more important than ever as journals navigate this new environment. I envision new review processes using artificial intelligence and the use of media in new ways to communicate with the coming generations of health professionals. This will be an exciting time to become involved with journals at all levels, and I believe Ernest Boyer who defined four attributes of scholarship would have to expand his categories of scholarship to encompass the coming changes [5, 6].

## References

1. Rodríguez JE, Amaechi O. Results of the family medicine journal reviewer demographic survey. Fam Med. 2024;56(9):531–3. https://doi.org/10.22454/FamMed.2024.768129.
2. Ioanidis JPA, Salholz-Hille M, Boyck KW, Baas J. The rapid massive growth of COVID-19 authors in the scientific literature. R Soc Open Sci. 2021;8:210389.
3. Durning SJ, Carline JD, editors. Review criteria for research manuscripts. 2nd ed. Washington, DC: The Association of American Medical Colleges; 2015.
4. Meyer HS, Durning SJ, Sklar DP, Maggio LA. Making the first cut: an analysis of academic medicine editors' reasons for not sending manuscripts out for external peer review. Acad Med. 2018;93:464–70.
5. Boyer EL. Scholarship reconsidered: priorities of the professoriate. Princeton: Carnegie; 1990.
6. Boyer EL. The scholarship of engagement. J Public Serv Outreach. 1996;1:11–20.

**Open Access** This chapter is licensed under the terms of the Creative Commons Attribution 4.0 International License (http://creativecommons.org/licenses/by/4.0/), which permits use, sharing, adaptation, distribution and reproduction in any medium or format, as long as you give appropriate credit to the original author(s) and the source, provide a link to the Creative Commons license and indicate if changes were made.

The images or other third party material in this chapter are included in the chapter's Creative Commons license, unless indicated otherwise in a credit line to the material. If material is not included in the chapter's Creative Commons license and your intended use is not permitted by statutory regulation or exceeds the permitted use, you will need to obtain permission directly from the copyright holder.

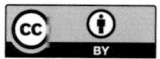

# Chapter 21
# Hospital Leadership Roles and Perspectives: Promotion and Leadership Development in Academic Medicine

Joseph R. Betancourt, Denice Cora-Bramble, and J. Emilio Carrillo

**Learning Objectives**
- List the different types of hospitals and key leadership roles within hospitals.
- Describe the state of diversity in hospital leadership positions.
- Reflect on the experiences and lessons learned from LHS+ identified hospital leaders.

## A Brief Overview of Hospitals

Hospitals are a major source of health care in the USA, housing healthcare professionals, advanced practice practitioners, nurses, among others, as well as medical and other equipments. According to the American Hospital Association, there are more than 6000 hospitals in the USA, but it is important to understand they are not all the same and can vary in size, focus, funding, mission, origin, services, and tax status, to name a few (Institute for Diversity, 2015). As such, hospitals can be classified based on several factors such as the following:

---

J. R. Betancourt (✉)
The Commonwealth Fund, New York City, NY, USA
e-mail: jschiff@cmwf.org

D. Cora-Bramble
George Washington University School of Medicine, Washington, DC, USA

J. E. Carrillo
Weill Cornell Graduate School of Medical Sciences, New York City, NY, USA

1. The services they provide or who they provide them to, including general hospitals which provide a broad range of services, or specialty hospitals, which have a specific focus (e.g., Children's Hospitals, Psychiatric Hospitals, Orthopedic Hospitals, Rehabilitation Hospitals, Veterans Hospitals)
2. Their location, including urban (city or densely populated population area), rural (sparsely populated areas), and community-based (suburban)
3. Their tax status, including for-profit (where revenue helps generate profit for shareholder investors, and taxes are paid to the government) or not-for-profit (where any profits must be reinvested for services and there is tax-exemption in lieu of activities that benefit the community)
4. Their level of care—such as acute care, tertiary or quaternary care—designations that aim to delineate the level of specialty services provided (higher along the scale indicates hospitals that take on more specialized care with greater acuity)
5. Their funding source, including whether they are private (and billing provides primary revenue) or public (meaning they accept government subsidies to provide care to the uninsured)
6. Their commitment to training, including whether they are academic (meaning they train medical students or residents) or nonacademic
7. Their tie to a larger health system, including whether they are integrated into a system with other hospitals or independent or freestanding
8. Their affiliation to, or religious origins, including whether they were funded and are under the direction of the principles of a particular organized religion (e.g., Catholic, Baptist, Adventist, Jewish)

The key here is that these classifications are not mutually exclusive. By this, we mean that one hospital can fit various characteristics (private, not-for-profit, academic, urban, or private, for-profit, specialty, etc.), although the large majority of hospitals in the USA are private, general, not-for-profit, and affiliated with a larger health system.

## Hospital Leadership Positions

Hospitals are complex organizations that are managed by a leadership team, providing oversight on a key set of critical functions and operations. Leaders on the team are often referred collectively as working in the "C-Suite," as a handful of key positions begin with "Chief" in their title. In some institutions, these individuals can also have the title of executive vice president, senior vice president, or vice president. Whereas hospitals may vary in their leadership structure, there are key positions that almost all hospitals have in common. Here is a brief, basic overview of key leadership positions at hospitals and the areas they oversee.

*The President and Chief Executive Officer* (CEO) are the top leaders who provide oversight and direction over hospital strategy and operations. The president is hired by and is accountable to the board of trustees of the hospital.

*The Chief Operating Officer* (COO) is often the second in charge, supporting the president in all efforts, and frequently overseeing hospital operations and managing others on the leadership team.

*The Chief Financial Officer* (CFO) is the leader who provides oversight of hospital finances and budget.

*The Chief Medical Officer* (CMO) oversees medical affairs that often include medical policy, professional conduct, and other relevant clinical issues.

*The Chief Nursing Officer* (CNO) is the lead nursing executive, providing leadership for the nursing staff, and often other patient care services.

*The Chief Quality Officer* (CQO) oversees all efforts related to quality measurement, improvement, patient safety, and patient experience.

*The Chief Human Resources Officer* (CHRO) provides leadership and management of human resources, including setting and overseeing policies and practices for all employee and employment matters.

*The General Counsel* provides leadership for all of the hospital's legal matters and can lead this work with a small internal team and/or oversee external teams who provide support in this area.

*The Chief Development Officer* (CDO) provides leadership on matters relating to philanthropy and fundraising for the hospital.

*The Chief Academic Officer* (CAO) provides leadership of all educational, training, and research areas at a hospital.

*The Chief Diversity and Inclusion Officer* (CDIO) oversees efforts related to diversity and inclusion at the hospital.

*The Chief Health Equity/Community Health Officer* oversees efforts in the areas of health equity (equity in the delivery of clinical care) and community health (community-based efforts to improve health and well-being of communities).

All hospital leadership teams include every position described above, except some may not have a CDO if fundraising isn't a major focus. Additionally, non-academic hospitals will not have a CAO. The CDIO and Chief Health Equity or Community Health Officer positions are variable as well. Although these positions have been increasing in recent years, not all hospitals have formal leaders in the C-Suite overseeing these portfolios of work as these areas may not be an area of emphasis or formal priority. As such, there may not be "formal" leaders to guide this work.

## The Work of a Leadership Team

Hospitals leaders work together to execute a strategy and oversee operations. This work is guided by the President/CEO, who, as described above, reports to the Board of Trustees. The Board will meet regularly with the President and leadership team as dictated by their governance role, and they have overall responsibility for all matters pertaining to the hospital. These include those related to quality, finance, accounting and integrity, human resources and compensation, and investment, to name a few. The President/CEO, in turn, will meet routinely with their C-Suite leaders to develop strategy, create an execution plan, and manage operations. Goal setting usually occurs prior to the beginning of a new fiscal year. Hospital leaders have their performance monitored, and they are held accountable for achieving their agreed-upon set of goals. Base compensation and financial incentives are included to encourage achieving said goals. Over the course of the year, the President/CEO will convene with the leadership team (often referred to as the "Executive Leadership Team" or some similar term) to monitor progress, address new and emerging issues, and set new goals as needed and dictated by any situations that emerge. This usually occurs weekly. The President/CEO, in addition to meeting with the team regularly, will usually and routinely also do one-on-ones with each individual on the leadership team to review each area in more detail. This might occur every week, or every 2–4 weeks, depending on the leader and what they oversee for the hospital (the President/CEO may meet weekly with the COO, CFO, and CMO, for instance, and less routinely with others).

## Diversity in Hospital Leadership

Diversity in leadership is essential in all sectors of healthcare delivery, especially in the context of healthcare disparities and the national pursuit of health equity. An extensive body of research has demonstrated the impact of diversity in health care, including on the care and experience of diverse patients [1, 2]. Like in other areas of health care, there is a significant lack of diversity in hospital leadership. In the last major survey period of the American Hospital Association's Institute for Diversity and Health Equity, minority representation among hospital leadership made little progress from 2011 to 2015; representation among CEOs remained at 9%, Board Members at 14%, and executive leadership was 12% in 2011 and 11% in 2015 [3]. Some progress has been made at the level of first and mid-level managers, increasing from 15% in 2011 to 19% in 2015. Furthermore, Fig. 21.1 demonstrates that the majority of the diversity at the level of the Executive Leadership Team is found among Chief Diversity Officers [4]. The racial and ethnic background of Board Members and Executive Leadership, as seen in Fig. 21.2, demonstrates a stark underrepresentation of Laino/a/x/e individuals [4], despite this population being the largest, youngest, and fastest-growing minority group in the USA [5]. This data clearly calls out the dire need for LHS+ hospital leadership.

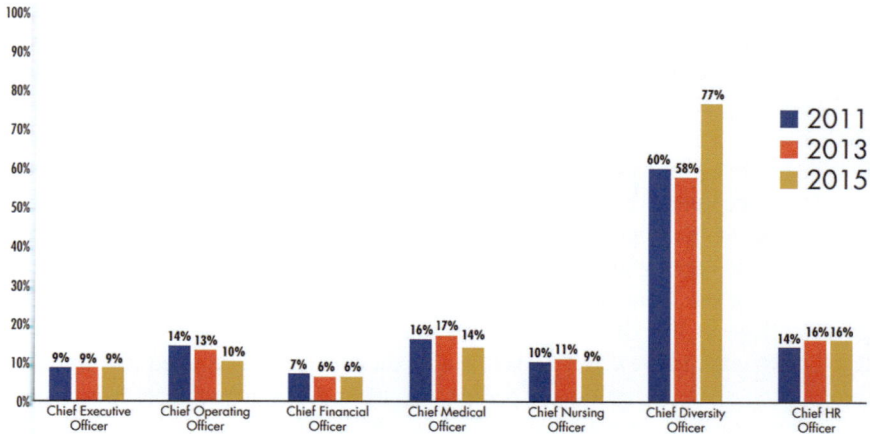

**Fig. 21.1** Minority representation in executive leadership positions [4]

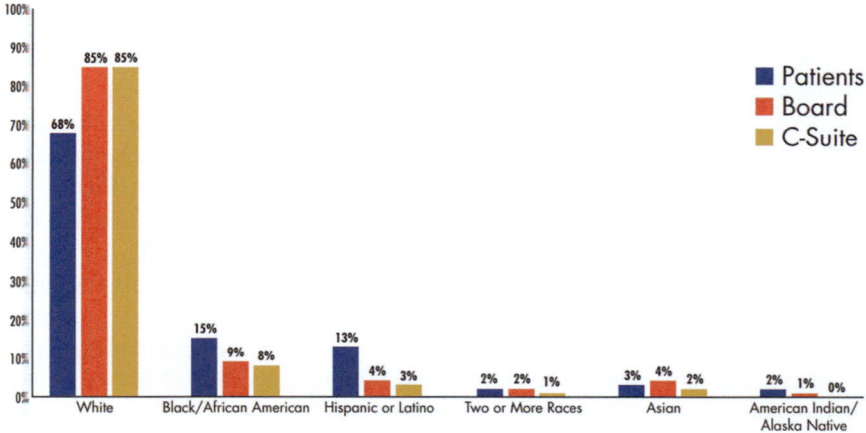

**Fig. 21.2** Minorities represented on hospital boards and executive leadership positions [4]

## Personal Narratives

As described above, LHS+-identified individuals are drastically underrepresented in hospital leadership. This section will provide some background and reflections from three successful LHS+ hospital executives. It will include a bit about their journey, key lessons learned, and their recommendations for how future leaders should prepare and the things they should be aware of if they are interested in pursuing a career in hospital leadership.

## Joseph R. Betancourt, MD, MPH

My grandparents came from Puerto Rico to New York City in the 1950s, working in the sweatshops in the garment district of Manhattan, clearing rooms at the YMCA, and becoming small business owners of a bodega in Spanish Harlem. My parents came over as children and faced the challenges of being recent immigrants, having limited English proficiency, and the discrimination that goes along with this. Despite all of this, they persevered, neither achieving a college education, but both dogged about stressing the importance of education. Caring for those who were vulnerable around us and organizing the community for social justice were early and formative exposures for me. Thanks to the sacrifices of my family, I was fortunate enough to go to college at the University of Maryland, and progress to medical school at Rutgers-Newark in New Jersey. While a medical student, I realized two important things. First, there weren't many people who looked like me, or came from where I came from, or who were bilingual. This quickly made me realize my culture, my language abilities, and my lived experience were unique assets in the clinical environment, especially in the care of diverse populations. Second, and connected to this and my family's experience, I realized that these assets came with incredible responsibilities. If people like me weren't going to step up and lead for our communities, who would? It became clear to me that I had to impact more than the patients I cared for; I needed to figure out how I could have bigger impact and scale to truly help our communities. This is where the fire to be a leader was sparked and what motivated me on a journey to learn everything I could to be an effective and thoughtful leader—including getting opportunities and learning so much from my coauthors. This journey began with a transformational leadership experience—the Commonwealth Fund-Harvard University Fellowship in Minority Health Policy after my internal medicine residency. It then progressed to my joining the Massachusetts General Hospital (MGH) and founding the Disparities Solutions Center. It culminated with my becoming Vice President and Chief Equity and Inclusion Officer, and then shortly thereafter, Senior Vice President for Equity and Community Health at MGH. In this last capacity, I oversaw a $25 M budget and a team of about 140. It is from this more than two decades of experience, and incredible mentors, collaborators, and colleagues, that I humbly share my key leadership lessons for those aspiring to be hospital leaders—and leaders in general. I'll begin with some foundational lessons:

*Information is everywhere—access it*

We live in a unique time. When I was an aspiring leader, I had to peruse bulletin boards for opportunities, read leadership books, and perhaps make a phone call to a leader who I admired in hopes that I might get some of their time and attention and learn from them. Today, information is everywhere. You can learn about leadership all over the internet, hear podcasts, watch videos on Youtube, and even read Twitter threads. Similarly, leaders are just an email away, easy to find, and often eager to help and connect. The first lesson here is take advantage of the information available to you and the unprecedented connectivity you have at your fingertips. Formal learning is one thing, but we are in an age of teaching ourselves and truly accessing the experts. Take advantage of this as you aim to build your leadership skills.

*Learn the Healthcare Leadership Landscape*

In this chapter, we try to provide you with an overview of the leadership landscape within hospitals. The truth is, leadership in health care is broad, and there are opportunities everywhere, including in health plans, community health centers, private industry, and public health, to name a few. It is important to be a diligent student of health care and healthcare leadership, so you can sharpen your approach and find the best fit for you.

*A successful career is at the intersection of passion, strengths, and organization of daily work.*

The most important thing you can do as you drive toward a fulfilling professional life is early self-exploration. A fulfilling career is one where you are doing work that you are passionate about; where most of your time at work is spent leveraging your areas of strength; and where you enjoy the ways your workdays are organized. Early in your career, you may not have these sorted out. Certainly, you may know what you are passionate about, but you still may not know your strengths, or how you like your days organized. Ultimately, you learn this over time, but trying a lot of things, through trial and error, and by talking to leaders who you admire and learning about their day to day. Once you discern your passion, your strengths, and how you work best daily, you can begin to build toward a career that maximizes all of these for you.

I'll now conclude with the key skills I have learned over the years and that I believe are essential for executive leadership:

*Understand structures, centers of power, and drivers of your organization*

As a leader, it is important you understand your organization—both formally and informally. You must understand the formal structures, such as the organizational chart, but you also must understand the informal centers of power, drivers of the organization, and what the key currencies that lead to success.

*Communication skills are key*

Clear, concise yet comprehensive and passionate communication is everything in leadership and necessary in all aspects of the work. You will want to find your voice over time, master your communication style, and don't be afraid to be passionate while being clear, concise, and comprehensive. Again, this takes years to perfect and evolves over time as you see styles that you can emulate while customizing to your own voice and experience.

*Lead through listening, and make people feel valued and respected*

The single most important skill in leadership is listening. Lead by listening. Not only can you learn key things that can make you and your organization better but by listening you make your colleagues feel valued, respected, heard, and much more likely to follow your leadership and vision. You must listen genuinely, actively, and deliberately and demonstrate that what you heard has helped shape your perspectives, and your leadership vision.

*Build and sustain trusting relationships and go out of your way for people and your team*

Leadership is about trust. For people to follow you, they have to trust you and your vision. Building trust by earning trust is a critical skill, and building trusting relationships is a key ingredient in building loyalty. One way this can be achieved routinely is to go out of your way for people, for all people, and to do it when it is not expected. You shouldn't do this for show, and you should do this to demonstrate selflessness, and the importance of sacrifice as you lead.

*Be values-driven, consistent, and equitable*

Respect from your peers comes from being values-driven, consistent, and equitable. Even if people do not agree with your decisions, they will follow your lead if they believe you are doing the right things for the right reasons.

*Be strategic, tactical, and effective at operations*

Leading with vision is important, but being strategic, tactical, and effective at operations and delivering on outcomes is what really sustains leadership. Ultimately, leadership is producing results, and this cannot be done if there isn't a focus on operations and details.

*Inspire teams to believe in you and see themselves as helping shape, and be part of the vision*

Inspiring others to change is essential, as change is hard, and others need to see themselves in the change, and feel there is something much better for all on the other side. Helping people feel like they are shaping the vision really facilitates organizational change.

*Share your journey and mentor and help develop and grow the individuals on your team*

It is important to share your journey, especially if it is relevant to the work you are trying to lead. Additionally, it is critical to mentor others into leadership positions and help grow them as individuals and key members of your team.

*Lead with integrity, transparency and be genuine, humble, and human*

Integrity, honesty, humility, transparency, and being genuine and human are key leadership principles. These are not platitudes; they are characteristics that when real, and deliberate, will improve your leadership capacities.

*Be available, accessible, and approachable*

Leading "on the ground" means being available, accessible, and approachable. This takes time, and deliberate effort, but the dividends you reap will be a sense of connectedness with your team, as opposed to the common "otherness" of lofty leaders. Eliminating hierarchies, and being flatter in your organizational approach, facilitates leadership and builds loyalty.

*Try to not take things personally*

Leadership often requires a thick skin. Learning to not take things personally—harder than it sounds—is a key leadership survival skill. As a leader, you often represent multiple things, not just yourself, and as such, you can become a vessel for many emotions from individuals across the organization. Realizing this allows you to sustain your efforts and avoids the expenditure of energy in battles that aren't necessarily about you, but what you represent.

*Balance in work/life*
Your energy and drive need to be replenished consistently by balancing work with joy. Being planful about finding joy—in any activity that does that for you—is important, because it will not happen by chance. Sometimes the grind of work takes the joy out of you, even when you are passionate about the work you do. Finding balance and finding joy are critical to leadership.

### Denice Cora-Bramble, MD, MBA
How would I define my career journey in a nutshell? Success against all odds. At times, the challenges, emotions, and soul wrenching experiences of leadership are not easily captured with data or even expressed with words. The pearls of my leadership journey developed over time, as pearls do in nature, a natural defense, layers against an irritant, eventually creating what is known as "mother of pearl." I can't say that I saw the pearls forming in my life, nor did I fully appreciate their beauty and importance.

My first pearl developed in my early years after migrating from Puerto Rico to enroll at George Washington University at the tender age of 16. I had an adolescent's heart with a semiformed identity and a relentless dream to become a pediatrician. My language challenges were not apparent to others but were an added hurdle for me. I listened to my professor's lectures in English and went through the exhausting mental gymnastics of translating them into Spanish while taking notes in class.

On campus I felt most at home at sundown when the Black- and Brown-faced housekeeping staff sat outside the dorms to wait for their shifts to begin. I felt like a drop of melanin in a sea of vanilla. The academic rigors, the Latino-Anglo cultural clash, my sheer naivete and a constant longing for home led to a seemingly endless river of terrifying freshman tears.

There is a bird in my native Puerto Rico, called the "pitirre" or gray kingbird. Despite its small size, it is known for his courage, perseverance, and unwavering ferocity, even when facing challenges from much bigger birds of prey. Like the "pitirre," I tackled Goliath-sized challenges with the innocence and insecurity of youth. My first pearl taught me the value of relentless perseverance, quivering courage, and soul-piercing faith.

A second pearl began forming during residency, when I delivered our first child. The birth of two sons followed during the early and mid-career phases of my leadership journey. Keeping all the balls in the air, or at least not dropping the important ones, was a central theme as I juggled my roles as a mother, wife, and pediatrician. Those three pillars at times were symmetrically balanced, and at others, symmetry was only an illusion in search of the user's manual.

My maternal role was reversed when I enrolled in business school at the age of 40 with three kids in tow. I laughed when the kids boldly asked me whether I had finished my homework! I learned to prioritize and to schedule my faculty meetings after the basketball schedule was finalized, so that I would not miss the games, particularly the playoffs. I mustered the nerve to not be apologetic with my bosses when I had to attend a teacher's conference. I learned not to sweat the small stuff and to use the asymmetric pillars as teaching moments for our kids. There were professional opportunities that I had to decline, but I did so without regrets or remorse. This precious second pearl shouted its wisdom: There is no "do over" with raising kids, so one must prioritize them and be there for them. Always. They will remember.

I stumbled on my third pearl, when I was recruited as the first Black Chief Medical Officer in Children's National Hospital's 150-year history. What does it mean to be the first? To be an "N" of one? How does one lead under these circumstances? On some days, it felt like I was swimming in a fishbowl, with my successes and failures transparently visible and on display for all to see. I carried the invisible backpack of bias and racism that other Black and Brown leaders carry but learned to thrive in spite of the load.

My leadership training, beyond the school of hard knocks, was instrumental in preparing me for this difficult yet rewarding CMO role. I was competitively selected as a Kellogg National Leadership Fellow and was given a unique career defining opportunity and funding to learn about global leadership as I traveled to South America, Europe, and other countries. I enrolled in the MBA program at Johns Hopkins University, as part of my Kellogg Fellowship individual learning plan. Courses such as negotiation, leading and managing change, and others, were critically important in preparing me for the CMO position. The important leadership enabler, being comfortable in one's own skin, is the most difficult to learn and hardest to teach others. How do I define the phrase, "being comfortable in one's own skin"? I found the answer in the third pearl and learned to be true to my unique leadership style, to be authentic, and to bring all of me to the role; to be bold and courageous in confronting bias and racism; and to never compromise my ethical principles.

Academic walls were the irritants for my fourth pearl. As a woman and a woman of color that has reached the pinnacle of her career, I have many academic wall stories to share. The beauty of this pearl is in how I responded to the word "no:" no to promotion, no to the grant, no to the award, and no to the position. An academic career can be immensely rewarding. Mine certainly has been. But embedded in the rewards, I found the irritant grains of sand. The word "no" must not shake one's self-esteem nor should it make one feel like an impostor. The fourth pearl is that "no" need not be the end of the road. It is merely an inflection point, time to regroup, to reconsider, to reexamine, or a time to press on.

My patients helped form my fifth and final pearl. I have been privileged to work side by side with world renowned clinicians, researchers, educators, and advocates. But my patients' voices and our clinician-patient journeys helped shape who I am today as a leader: the illegal immigrant who was raped by her "coyote" during her journey across the Rio Grande, the adolescent with three concomitant sexually transmitted infections, and the crack baby abandoned in the hospital by his mother. These patients and many others presented with clinical issues, but their social and financial barriers seemed insurmountable. Their silent voices shout out asking all of us to be their tireless advocate, their bridge, asking us to open doors for them, to provide for their needs, and to use our collective power and voice to help them.

**J. Emilio Carrillo, MD, MPH**

Hospitals are an integral part of the community. Hospitals touch people at the time of their greatest joys and their greatest sorrows. They provide health care at every stage of a person's life and anchor the community. Besides providing health care, the hospitals are often the largest employers in a community. In particular, the New York municipal hospitals are situated at the heart of many Latino communities. The municipal hospitals in New York have traditionally opened their doors to all regardless of immigrant status or ability to pay.

During the early 1990s, I had the privilege of running the NYC Health and Hospitals Corporation. This is the largest municipal health system in the country, serving all including the poor and disenfranchised. I had the opportunity to build on generations of doctors and staff who have advocated for the right of every human being to have access to caring, comprehensive, and high-quality health services.

I steered the corporation through a critical period in the City's history when a financial crisis, crime, drugs, and AIDS challenged the City's healthcare infrastructure. We navigated these challenges by partnering with the unions and the community and making the hospitals reflect the communities they serve. Primary care joined hospital care at the forefront of healthcare services. Primary care became its own fiscal and operational center allowing for greater growth and creativity. Similarly, the seeds were planted for a municipal managed care plan which would protect the interests and needs of our communities.

Talent was looked for and recruited in communities not previously represented. Diversity and inclusion were practiced decades before society understood the importance of broad representation by those communities that are served. The Central Office team grew to include representation from the Latino, African American, Afro Caribbean, and Chinese communities. We built the first diverse team to run and strengthen the Corporation.

Two members of the team went on to become future Presidents of the Corporation.

Cultural competency became a key driver of health care. A strong push was made to enhance the language and cultural capabilities of Bellevue Hospital's Psychiatric services. Physician diversity and inclusion were advanced as were the capacity to provide interpreter services and culturally appropriate care. The interpreter services were added or expanded throughout the other municipal hospitals.

Other hospitals in New York also opened their doors to cultural competence and created a wide diversity of programs from staff training to cafeterias serving food reflective of the communities served.

## Skills-Based Exercise

Create an "elevator pitch"—a brief, 2-min summary that is clear and concise—that describes why you are interested in a hospital leadership position, and what leadership skills you would bring to that position.

## Reflection Exercise

Given what you have learned about hospital leadership, is there a position that seems appealing to you? If so, why? And what it would take for you to build your skills and experience to prepare yourself for such a position?

## Conclusion

Latino/a/x/e leadership in health care is essential to the future of our nation. Given the important role hospitals play in caring for patients, training healthcare professionals, and providing the environment for clinical research, there are ample opportunities for leadership. Furthermore, there are multiple leadership positions, and a variety of hospitals to choose from, and drive toward. In this chapter, we aimed to illustrate the hospital landscape, highlight the importance of diversity in leadership, and describe our journeys, sharing lessons learned along the way. Our hope is that those who read this material will not only be inspired to pursue a position in hospital leadership but also be informed on how to get there and how to be successful once you arrive.

## References

1. Dreachslin JL, Hobby F. Racial and ethnic disparities: why diversity leadership matters. J Healthc Manag. 2008;53(1):8–13. https://pubmed.ncbi.nlm.nih.gov/18283965/
2. Dreachslin JL, Weech-Maldonado R, Gail J, Epané JP, Wainio JA. Blueprint for sustainable change in diversity management and cultural competence. J Healthc Manag. 2017;62(3):171–83. https://doi.org/10.1097/JHM-D-15-00029.
3. Livingston S. Racism still a problem in healthcare's C-suite. Modern Healthcare. 2018, February 24. https://www.modernhealthcare.com/article/20180224/NEWS/180229948/racism-still-a-problem-in-healthcare-s-c-suite
4. Institute for Diversity in Health Management & Health Research & Educational Trust. Diversity and disparities: a benchmark study of U.S. hospitals in 2015. 2016. https://ifdhe.aha.org/system/files/media/file/2020/03/Diverity_Disparities2016_final.pdf
5. U.S. Census Bureau. 2020 census results. 2021. https://www.census.gov/programs-surveys/decennial-census/decade/2020/2020-census-results.html

**Open Access** This chapter is licensed under the terms of the Creative Commons Attribution 4.0 International License (http://creativecommons.org/licenses/by/4.0/), which permits use, sharing, adaptation, distribution and reproduction in any medium or format, as long as you give appropriate credit to the original author(s) and the source, provide a link to the Creative Commons license and indicate if changes were made.

The images or other third party material in this chapter are included in the chapter's Creative Commons license, unless indicated otherwise in a credit line to the material. If material is not included in the chapter's Creative Commons license and your intended use is not permitted by statutory regulation or exceeds the permitted use, you will need to obtain permission directly from the copyright holder.

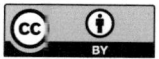

# Chapter 22
# Considerations in Switching Institutions for Career Advancement: Background of the Road Traveled

David A. Acosta

> **Learning Objectives**
> - Describe considerations in switching institutions for career advancement.
> - Describe the challenges and opportunities inherent in career shifts.
> - List better practices in navigating transitions between institutions.

## Introduction

My journey after completing my residency training in Family Medicine (FM) and Community Health began in a small rural town with a population of 7000 (county draw of 22,000) located 85 miles from the nearest regional medical center. I became one of the two medical directors for three Federally Qualified Health Centers that served a large migrant farmworker population. After 8 years of practice and serving as a FM clinical preceptor for the University of Davis School of Medicine, I made the decision to enter academia and made my first switch to another institution. I was recruited to join the faculty of a FM residency program affiliated with the University of Washington School of Medicine (UWSOM) and housed in a large metropolitan health system. In my second year, I was promoted to associate residency program director and fellowship director of a new rural family medicine fellowship program. After 14 years, I was recruited to become the inaugural assistant dean of multicultural affairs at the UWSOM in Seattle who was a physician and the first LHS+ assistant dean in the School of Medicine—my second switch to another institution and health system. After serving for 10 years, I was recruited to the University of California Davis Health System to serve as their inaugural Chief Diversity and Inclusion Officer (CDIO) and first LHS+ executive to serve in the C-suite—my

---

D. A. Acosta (✉)
American Medical Colleges, Washington, DC, USA

third switch. After 4 years of service, the Association of American Medical Colleges (AAMC) recruited me to my present job as CDIO—my fourth and, hopefully, final switch. Here too I was the first LHS+ CDIO to serve at the AAMC.

## Restless in Seattle

Early in my career, I found myself becoming restless after 4 years of practice—a time that made me reflect on my personal life as a Latino, my career, and professional development. At first this, restlessness concerned me that this was abnormal behavior, and it made me wonder if everyone experienced this phenomenon. Questions that spun around in my head included: "Is there something better out there than what I'm doing now?" and "Is what I'm doing as good as it gets?" and "What's making me feel this way?"

Since that experience, that feeling of restlessness recurred every 4 years. I soon began to realize that for me this was a natural phenomenon. Always questioning and challenging myself was in my Latino DNA, and I now have come to the conclusion that it has made me become a better person, a better clinician, a better medical educator, and a better administrator. Exploring "what else was out there" pushed me forward to new limits and enabled me to expand my horizons in ways that I could not have done if I stayed in one place. Now that I look back on my career, I ask, "what lessons have I learned along the way?" "What lived experiences and lessons can I share as a Latino in switching institutions for career advancement?"

## Lesson #1: Weighing the Balance—Inhibitors Versus Catalysts of Success

### Inhibitors of Success

Sometimes inhibitors (barriers, challenges) can be the driver that push you to begin exploring elsewhere. For example, the diversity, equity, and inclusion (DEI) framework I had developed for the UWSOM—an interprofessional model that expanded across all health science disciplines at the UW that included nursing, public health, pharmacy, social work, and medicine and the medical center, where DEI was the central element that was interconnected with all the disciplines—did not land well with the dean of the SOM. The dean and I did not see eye to eye on this opportunity. He was not interested and felt strongly that DEI work should remain solely within the medical school (the inhibitor). There was another inhibitor that influenced my decision. Although I was promoted to become the inaugural CDIO at the UWSOM in my final year, I was never invited to join and participate in the dean's C-suite meetings with the other chief officers. As a result, I began to explore and applied to other available job positions around the USA. I soon discovered that many other medical schools were intrigued by the DEI framework I developed and were very interested in adopting that framework for their institution. This was the catalyst and the validation I needed to switch institutions. As a result, I chose to join the UC Davis SOM and Health System.

## *Catalysts for Success*

Catalysts can also be the driver to push you to explore. For example, for me personally, it was about exploring something meaningful other than what I was presently doing, exploring something that could be a "game changer" given the events that were happening when I decided to explore (e.g., the 2016 election). Catalysts can be a personal call to action. I felt that if I wanted to do something meaningful for the greater good, especially for the Latino communities like the one I came from, I needed to be intentional and "go into the belly of the beast to slay the dragon." Hence, my move to Washington, D.C., to work for the AAMC.

In addition, future aspirations (e.g., professional development, personal growth) can also serve as significant catalysts and drivers of change. I asked myself, "Could I grow professionally and personally as a Latino if I stayed at the UWSOM?" After exploring other job prospects (I interviewed at three different academic health centers), I finally accepted the fact that I was not going to grow professionally at the UWSOM due to the dean's set of limits that he imposed.

## Lesson #2: Benefits vs. Risks of Switching Institutions

Finally, it is important to consider both the benefits and the risks associated with switching institutions.

## *Benefits*

One of the biggest benefits that came from switching institutions was that it was "therapy" for my restlessness. It confirmed for me that sometimes there *are* better places than the one you are presently employed at. The other added benefit is that it created the opportunity to test my ideas, any new concepts I had developed, e.g., asking myself, "Will these ideas work in other institutions?" For example, switching institutions provided the "true test" for the new DEI framework that I developed at the UWSOM, e.g., "would it work at UCDSOM? Could I operationalize the framework in a shorter time frame at UCDSOM, since I had a better idea on how to get stakeholder buy-in?" Initially, my efforts took literally 10 years to develop and implement this framework at the UWSOM. It took only 3 years at UCDHS.

Lastly, switching institutions brought on new challenges for me and an opportunity to advance my learning (influenced my professional development and my leadership development):

Learning how to be *nimble* in a new setting
Learning how to be a *change agent* and understanding the importance of change management (understanding that any DEI initiative is a change initiative)
Learning about *transformational leadership* and how important this leadership style was in creating transformative changes in the system to disrupt the status quo
Learning how my *cultural identity* as a Latino influenced my leadership style

## *Risks*

And again, there are several risks to consider. Changing institutions too frequently can be interpreted as a "red flag" in some circles (by recruiters, by search committee faculty reviewing your resume) and can make administrative leadership weary of you. The stress that accompanies moving can place a huge burden on your spouse, your significant other, and your family, e.g., stress of moving, stress of adapting to a new community (especially if it's far away from extended family members), stress of your children needing to leave their friends and their school and transitioning to a whole new school, etc. These are such important factors to discuss. I strongly believe that the decision you make about transitioning to another institution in a different location must be a joint decision if you are going to succeed professionally and personally. In addition, the institution needs to not only recruit you, but they also need to recruit your spouse (or your significant other) if they plan to successfully recruit you. The good news is that most institutions recognize this as a key factor in their recruitment efforts. For example, both the UCDSOM and AAMC took the time to reach out to my spouse to understand her needs and desires. AAMC set up a professional agency to work with her and introduced both of us to the local community (including the local LHS+ community).

The other risk you need to consider is discovering that you're not as adaptable and as resilient as you thought you were. Definitely a true reality check! At the same time, you may discover that the institution that is recruiting you is not being as forthcoming as you thought and hoped for.

## **Better Practices to Consider**

So here are some better practices to consider when you are considering switching institutions. Allow me to share some of the lessons that I have learned over the years:

*It's OK to explore*! You're never going to know if things are better than the present place of employment unless you go outside your walls. Give yourself permission to do so.

*Be realistic and honest* with yourself. Are you the problem? Is this why you're having difficulty with the institution that you are presently at? In some cases, it sometimes is too easy to blame the institution for the issues that you're facing. Or is it truly the institution that is the problem? Is this why you're having difficulty?

*Visualize what success looks like.* It's equally important to envision what success looks like for you. And remember, that vision can and does change over time. Several factors from your personal life, e.g., the relationship in your marriage, your spouse's or significant other's job opportunities aspirations, extended family issues like the care of one of your parents, the children (their schools, the extracurricular activities) as well as your professional life, can have significant impact on influencing that vision over time. Realize that this *is* normal and it's easier to grasp if you can anticipate it.

*Pros and Cons.* When you have found a place that you're considering transitioning to, be sure to list your pros and cons—the *absolute* contraindications, e.g., things you are not willing to give up (on both the personal and professional level). From a personal level, this included my cultural identity as a Latino. These absolute contraindications are the *nonnegotiable* things on your list. Don't forget to include the *relative* contraindications, e.g., things that you may be willing to sacrifice or give up. These are the *negotiable* items on your list.

*Location is everything.* It is true what real estate agents swear by—location, location, location! This includes the landscape and the terrain you want to live in. Geographic location is important to consider and what will make you happy. What type of environment do you want to come home to after a long grueling day at the office, clinic, or hospital? What environment allows you to defuse? Location also includes the political, social, and economic climate of the community you choose to live in. Is it important to you to live in a Latino community? It also includes job opportunities for your spouse or significant other, education opportunities for your spouse, significant other, and/or your children. This also includes the demographics of your community and of the institution you're planning to work at.

*Visit the institution and community you have your eye on more than once.* Campuses and communities change from day to day. It's not uncommon to experience it on a good day, but what's it like on a bad day? Is that something you're ready to deal with?

*Joint decisions.* It seems obvious, but sometimes you just have to hear it again and again. Be sure that if you are in a relationship that you make this a joint decision and not a unilateral decision.

*Document, document, document.* It's important that you document *everything* that you were told by your recruiters, by the leaders you met during your interviews. It's too easy to forget the details of the many conversations you had and of the promises that were made. Talk is cheap. Write some of these details down that you can refer to once you get to the negotiation phase.

*Contract negotiations.* There's a simple rule of thumb to follow—*everything* for the most part is negotiable. Don't let people tell you otherwise. Once you have your contract in hand, be sure that you read it in its entirety and never assume anything. This is not a time to "skim" the contract. If there is language or content in the contract that you do not understand, do not sign anything until you have a clear idea of what these terms mean. In some cases, it is worth hiring a contract lawyer to review the contract if you're not used to reviewing contracts (average cost is about $350).

*Your value and assets.* Next rule of thumb—do not underestimate your worth. We often underestimate our own value and the assets we bring to the table and frequently undercut ourselves when it comes to salary negotiations.

*Do your homework.* Don't trust everything you are told by your future employer. Check the information out with others at the institution. Ask them what their lived experiences at the institution are? Ask if you can talk to faculty/administrators that have left the institution?

*Identify your allies early.* These are individuals who you connect with and feel that you can trust. They eventually will provide the support you need in the early phase of your transition and look out for you long term. Be sure to reciprocate when necessary.

## Conclusion

The complexities associated with switching institutions and transitioning to a new workplace environment to advance your career in academic medicine can be daunting and at the same time exhilarating. Key lessons learned from a variety of experiences emphasize the importance of self-awareness and self-reflection, discovering how adaptable you may or may not be, and being intentional about discovering new opportunities will be critical to your professional and personal development and success. As you begin your exploration, be cognizant of those elements that may be inhibitors to your success as well as those that may be catalysts that drive your success. Evaluating the benefits and the risks associated with switching institutions is equally important to consider in your search to enhance your career and the meaningful impact that you can have and want to make. In the long run, this is about believing in what defines you professionally and personally, celebrating the accomplishments you have made and those that validate you, and never underestimating the contributions and value that you bring to the table.

> Success…can only come if you continue to believe in yourself, manage adversity with grace and continue forward with a stronger sense of purpose. John Baldoni

**Open Access** This chapter is licensed under the terms of the Creative Commons Attribution 4.0 International License (http://creativecommons.org/licenses/by/4.0/), which permits use, sharing, adaptation, distribution and reproduction in any medium or format, as long as you give appropriate credit to the original author(s) and the source, provide a link to the Creative Commons license and indicate if changes were made.

The images or other third party material in this chapter are included in the chapter's Creative Commons license, unless indicated otherwise in a credit line to the material. If material is not included in the chapter's Creative Commons license and your intended use is not permitted by statutory regulation or exceeds the permitted use, you will need to obtain permission directly from the copyright holder.

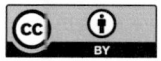

# Chapter 23
# Considerations for Lideres of Tomorrow

Francisco Lucio, Wined Ramirez Lopez, Cristhian A. Gutierrez-Huerta, and Arturo Saavedra

**Learning Objectives**
- Describe the importance of accreditation in academic leadership.
- Consider opportunities in hospital and clinical leadership.
- Describe the importance of law, policy, and advocacy in leadership.
- Recognize the role of community engagement in effective leadership.
- Assess the impact of technological advances on future leadership needs.

## Introduction

There are a multitude of considerations for the LHS+ (Latina/o/x/e, Hispanic, or of Spanish Origin+) *lideres* of tomorrow. Health care is a dynamic field that is constantly changing whether it is merging of hospital systems, shifting population

F. Lucio (✉)
Health Care Advancement, University of Arizona, Phoenix, AZ, USA
e-mail: flucio@arizona.edu

W. R. Lopez
School of Medicine, Universidad Central Del Caribe, Bayamon, Puerto Rico
e-mail: wined.ramirez@uccaribe.edu

C. A. Gutierrez-Huerta
Medical College of Wisconsin, Milwaukee, WI, USA
e-mail: president@lmsa.net

A. Saavedra
VCU School of Medicine, VCU Health System, Richmond, VA, USA
e-mail: Arturo.Saavedra@vcuhealth.org

demographics, new law and policy implications, or technological advances. Each area of change has direct impacts on the awareness and skill necessary for *lideres* to successfully navigate. In this chapter, we focus on select areas that *lideres* of tomorrow should develop for effective leadership.

## Accreditation

For the *lideres* of tomorrow, accreditation must not be seen as a bureaucratic hurdle but as a strategic framework for transformation. From an LHS+ lens, both learners and faculty must consider how accreditation standards set by the Liaison Committee on Medical Education (LCME) and Commission on Osteopathic College Accreditation (COCA) shape institutional priorities, particularly in areas such as curriculum design, faculty development, student support, and leadership representation. Maintaining compliance is not just about meeting requirements but an opportunity to evaluate success through measurable outcomes and long-term impact. A Continuous Quality Improvement (CQI) mindset is essential to ensure that changes are approached in a way that serves to elevate and develop sustainable data-driven improvements for LHS+ communities. Student success is the ultimate metric of institutional quality, and it is inextricably linked to the success of faculty and staff who support them. When faculty and staff are recruited, developed, and supported as *lideres*, they create an academically rigorous environment that anchors student achievement and, by extension, institutional success.

To meet compliance, medical schools must demonstrate that they appoint, renew, promote, and support faculty through structured faculty development pathways and leadership opportunities, aligning with LCME Elements 4.2 (Faculty Appointment Policies) and 4.5 (Faculty Professional Development) [1]. Clear guidelines for promotion, scholarly productivity, and leadership opportunities are essential, whether faculty pursue clinical, educator, or researcher tracks. Providing this structure fosters long-term faculty success and institutional stability (Standard 4), which directly impacts the learning environment for learners [1].

A positive culture and climate for developing the next generation of *lideres* should recognize scholarly and community engaged activities or relevance for LHS+ communities. For example, the development of bilingual medical tracks not only aligns with LCME standards related to curricular content (Standard 7) but also enhances educational opportunities for students serving Hispanic and other linguistically diverse populations [1].

Furthermore, the role of medical educators in scholarly publishing and editorial leadership underscores the need for representation in academic literature. Encouraging faculty and learners to engage in peer-reviewed contributions strengthens institutional research capacity and aligns with LCME expectations for faculty scholarly productivity (element 4.3) and student research opportunities (Element

3.2) [1]. Similarly, hospital leadership roles reinforce the importance of integrating clinical training with academic leadership.

A key priority is to cultivate leadership that supports faculty and learners across diverse career paths reinforcing Element 4.1 (Sufficiency of Faculty) and Element 8.4 (Evaluation of Educational Program Outcomes) by ensuring that faculty receive adequate training and support in their roles. The development of bilingual medical tracks, for example, not only aligns with LCME standards related to curricular content (Standard 7) and diversity programs/partnerships (element 3.3) but also enhances educational opportunities for students serving Hispanic and other linguistically diverse populations [1].

It is important to note that accreditation standards and elements are reviewed and updated annually (https://lcme.org/publications/). It is imperative for competent *lideres* to be cognizant of changes and engage in proactive analysis of how modified standards can be addressed through an LHS+ lens. Incorporating CQI strategies to monitor, assess, and enhance responses to evolving accreditation expectations ensures that both faculty and student success are sustained, and LHS+ communities are represented.

## Hospital and Clinic Leadership

According to the most recent US Census and press releases, Hispanics accounted for greater than 70% of population growth and currently make up about 20% of the population [2]. As a result, our ability to care for patients equitably and with cultural competence requires mentorship of *lideres* and promotion into careers in hospital and clinical leadership. Ensuring language proficiency and communication with healthcare teams, representation in clinical trials and workforce development are stated goals of the US Department of Health and Human Services (HHS) [3]. Hispanics will not only be patients but also employees and a very important aspect of the entire arc of medical care, before presenting to the hospital and after discharge. When one considers nursing home opportunities, care management, social work, and the entire continuum of care, *lideres* have a unique opportunity to add value to the enterprise and ensure the health of all communities.

Clinics and hospitals present an outstanding opportunity for LHS+ individuals to lead. There are several roles that may be of interest including medical directorships, quality and safety officers, chief medical officers, as well as executive leadership roles such as chief operating officer and chief executive officer. All of these roles require skill sets that include the ability to communicate clearly and transparently, the ability to collect and interpret data, the necessity to craft a vision, and create accountable systems and reward success. Whether in the outpatient or inpatient setting, these roles allow us to improve access and quality of care for all populations.

Additional training in public health, health administration, business, or financial analysis may increase the chance of success in these roles. These additional degrees are not required of clinicians however, as much as a deep sense of service and commitment. Shadowing experiences may help students and young professionals decide if these roles are aligned with their professional interests. Interestingly, these roles often transcend clinical training and present an opportunity to collaborate with diverse teams and various scopes of practice.

As medical delivery systems become more complex, there is a need to develop individuals with multiple concurrent interests. Our healthcare leadership teams will always rely on clinical managers to ensure that we care for diverse populations in the setting of resource constraint by displaying relentless commitment to the best quality of care. Whereas population health science continues to evolve, the need to care for each individual patient with respect and compassion will never expire. One thing is for sure: Regardless of leadership role, our teams must always remember to keep the patient at the center of all we do. LHS+ individuals are well poised to contribute admirably in this wonderful endeavor.

## Law, Policy, and Advocacy

Law, policy and advocacy are distinct areas important to gain knowledge and skill in to become a well-rounded leader in academic medicine. Academic medicine is composed of a dynamic interplay among hospitals and other clinical sites, colleges and universities, employed and volunteer faculty, undergraduate and graduate medical education trainees, public and private research funders, and formal and informal partnerships with community organizations, business, and government. This complex set of actors, institutions, and systems is governed to differing degrees by distinct laws and -policies.

Whether it is rules related to hospital regulations, compliance, patient privacy, medical malpractice, or employment laws, etc., it is critical to have an understanding of legal do's and don'ts. It is not realistic nor necessary that every academic medicine leader has a law degree—although many more MD/JD programs are being offered—but, seeking opportunities to gain more knowledge about different areas germane to your position is prudent. This can be accomplished by attending or hosting Grand Rounds focused on legal issues in medicine, attending professional development sessions at your professional association conferences and symposia, or working closely with your institutional general counsel to gain better understanding of the unique legal issues that arise in your academic role.

More recently, leaders in academic medicine have faced the challenge of responding to social issues such as whether DACA (Deferred Action for Childhood Arrivals) applicants are eligible for admission to medical school, the Black Lives Matter movement, and the anti-Diversity, Equity, and Inclusion (DEI) assault, to name a few. These and other similar issues squarely impact the LHS+ population who continue to face inequitable physical and mental health outcomes flowing from unjust laws, policies, and practices rooted in prejudice and discrimination [4]. The better you are able to understand the nuance and legal parameters of policies and practices, the better you will be able to communicate or negotiate with your institutional general counsel and other leaders, advise those you lead, make decisions, and advocate on behalf of those most impacted.

There is a rich history of advocacy from the academic medicine community—especially from students—to change practices such as smoking on airplanes to expanding civil rights [5]. As a leader in academic medicine students and faculty will seek your guidance and support on a wide variety of advocacy matters. Fortunately, advocacy is a skill that can be developed.

The ability to influence legislation, policies, and public opinions is a skill that can be refined through various means. One way to refine your advocacy skills is through media training. Media training may come in the form of a workshop or a more formal training program such as the Stanford Global Health Media Fellowship [6]. Media training may involve learning the ability to work effectively with various media outlets including television, podcasts, radio, or print media both in English and Spanish. Additionally, developing the ability to communicate technical science to lay people in an understandable and persuasive manner may be the most important advocacy skill. Legislative visits are another avenue to build your advocacy skills. Visits can be with city, state, or federal legislators and their aides who can benefit from your perspective on a number of healthcare issues. Finally, professional development opportunities may exist through your professional association advocacy and policy committees.

*Lideres* will need a diverse tool belt to advance academic medicine to new heights. LHS+ *Lideres* bring unique cultural perspectives to reach patients, the public and government leaders. Leveraging opportunities with community engagement, accreditation, hospital leadership, and advocacy skills will ensure the *lideres* of tomorrow maximize the promise of academic medicine to advance clinical care, education, and research for a healthier society.

## Community Engagement

LHS+ *lideres* are uniquely motivated to serve their communities of origin. This means that engaging and connecting with the local community is not only a strategic approach for community buy-in and research capability, but one grounded as a source of professional motivation for *lideres*. Furthermore, placing *lideres*, who are representative of these communities, into engagement and outreach activities will improve rates of clinical mistrust in these vulnerable populations. Thus, the idea to connect *lideres* to the community will help improve health outcomes for these groups and be a potential source of professional and academic development.

The changing landscape of the population is also an important observation and one that will require updating access to and how quality care is provided to these communities. The rate of US-born Latinos is far outpacing the rate of first-generation Latino immigrants leading to the realization that most Latino adults in 20 years will be US-born [7]. To address this change, individuals should be surveyed and people representing every aspect of this diaspora should be invited to share their perspective to future LHS+ *lideres*. *Lideres* should take the diversity of the group into account and apply necessary changes to their clinical and academic practices. Moreover, it is crucial to realize that although the immigrant population is in decline, this population still has a significant clinical burden and requires a uniquely crafted culturally competent quality of care.

## Technological Advances

The next 10–20 years will see dramatic shifts in health care. The advancement and implementation of artificial intelligence (AI), robotics technology, and medical research advances will necessitate an updated workforce and updated *lideres* to train the next generation. New solutions (AI-assisted language translation, improved telemedicine options, diagnostic and procedural tools, etc.) and familiar problems (cost, access, AI bias, etc.) will arise that may simultaneously exacerbate and mitigate health equity for the LHS+ population. The *lideres* of tomorrow must remain up-to-date in knowledge and application of new technologies, flexible, and continue to be guided by the values that seek to uplift all communities. As technology continues to develop and applied to medical education and patient care, some questions for *lideres* to consider are the following:

1. Is the data that is shared secure and safe?
2. Does the introduction of this technology enhance or erode the patient-physician or learner-teacher relationship?
3. Who is excluded or whose access is limited if new technology is implemented?
4. What is the potential for bias in the outputs?
5. How can this technology mitigate health inequities in LHS+ communities and all communities?

*Lideres* of tomorrow will face a different world, but a focus on values-driven decision-making will guide our *lideres* to a healthier and better future.

## References

1. Liaison Committee on Medical Education. Data collection instrument for full accreditation surveys: academic year 2026–2027. Association of American Medical Colleges & American Medical Association. 2025, May. Retrieved from https://lcme.org/publications/
2. Bureau UC. New estimates highlight differences in growth between the U.S. Hispanic and Non-Hispanic populations. Census.gov. 2024, June 28. http://www.census.gov/newsroom/press-releases/2024/population-estimates-characteristics.html#:~:text=Hispanics%20of%20any%20race%20grew,of%201.64%20million%20in%202023
3. HHS fact sheet: advancing health equity for Hispanics. 2023, September. https://www.hhs.gov/sites/default/files/hhs-fact-sheet-advancing-health-equity-for-hispanics.pdf

4. Brenes F. Hispanics, mental health, and discriminating policies: brief report. Hisp Health Care Int. 2019;17(4):178–80. https://doi.org/10.1177/1540415319875103.
5. Schreidah CM, Robinson LN, Pham DX, Balaji D, Tinsley MS. The case for advocacy curricula and opportunities in medical education: past examples to inform future instruction. Acad Med. 2023;99(5):482–6. https://doi.org/10.1097/acm.0000000000005615.
6. Krohn KM, Yu G, Lieber M, Barry M. The Stanford Global Health Media Fellowship: training the next generation of physician communicators to fight health misinformation. Acad Med. 2022;97(7):1004–8. https://doi.org/10.1097/acm.0000000000004630.
7. Funk C, Lopez MH. A brief statistical portrait of U.S. Hispanics. Pew Research Center. 2022, June 14. https://www.pewresearch.org/science/2022/06/14/a-brief-statistical-portrait-of-u-s-hispanics/

**Open Access** This chapter is licensed under the terms of the Creative Commons Attribution 4.0 International License (http://creativecommons.org/licenses/by/4.0/), which permits use, sharing, adaptation, distribution and reproduction in any medium or format, as long as you give appropriate credit to the original author(s) and the source, provide a link to the Creative Commons license and indicate if changes were made.

The images or other third party material in this chapter are included in the chapter's Creative Commons license, unless indicated otherwise in a credit line to the material. If material is not included in the chapter's Creative Commons license and your intended use is not permitted by statutory regulation or exceeds the permitted use, you will need to obtain permission directly from the copyright holder.

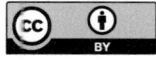

# Index

**A**

Academic department, 183
Academic faculty track, 46
   academic performance reviews and critical conversations, 48
   contextual factors, 47, 48
   decision making, 29
      academic medicine, 29
      adjunct and visiting faculty, 34
      areas of focus/excellence, 35
      choosing, 37, 38
      clinical faculty, 34
      cultural backgrounds, lived experiences and legacies, 30
      faculty appointments, tracks and ranks, 33
      faculty member, 32
      lecturer/instructors, 35
      medicine and research, 30
      personal narratives, 40–42
      personal strengths and impacts faculty, 30
      professional goals chart, 39
      promotion and/or tenure criteria, 36, 37
      tenure-track faculty, 33, 34
      track types, summary of, 35, 36
      values, passions and goals, 30, 31
   health sciences, 46
   literature review, 46
   personal narrative, 56, 57
   professional identity, 48
   review and approval process, 51, 52
   skills exercise, 53, 54
   switching tracks, impetus for, 49
   switch making, benefits and risks of, 49–51
   track-switching experiences, 47
Academic Health Center, 210
Academic health system, leadership positions, 234
Academic leadership, Hispanic, 21–22
Academic medical center, 170, 174, 180, 218
Academic medicine, 135, 205
   benefits of inclusion
      cultural and linguistic concordance, transforming clinical care through, 4
      DEI and institutional impact, 4
      enriching education and mentorship, 4
   benefits of LHS+ inclusion
      challenges and opportunities, 5
      opportunities, 5–7
   career in, 150
   DEI, 227, 228
   Hispanics importance
      academic community, building, 20
      academic leadership and creating change, 21–26
      acculturation process for, 18, 19
      demographic shift in U.S., 15, 16
      equity in health professions and, 16, 17
      Hispanic faculty acculturation, 19, 20
      need in, 17, 18
   LHS+ representation in leadership positions in, 82
      COVID-19 pandemic, health injustices by, 84
      invisibility of academy and for future, 84, 85
      population, changing demographics of, 82, 83

Academic medicine (cont.)
  promotion and leadership development, 347, 348
    balance in work/life, 355
    communication skills, 353
    diversity in hospital leadership, 350
    executive leadership, 353
    healthcare leadership landscape, 353
    integrity, transparency and be genuine, humble and human, 354
    journey and mentor, 354
    lead by listening, 353
    leadership team, work of, 349, 350
    personal narratives, 351, 352, 355–357
    positions, 348, 349
    strategic, tactical, and effective at operations, 354
    trusting relationships, 354
  researcher track in, 150
Academic performance reviews, 48
Academic portfolio, 110–112
Academic track, 133
Accomplishment evaluation, 37
Accountability, 176
Accreditation, 370, 371
Accreditation Council for Graduate Medical Education (ACGME), 108, 249–252, 255–258, 265
Acculturation process, for academic medicine, 18–19
Active learning, *MedEdPORTAL*, 318
Active service participation, 120
Adjunct faculty, 34
Administration/clinical coordination, 124
Admissions
  application process, 271
  dean, roles and responsibilities, 274, 275
  definition, 270
  leadership roles and structures, 273–274
    committee chair, 273, 274
    dean, 274
    professional staff, 274
  LHS+-focused pathway programs and partnerships, 273
  LHS+ students, 275–277
  personal narrative, 279–280
  process, 271
  resources, 277–278
  roles, 271
Adverse Childhood Experiences (ACEs), 305, 306
Advocacy, 7
  *lideres*, 372–373

American Anthropological Association (AAA), 164
American Association for the Advancement of Science (AAAS), 165
American Association of Colleges of Osteopathic Medicine, 82
American Association of Medical Colleges (AAMC), 170, 224, 250, 252, 258, 364
  COD Fellowship, 197
  Group of Faculty Affairs, 287, 298
  Health Executive Diversity and Inclusion Certificate Program, 230
  leadership development programs, 94
  Standpoint Survey, 290
American Medical Association (AMA), 131
American Osteopathic Association, 82
Annika Rodriguez Scholars Program, 163
Appropriate size, *MedEdPORTAL*, 319
Approval process, 51–52
Artificial intelligence (AI), 374
Assimilation, 19
Associate Dean for Academic Affairs, 208
Association for American Medical Colleges (AAMC), 25, 98, 132, 164, 173, 196
Author Development Program, 324

**B**
Beth Israel Deaconess Medical Center (BIDMC), 186
Bias, 116
Black Chief Medical Officer, 356
Bordas' Latino leadership, 203
Boyer's expanded model of scholarship, 314
Building the Next Generation of Academic Physicians (BNGAP), 286, 296

**C**
California University of Science and Medicine (CUSM), 10
Candidate, search firm, 62–63
Career advancement, 118
  switching institutions for, 361, 362
    benefits vs. risks of, 363, 364
    catalysts, 363
    inhibitors versus catalysts of success, 362, 363
    practices, 364–366
Career development, 51
Career Management Life Cycle Model, 287

Index 379

Career path, 146
Career planning, educator track, 139–142
Catalysts, career advancement, switching institutions, 363
CDIO, *see* Chief Diversity and Inclusion Officer
Centers for Disease Control, 163
Centro de Salud Familiar 'La Fe, 211
Chair of the Department of Pediatrics of PSM, 208
Chairperson position, 170, 171, 173
Chair responsibility, 172
Change, 175
Chief Academic Officer (CAO), 349
Chief Development Officer (CDO), 349
Chief Diversity and Inclusion Officer (CDIO), 349, 361, 362
Chief Executive Officer (CEO), 348
Chief Financial Officer (CFO), 349
Chief Health Equity/Community Health Officer, 349
Chief Human Resources Officer (CHRO), 349
Chief Medical Officer (CMO), 227, 349
Chief Nursing Officer (CNO), 349
Chief Operating Officer (COO) of health systems, 227, 349
Chief Quality Officer (CQO), 349
Clinical and Translational Science Award (CTSA), 163
Clinical Associate Professor, 50, 119
Clinical care, through cultural and linguistic concordance, 4
Clinician-educator pathways, 241
Clinical-educator track, 107
  promotion guidelines for, 108
Clinical faculty, 34
Clinical learning environment (CLE), 250, 252, 256, 257, 261, 265
Clinical pathway, 103, 104
Clinical Teacher, 135
Clinical track
  academic portfolio, 111, 112
  academic track, 117
  academic, educational or teaching portfolio, 110, 111
  administration/clinical coordination, 124
  assistant, LHS+ faculty navigation journey from, 105–107
  career advancement, 118
  clinical educator track, promotion guidelines for, 108
  clinical pathway, 103, 104
  clinical research and scholarship, adequacy in, 118
  criteria for promotion, 120
  curriculum vitae, 110
  decision process, 114
  education, philosophy, 121, 122
  educational scholarship, 123, 124
  evaluations, honors and awards for teaching, 124
  letters of recommendation, 112, 113
  LHS+ faculty, challenges for
    diversity tax, 116
    institutional culture, 117
    patient satisfaction, 116
  LHS+ lens, corrective/proactive protocol, 114, 115
  medical school curriculum
    curriculum development, 122, 123
    education committees, 123
    faculty advisor/mentor, 123
    responsibilities, 122
    spine intervention service, 123
  patient satisfaction scores, 119
  personal narrative, 121, 125–128
  professional development, 124
  promotion process, 108, 119, 120
    packet contents, 109, 110
  rank, LHS+ medical school faculty by, 105
  regional/national educational programs, 124
  review process, 113
  surgical residency, 119
Clinic leadership, *Lideres*, 371–372
Co-dependent model of education, 260
Cohesiveness, promotion of, 154, 155
College of Medicine, 194
Commission on Osteopathic College Accreditation (COCA), 370
Committee member, search Firm as, 63–64
Commonwealth Fund-Harvard University Fellowship, 352
Communication, 175
Community-Based Participatory Education (CBPE) model, 160
Community engagement, 141
  *lideres*, 373, 374
Community Health, 361
Community Medicine, 204
Contextual factors, 47, 48
Continuous Quality Improvement (CQI), 370, 371
Corrective/proactive protocol, LHS+ lens, 114–115

Council on Graduate Medical Education (COGME), 132
COVID-19 pandemic, 132, 230
   health injustices by, 84
CQI, *see* Continuous Quality Improvement
Creative Commons licenses, 329
Crisis management, 175
C-Suite, 348
Cuban immigrants, 187
Cultural balance, 91
Cultural competence, 7, 141, 255, 256, 259, 357
Cultural identity, power and role, 90–91
Culture, 19
Curriculum development, 122
Curriculum vitae (CV), 110
   high-quality, 67–69
      academic portfolio, 70
      personal narratives, 76–79
      skills exercise, 75
      template exercise, 75
      themes, 75
   self-audit, worksheet, 139

**D**

Danforth Scholars Program, 163
De colores, 91
Dean
   for admissions, 274
   roles & responsibilities, 274, 275
Dean for Students Affairs
   definition, 304
   educational equity, 305–307
   professional development opportunities, 307, 308
   rewarding and challenging aspects, 305
   role and responsibilities, 304
   self-reflection, 307
   strengths, 307–309
   values, 307–309
Dean of faculty affairs and development (DOFAD)
   AAMC Standpoint Survey, 290
   compensation, 291, 292
   faculty needs assessment survey, 290
   faculty orientation and onboarding, 291
   hospital systems and academic institutions, 291
   implications, 291
   LHS+, 285, 286
   national scholarly meetings, 296–297
   networking, 297
   personal narrative, 297–300
   promotion, 288, 289
   recruitment, 290
   reflection exercise, 292–295
   roles and responsibilities, 287
   shared governance/committees, 289
   skills-based exercise, 295
   societies/organizations, 295, 296
Dean of Graduate Medical Education (GME), 227
Dean of School and Medicine, 216, 220
Dean of the School of Nursing, 212
Decision process, 114
Deep contemplation, 55
Deferred Action for Childhood Arrivals (DACA), 372
Demographic shift, 15–16
Department chair, 170, 171
   job application and interviews, 176, 177
   job offer negotiation, 178
   LHS+ faculty, 87
   modified AAMC faculty roster, 170
   need for, 171
   personal and professional prerequisites, 173
   personal considerations, 175, 176
   personal narratives, 181–190
   preparation, considerations and qualifications in, 173, 174
   reflection exercise, 179
   role, readiness framework, 180
   roles and responsibilities, 171, 172
   skills exercise, 179–180
   strengths, candidates, 178, 179
Department of Health of Puerto Rico, 206
Department of Pediatrics, 208
Design and Division of Library, 204
Designated Education Officer (DEO), 250
Designated institutional officer (DIO), 207, 214, 250–252, 254–258, 260–261, 265
DHHS Secretary of Health, Health Policy Fellowship, 225
Disproportionate allocation of resources, 305
Distribution of Efforts (DOE), 45, 48
Diversity, equity and inclusion (DEI), 4–5, 73, 104, 174, 187, 224, 362
   academic health system, leadership positions in, 234
   academic medicine, leadership levels in, 227, 228
   future of, 233
   keys to success, 231

Index 381

leadership, 233
Medicine and Medical Education, 224–226
personal narratives, 229–231
principles, 228
  feedback, 228
  kindness, compassion and grace, 229
  massive diverse network of support, 228
  mission matters, 228
  pay attention, 228
  problems, 228
strategic plan committee members or stakeholders, 232
strategic planning, 232
Diversity tax, 116
Division of Ethics, Humanities, Arts, 204
Division of Family Medicine, 204
Division of Internal Medicine, Division of Policy, Research and Community Development and Research, 204
Due process, 257

**E**
Early-career faculty, 106
Economic growth, 158
Editor in Chief (EIC), 342–344
Editorial leadership, 370
Educational equity, 5, 305–307
Educational leadership, 227
Educational portfolio, 110–111
Educational scholarship, 123, 124
  *MedEdPORTAL*, 314, 315, 327
  self-evaluation, 318
Educational Summary Report (ESR) methods, 323
Educator track, 132, 133
  advancing by rank, 136
  associate professor criteria, 136
  career planning for, 139–142
  CV audit with criteria comparison, 138, 139
  CV self-audit, worksheet for, 139
  Hispanic/Latino health disparities, 135
  LHS+ specific faculty development programming, 137
  missions, 134, 135
  missions, considerations, 137
  personal narratives, 142–146
  professional priorities, 133
  reflection and skills exercise, 137, 138
  research activities, 135
  research categories, 136

  teaching activities, 134
  Universidad Central Del Caribe School of Medicine, 133, 134
Eligibility criteria, 275, 276
El Paso Neither community, 217
El Paso regent, 217
El Paso School of Medicine, 218
Emotional intelligence, 175
Emotional leadership theory, 155
Empowerment and Resources Seminar, 118
Engagement/commitment, 155
Equity, diversity, and inclusion (EDI), 284, 286, 290
Equity, health professions and academic medicine, 16–17
Executive leadership, 88–90
  cultural/climate assessments, 89
  self-reflection, questions for, 89, 90
Executive Leadership in Academic Medicine (ELAM) program, 196, 209, 225, 350

**F**
Faculty advisor/mentor, 123
Faculty Affairs, 285
Faculty career development, 285
Faculty life cycle, 287, 293
Faculty needs assessment survey, 290
Faculty Physician Advisory Council (FPAC), 6
Faculty ranks, 36
Family Medicine (FM), 127, 361
Federally Qualified Health Center (FQHC), 211, 361
Florida International University School of Medicine (FIU), 204
Foster School of Medicine, 220
Four-Year Medical School, 217

**G**
General Counsel, 349
Graduate Medical Education (GME) programs, 81, 207
  accreditation and compliance, 257
  accreditation of sponsoring institution, 258
  ACGME accreditation standards, 250, 251
  additional education through degrees or certificate programs, 258
  assisting with individual program functions, 256
  assist with creation of new programs, 257
  attendance at courses, 258

Graduate Medical Education (GME) programs (cont.)
   CLE, 250
   cultural competence, 256
   definition, 249, 250
   DIO, 250, 251, 260–261
   due process, 257
   financial oversight, 258
   finding mentors, sponsors, coaches, advisors, and allies, 259
   leadership skills, 258
   LHS+ academic professionals progress, 251, 261, 262
   medical school LHS+ Faculty, 252
   mentors, role of, 262–263
   mission, vision, and institutional strategy, 256
   model of education, 260
   non-clinical service activities, 258, 259
   overall educational faculty development, 257
   PD and PC development, 257
   personal narratives, 263–265
   requirements, 256
   roles and development pathways, 252–255
   Sponsoring Institution, 250
Graduate residency education (GME), 174
Graduate School Biomedical Sciences, 220
Gray kingbird, 355

## H
Harvard Macy Medical Education Program, 198
Harvard Medical School, 165
Harvard School of Public Health Clinical Scholars Program, 215
Health disparities, 141, 305, 306, 308, 309
Health equity, 3, 226, 305, 309
Health inequity, 305, 309
Health injustices, COVID-19 pandemic, 84
Health Occupations Management (MBA/HOM), 197
Health policy, 42
Health professions, equity in, 16–17
Health Sciences Center, 220
Hidden curriculum, 164
High-quality academic portfolio, 70
High-quality CV, 67–69
Hispanics, 2
   academic medicine
      academic community, building, 20
      academic leadership and creating change, 21–26
      acculturation process for, 18, 19
      demographic shift in U.S., 15–17
      Hispanic faculty acculturation, 19, 20
      need in, 17, 18
Holistic practice, 271
   core principles, 270
   definition of, 270
Hospital leadership, 347, 348
   balance in work/life, 355
   communication skills, 353
   diversity in, 350
   executive leadership, 353
   healthcare leadership landscape, 353
   integrity, transparency and be genuine, humble and human, 354
   journey and mentor, 354
   lead by listening, 353
   leadership team, work of, 349, 350
   *Lideres*, 371, 372
   personal narratives, 351, 352, 355–357
   positions, 348, 349
   strategic, tactical, and effective at operations, 354
   trusting relationships, 354
HRSA funded program, 213

## I
Idealized influence, 92
Inspirational motivation, 92
Institutional culture, 117
Institutional designated officers (DIOs), 227
Intellectual stimulation, 92
Intensive care, 145
Interim Assistant Dean, 214
Interprofessional education, 322
Interviews, 176–177

## J
Job application, 176, 177
Job offer negotiation, 178
Journal evolution, *MedEdPORTAL*, 315–317

## K
Kellogg Community Partnership Program, 214
Kern's Six-Step Approach, 160
Kirkpatrick evaluation model, 328
Korean war, 41

## L
Language skills, 141
Latina/o/x/e Dean, 200–203

# Index

Latina/o/x/e, Hispanic, or Spanish Origin+ (LHS+), 170, 223
  academic medicine, benefits of inclusion
    challenges and opportunities, 5
    cultural and linguistic concordance, transforming clinical care through, 4
    DEI and institutional impact, 4
    enriching education and mentorship, 4
    opportunities, 5–7
  academic professionals progression, 251
  corrective/proactive protocol, 114, 115
  cultural competency, 7
  educators, 132
  experience, 306
  faculty, challenges for
    diversity tax, 116
    institutional culture, 117
    patient satisfaction, 116
  faculty navigation, 105–107
  focused pathway programs, 273
  health education, *MedEdPORTAL*, 325–327
  identity, 245
  institutional impact, 8
  leadership and advancement opportunities for advancement for, 92
    AAMC, 93
    agreed-upon faculty development framework, 93
    organized medicine, 93
    U.S. hospitals and healthcare organizations, 93
  leadership and advocacy, 7
  medicine and academic medicine, 3, 4
  personal awareness, 7
  personal development, 7
  physical medicine and rehabilitation, 9
  physicians/scientists, 158
  students, 270, 271, 275–277, 279, 280
  in U.S. medical schools, 2, 3, 81, 85, 86
    AAMC leadership development programs, 94
    academic medicine, leadership positions in, 82
    academy and for future, invisibility of leaders in, 84, 85
    advancement opportunities for advancement for, 92, 93, 95
    American Association of Colleges of Osteopathic Medicine, 82
    American Osteopathic Association, 82
    challenges, 87–89
    COVID-19 cases, hospitalizations, 84
    cultural and language barriers, 82
    cultural identity, power and role of, 90, 91
    department chairs in, 87
    faculty and leaders, data for, 85–87
    faculty by rank, 86
    FT women faculty, 86
    group level, 95, 96
    health injustices, 84
    Hispanic population, 83
    individual level, 95
    institutional level, 96
    key and executive leadership, 88–90
    Latino leadership and transformational leadership, 92
    medical school deans in, 87
    personal narratives, 97–100
    population, changing demographics of, 82, 83
    power of, 91, 92
    race/ethnicity, department chairs, 87
    Ten Latino leadership principles, 91
Latino/a/x/e leadership, 358, 373
Latino DNA, 362
Latino/Hispanic adults, 2
Latino leadership, 201–202
Latino Medical Student Association (LMSA), 6, 9, 159–161, 163, 286, 296, 324
  Faculty Physician Advisory Council, 118, 324
Latino-style optimism, 203
Law, *lideres*, 372, 373
LCME, *see* Liaison Committee on Medical Education
Leadership, 7
  development, 22
  types of, 155
  LHS+ representation in
    academic medicine, 82
    COVID-19 pandemic, health injustices by, 84
    invisibility of academy and for future, 84, 85
    population, changing demographics of, 82, 83
  skills, 195, 258
  training, 196
  transition, 62
Letters of recommendation, 112, 113
Liaison Committee on Medical Education (LCME), 108, 208, 209, 217, 370
Licensing of medical schools (LCME), 225

Lideres, 369
   accreditation, 370, 371
   community engagement, 373, 374
   hospital and clinic leadership, 371, 372
   law, policy and advocacy, 372, 373
   researcher track, 159, 160
      future directions, 161
      outcomes and impact, 160
      program design and implementation, 160
   technological advances, 374
LIDEReS – LHS+ Identity Development, 118
Limited English proficiency (LEP), 323
LISTOS, *see* LMSA Instruction, Support, Training & Orientation Session for Advisors
LMSA, *see* Latino Medical Student Association
LMSA Instruction, Support, Training & Orientation Session for Advisors (LISTOS), 74

# M
Marginalization, 19
Massachusetts General Hospital (MGH), 352
Massachusetts General Hospital (MGH) Institute of Health Professions, 198
Master of Public Health (MPH), 163, 198
Master of Science in Health Professions Education degree program, 198
Master's degree in Business Administration (MBA), 197
Master's degree in medical management (MMM), 198
Master's degree in public administration (MPA), 197
*MedEdPORTAL*, 6, 135, 245, 313, 314
   AAMC Electronic Residency Application System, 322
   active learning, 318
   aligning educational scholarship, 327
   aligns with core values, 332
   appropriate size, 319
   Boyer's Expanded model of scholarship, 314
   educational objectives, 320, 321
   educational scholarship, 314, 315, 330
      self-evaluation, 318
   engagement and inclusivity, 333
   ESR templates, 320, 321
   journal, 315–317
   journal evolution, 315
   Kirkpatrick Evaluation Model, 328
   learning objectives, measurable verbs for, 328
   LHS+ health education, 325–327
   peer review, educational activities, 320
   personal narratives, 329–331
   problem/gap/hook framework, 321
   publications, 322, 330
      LHS+ communities, 326
   scholarly publishing, expanding access to
      Author Development Program, 324
      diversity, equity, and inclusion, 324
      prospective authors, mentorship and guidance for, 325
   submissions, 323
      characteristics of, 317
   sufficient evidence, 319
   traditional publishing, 333
   uniqueness, 319
   US peer-reviewed journal, 323
   writing learning objectives, 327
Media training, 373
Medical delivery systems, 372
Medical education, 131, 135
Medical journals, 340, 344
Medical Organization for Latino Advancement (MOLA), 324
Medical School Admission Requirements (MSAR), 276
Medical school curriculum
   curriculum development, 122, 123
   education committees, 123
   faculty advisor/mentor, 123
   responsibilities, 122
   spine intervention service, 123
Medical School Dean, 194
   AAMC, 196
   AAMC Council of Deans Fellowship Program, 197
   ELAM, 196
   formal training opportunities and degree programs, 197
   Harvard Macy Medical Education Program, 198
   human resources, 198
   know yourself, 195, 196
   Latina/o/x/e Dean, 200–203
   leadership training, 196
   LHS+ faculty, 87
   MBA, 197
   medical management, 198
   personal narratives, 203–220
   personal preferences, 194
   school-wide committees, 198
   skill requirements, 195

training through committee service, 199
Medical School Decanal Administrative Hierarchy, 239
Medical School in North America, 204
Medical schools, 104
Medicine and Medical Education, 224–226
MEDLINE indexing, 329
Mental health, 141
Mentorship, 4, 5
Middle States Commission of Higher Education (MSCHE), 208
Minority Health Policy, 352
Misinformation, 140

## N
National and international recognition, 106
National Association of Community Health Centers, 214
National Boricua-Latino Health Organization (NBLHO), 163
National Committee Service, 198
National Health Service Corps Scholarship Program, 211, 212
National Hispanic Medical Association (NHMA), 159, 163, 324
National Hispanic Science Network, 159
National Institute on Minority Health and Health Disparities (NIMHD), 163
National Institutes of Health (NIH), 68, 159
National Institutes of Health Office of Intramural Research Hispanic Health Research Scientific Interest Group, 159
National Science Foundation (NSF), 159
Nature vs Nurture aspect of leadership, 188
New England Journal of Medicine, 215
New Orleans Muslim community, 164
New York University (NYU) School of Medicine, 230
NHLBI K award, 225
NIH Loan Repayment Program, 163
Non-clinical service activities, 258, 259
Non-tenure clinical series track, 54
Northeast Consortium on Cross Cultural Care, 225
NYC Health and Hospitals Corporation, 357

## O
OB GYN Department Chair, 11, 188
Office of Multicultural Affairs, 164
Organized medicine, 93, 96

## P
Partnerships, 271, 276
Paso del Norte Area Health Education center (PDN-AHEC), 212
Pathway programs, definition of, 270
Patient Safety/Quality Improvement (PS/QI) outcomes, 112
Patient satisfaction, 116, 119
Performance reviews, 48
Personal awareness, 7
Personal development, 7
Philadelphia Ujima™, 225
Physical Medicine and Rehabilitation (PMR), 264, 265
Physician/scientist, steps to, 151, 152, 163
Pitirre, 355
Ponce Health Sciences University (PHSU) School of Medicine, 205, 209, 210
Ponce School of Medicine (PSM) and Health Sciences, 206, 207, 209
Portfolio, high-quality academic, 70
President/CEO, 350
Principal Investigator, 227
Privademics, 57
Professional coaches, 174
Professional development, 124
Professional fulfillment, 31
Professional identity, 45, 48
Professional staff support, 274
Program coordinator (PC) development, 257
Program Director (PD), 253, 254, 257, 264
  development, 257
  Pediatric Residency Program, 206
Programmatic development, 171
Promotion, 285
  CV and portfolio for
    high-quality academic portfolio, 70
    high-quality CV, 67–69
    leadership activities, 74
    LHS+ related contributions, 73, 74
    maximizing research activities, 72
    operational work, 72, 73
    personal narratives, 76–79
    pursuing and achieving, 70–72
    skills exercise, 75
    template exercise, 75
    themes, 75
  guidelines for, 107
Promotion and tenure (P&T) committee, 69, 108, 113
Promotion packet
  contents, 109
  creating, 109, 110

Promotion process, 108
  researcher track, 156
Prospective authors, mentorship and guidance for, 325
P&T committee, *see* Promotion and tenure committee
Public Health, 42
Puerto Rico, 207

**Q**
Quality management, 171

**R**
Racism, 116
RAND Corporation, 204
Recommendation letters, 112–113
Recruitment process
  portfolio and executive presence in, 61, 62
    committee member, working with search firm as, 63
    committee, voice, 63, 64
    gate opener, 64
    insidious, innocuous slights, 64
    uncomfortable conversations, 63
    working with search firm as candidate, 62, 63
Regional/national educational programs, 124
Research categories, 136
Researcher track, 150
  in academic medicine, 150
  challenges, 157, 158
  cohesiveness, promotion of, 154, 155
  diversity, missing creativity from, 158, 159
  economic growth and competitiveness, 158
  engagement/commitment, 155
  leadership, types of, 155
  LHS+ physicians/scientists, 158
  LIDEReS in research, 159, 160
    future directions, 161
    outcomes and impact, 160
    program design and implementation, 160
  personal narrative, 161–165
  physician/scientist, steps to, 151, 152
  promotions on, 156
  research laboratory/research team, traits of, 153, 154
  research path, physician embark on, 150, 151
  social justice, 158
  sustainable research program, components of, 153

Research laboratory/research team, traits of, 153, 154
Research mentor, 152, 164
Research path, physician embark, 150, 151
Research residency programs, 150
Restlessness, 362
Review and approval process, 51, 52
Reviewer, serving as, 336
  associate editor, 338
  DEI, 339
  diversity, equity, and inclusion, 337
  editing, and writing, LHS+ identified individuals, 337, 338
  editor-in-chief of journal, 342–344
  journal editors, 336
  LHS+ identity, 339
  LHS+ identity, aspects of, 336
  medical journals, 339–341
  review process, 341, 342
Review process, 113

**S**
School-based health centers, 213, 214
Search firm
  as candidate, 62–63
  as committee member, 63–64
Secretary of Health at Health and Human Services, 204
Selection committee, 271
Selection criteria, 270, 275
Self-reflection, 307
Senior Associate Dean EDI, 231
Separation, 19
SF 32 self-perception of health questionnaire, 215
Simulated Minority Admissions Exercise Program, 225
Skills exercise, 53, 54
SMART format, 320
Social capital analysis, 306
Social connectedness, 306
Social determinants of health (SDoH), 204, 305, 306, 309
Social Drivers of Health, 305
Socialization, 32
Social justice, 158
Spanish Origin+, 2
Specialty/subspecialty professional organization's regular conference, 242
Sponsor, 20, 22, 26
Sponsoring Institution (SI), 250, 262
Stanford Global Health Media Fellowship, 373

Index 387

State of Texas, 216
State University of New York (SUNY) College of Optometry, 230
Stereotypes, 140
Student National Medical Association (SNMA), 9
Submission, *MedEdPORTAL*, 317
Sufficient evidence, *MedEdPORTAL*, 319
Surgical Critical Care fellowship, 186
Sustainable research program, 153
Switching institutions
    benefits vs. risks of, 363, 364
    career advancement, 361, 362
    practices, 364–366
Switching tracks, impetus for, 49
Switch making, benefits and risks, 49–51
Symbolic capital, 45, 50

**T**
Teaching portfolio, 110–111
Tenure-clock-stopping policies, 33
Tenure-track faculty, 33, 34
Texas Association of Community Health Centers, 214
Texas Tech Board of Regents, 217
Texas Tech system, 218
Texas Tech University Health Sciences Center El Paso, 220
Tools for Assessing Cultural Competences (TACCT), 225
Track types, summary of, 35, 36
Transformational leaders, 92
Transitional Year Program Director, 207

**U**
UCDSOM, 364
UCSF, 183
Undergraduate medical student education (UME)/Curriculum Dean, 174
    clinician-educator pathways, 241
    conferences and professional development, 242
    definition, 238–239
    LHS+ identity, 245
    MACRO functions, 240
    path, preparation for, 243, 244
    usual qualifications, 241, 242
    usual training and experience pathway, 243
Underrepresented in medicine (URiM), 252, 260, 262
Uniqueness, *MedEdPORTAL*, 319
University of Arizona, 165
University of Calgary, 219
University of California Davis Health System, 361
University of California San Francisco (UCSF), 182
University of Davis School of Medicine, 361
University of Minnesota, 226
University of Puerto Rico (UPR), 41
University of Texas El Paso (UTEP), 212
University of Washington School of Medicine (UWSOM), 361–363
Urban Health Education and Educational Research (UHEER), 225
US Department of Health and Human Services (HHS), 371
US medical schools
    LHS+ leadership in, 81
    AAMC leadership development programs, 94
    academic medicine, leadership positions in, 82
    academy and for future, invisibility of leaders in, 84, 85
    American Osteopathic Association and the American Association of Colleges of Osteopathic Medicine, 82
    challenges, 87–89
    COVID-19 cases, hospitalizations, 84
    cultural and language barriers, 82
    cultural identity, power and role of, 90, 91
    faculty by rank, 86
    FT women faculty, 86
    group level, 95, 96
    health injustices, 84
    Hispanic population, 83
    individual level, 95
    institutional level, 96
    key and executive leadership, 88–90
    Latino leadership and transformational leadership, 92
    LHS+ faculty and leaders, data for, 85–87
    LHS+ faculty, advancement opportunities for advancement for, 92, 93, 95
    personal narratives, 97–100
    population, changing demographics of, 82, 83
    power of, 91, 92
    race/ethnicity, department chairs, 87
    Ten Latino leadership principles, 91

Usual qualifications, 241, 242
UT Southwestern Medical Center (UTSWMC), 263, 264
UWSOM, *see* University of Washington School of Medicine

**V**
VA Caribbean Healthcare System PMR residency program, 265
Vida Medical Spanish Curriculum, 10
Visiting faculty, 34

**W**
Wellbeing, 141
Women's Health Center of Excellence (WH COE), 225
World Health Organization (WHO), 305

**Y**
YMCA, 352